MW01519739

Oral Cancer Metastasis

Jeffrey Myers
Editor

Oral Cancer Metastasis

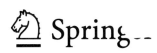 Springer

Editor
Jeffrey Myers
Department of Head and Neck Surgery – Unit 441
University of Texas
M D Anderson Cancer Center
Houston, TX 77030
USA
jmyers@mdanderson.org

ISBN 978-1-4419-0774-5   e-ISBN 978-1-4419-0775-2
DOI 10.1007/978-1-4419-0775-2
Springer New York Dordrecht Heidelberg London

Library of Congress Control Number: 2009930631

Printed on acid-free paper

Springer is part of Springer Science+Business Media (www.springer.com)

*This book is dedicated to Dr. Helmuth
Goepfert and Dr. Josh Fidler, who taught
me the clinical significance and the ways
to approach the study of oral cancer
metastasis. I am grateful to both of them
for providing me with the appropriate
"soil" for my germination and growth
as a head and neck "surgeon-scientist."*

Acknowledgements

I would like to thank Ms. Mariann Crapanzano for her expertise and dedication in editing this book, and Mrs. Rachel Warren and her team at Springer for their professionalism and support in producing this book.

Preface

Squamous cell carcinoma of the oral cavity (SCCOC) is one of the most prevalent tumors of the head and neck region. Despite improvements in treatment, the survival of patients with SCCOC has not improved significantly over the past several decades. Most frequently, treatment failure takes the form of local and regional recurrences, but as disease control in these areas improves, SCCOC treatment failures more commonly occur as distant metastasis. The presence of cervical lymph node metastasis is the most reliable adverse prognostic factor in patients with SCCOC, and extracapsular spread (ECS) of cervical lymph nodes metastasis is a particularly reliable predictor of regional and distant recurrence and death from disease. Decisions regarding elective and therapeutic management of cervical lymph node metastases are made mainly on clinical grounds as we cannot always predict cervical lymph node metastasis from the size and extent of invasion of the primary tumors. Therefore, the treatment of the neck disease in the management of SCCOC remains controversial. The promise of using biomarker-based treatment decisions has yet to be fully realized because of our poor understanding of the mechanisms of regional and distant metastases of SCCOT. This book summarizes the contemporary approaches to clinical and radiographic assessment and primary and adjuvant treatment of oral cancer metastases, and also explores the current status of investigations into SCCOC metastases and the potential of these studies to positively impact the clinical management of SCCOC in the future.

Contents

Contributors

Lee WT Alkureishi, M.D., M.R.C.S.
Department of Plastic and Reconstructive Surgery
University of Chicago Medical Center
5841 South Maryland Ave
Chicago, Illinois 60637
Lee_alkureishi@hotmaol.com

Carlos Caulin, Ph.D.
Assistant Professor
Department of Head and Neck Surgery
The University of Texas M. D. Anderson Cancer Center
1515 Holcombe Blvd.
Unit Number: 123
Houston, TX 77030

Zhong Chen, M.D., Ph.D.
Staff Scientist, Tumor Biology Section
Head and Neck Surgery Branch
National Institute on Deafness and Other Communication Disorders
National Institutes of Health
10 Center Drive, CRC Room 4-2732
Bethesda, MD 20892
chenz@nidcd.nih.gov

Donald Courter, Ph.D.
Fellow
Department of Radiation Oncology
Stanford University
875 Blake Wilbur Dr, MC 5847
Stanford, CA 94305-5847
qle@stanford.edu

Reza Ehsanian, Ph.D.
Tumor Biology Section, Head and Neck Surgery Branch
National Institute on Deafness and Other Communication Disorders
National Institutes of Health
10 Center Drive, Bethesda, MD 20892
ehsanianr@nidcd.nih.gov

Robert. L. Ferris, M.D., Ph.D.
Associate Professor Vice-Chair for Clinical Operations
Chief, Division of Head and Neck Surgery Departments of Otolaryngology and
Immunology Co-Leader, Cancer Immunology Program
University of Pittsburgh Cancer Institute
Pittsburgh, PA 15232
ferrisrl@msx.upmc.edu

Amato Giaccia, Ph.D.
Professor
Department of Radiation Oncology
Stanford University
875 Blake Wilbur Dr, MC 5847
Stanford, CA 94305-5847
giaccia@stanford.edu

Lawrence E. Ginsberg, M.D.
Professor of Radiology and Head and Neck Surgery
MD Anderson Cancer Center
Department of Diagnostic Radiology, Unit 370
1515 Holcombe Blvd.
Houston, TX 77030

Jennifer Rubin Grandis, M.D., F.A.C.S.
Vice Chair for Research
UPMC Endowed Chair in Head and Neck Cancer Surgical Research
Department of Otolaryngology
Professor of Otolaryngology & Pharmacology
University of Pittsburgh School of Medicine
Program Leader, Head & Neck Cancer Program
University of Pittsburgh Cancer Institute
American Cancer Society Clinical Research Professor
Eye & Ear Institute, Suite 500
200 Lothrop Street
Pittsburgh, PA 15213
jgrandis@pitt.edu

Paul M. Harari, M.D.
Jack Fowler Professor and Chairman
Department of Human Oncology

University of Wisconsin School of Medicine and Public Health
600 Highland Ave.
Madison, WI 53792

C. Wesley Hodge, M.D.
Radiation Oncology
Robert Boissoneault Oncology Institute
2020 SE 17th St
Ocala, FL 34471

Dr. Zhanzhi Hu
Affymetrix
3420 Central Expy
Santa Clara, CA 95051-0703

Shen Hu, Ph.D.
Assistant Professor
School of Dentistry & Jonsson Comprehensive Cancer Center
University of California, Los Angeles
10833 Le Conte Ave
Los Angeles CA 90095
shenhu@ucla.edu

Deepak Khuntia, M.D.
Associate Professor
Department of Human Oncology
University of Wisconsin School of Medicine and Public Health
600 Highland Ave.
Madison, WI. 53792

Quynh-Thu Le, M.D.
Professor
Department of Radiation Oncology
Stanford University
875 Blake Wilbur Dr, MC 5847
Stanford, CA 94305-5847
qle@stanford.edu

Jessyka G. Lighthall, M.D.
Department of Otolaryngology/Head Neck Surgery
Oregon Health & Science University
Portland, OR 97229

Stephen P. Malkoski, M.D., Ph.D.
Assistant Professor
Pulmonary Sciences and Critical Care Medicine
University of Colorado Denver School of Medicine
13001 East 17th Place
Building 500, 1st Floor East
Aurora, CO 80045

Rafael R. Mañon, M.D.
Clinical Assistant Professor, FSU College of Medicine
Assistant Professor, UCF College of Medicine
Department of Radiation Oncology
MD Anderson Cancer Center—Orlando
1400 S. Orange Avenue
Orlando, Fl 32806

Zvonimir Milas, M.D.
Clinical Fellow
Department of Head and Neck Surgery
University of Texas M D Anderson Cancer
1515 Holcombe Blvd.
Houston, TX
zmilas@mdanderson.org

Eugene N. Myers, MD, FACS, FRCS (Hon)Edin
Department of Otolaryngology
University of Pittsburgh Medical Center
Pittsburgh, PA 15213
Distinguished Professor and Emeritus Chair
Department of Otolaryngology,
University of Pittsburgh Medical Center
Pittsburgh, PA 15213
myersen@upmc.edu

Jeffrey Myers, M.D. Ph.D.
Ashbel Smith Professor and Deputy Chair
Department of Head and Neck Surgery – Unit 441
University of Texas M.D. Anderson Cancer Center
1515 Holcombe Blvd.
Houston, TX 77030
jmyers@mdanderson.org

Robert Newman, M.D.
University of Alabama at Birmingham
563 Boshell Building, 1808 7th Avenue South
Birmingham, AL 35294

Mark E. P. Prince, M.D., F.R.C.S.(C.)
Associate Professor
Otolaryngology - Head and Neck Surgery
University of Michigan
Department of Otolaryngology - HNS
1500 E. Medical center Drive
1904 Taubman Center
Ann Arbor, MI 48109

Ali Razfar
Department of Otolaryngology and Head Neck Surgery
University of Pittsburgh
Suite 500, Eye & Ear Building
203 Lothrop Street
Pittsburgh, PA
alr50@pitt.edu

Eben L Rosenthal, M.D.
Julius Hicks Professor of Surgery
Division of Otolaryngology
University of Alabama at Birmingham
563 Boshell Building
1808 7th Avenue South
Birmingham, AL 35294

Gary Ross M.D.
Consultant Plastic Surgeon
Honorary Senior Cliinical Lecturer
Depeartment of Plastic Surgery
The Christie, Wilmslow Road, Manchester, M204BX
glross@gmail.com

Sandro J. Stoeckli, M.D.
Professor and Chairman
Clinic of Otorhinolaryngology, Head and Neck Surgery
Kantonsspital St. Gallen
Rorschacherstrasse 95
9007 St. Gallen, Switzerland
sandro.stoeckli@kssg.ch

Carter Van Waes, M.D., Ph.D.
Senior Investigator and Chief, Head and Neck Surgery Branch,
National Institute on Deafness and Other
Communication Disorders
National Institutes of Health
10 Center Drive, CRC Room 4-2732
Bethesda, MD, 20892
vanwaesc@nidcd.nih.gov

Xiao-Jing Wang, M.D., Ph.D.
Professor
Department of Pathology
Institution University of Colorado Denver
12800 E. 19th Ave., Bldg. RC1N, Rm 5128, mail stop 8104
Aurora, CO 80045
xj.wang@ucdenver.edu

Amy S. Whigham, M.D.
Chief Resident
Department of Otolaryngology
Vanderbilt-Ingram Cancer Center
Vanderbilt University School of Medicine
2220 Pierce Avenue
654 Preston Research Building
Nashville, TN 37232

David T. Wong, D.M.D., D.M.S.C.
Felix & Mildred Yip Endowed Professor
Associate Dean of Research
Director- Dental Research Institute
Oral Biology & Medicine/Dentistry
University of California at Los Angeles
10833 Le Conte Avenue, 73-017 CHS
Los Angeles CA 90095

Wendell G. Yarbrough, M.D.
Ingram Professor of Cancer Research, Otolaryngology and Cancer Biology
Director, Barry Baker Laboratory for Head and Neck Oncology
Department of Otolaryngology
Vanderbilt University School of Medicine,
Nashville, TN 37232
wendell.yarbrough@vanderbilt.edu

Ge Zhou, Ph.D.
Assistant Professor
Department of Head and Neck Surgery
The University of Texas M.D. AndersonCancer Center
1515 Holcombe Blvd.
Houston, TX 77030
gzhou@mdanderson.org

Xiaofeng Zhou, Ph.D.
Assistant Professor
College of Dentistry/Center for Molecular Biology of Oral Diseases
University of Illinois at Chicago
801 S. Paulina Street
Chicago IL 60612
xfzhou@uic.edu

Chapter 1
Oral Cancer Overview: The Significance of Metastasis and Surgical Management of the Neck

Eugene N. Myers

Abstract Squamous cell carcinoma of the oral cavity has the propensity to metastasize to the cervical lymph nodes even in the early stages. The presence of lymph node metastasis is the most significant independent variable in determining survival of patients with cancer of the head and neck. Therefore, the diagnosis and management of cervical lymph node metastasis is one of the most important responsibilities of the head and neck oncologist.

The management of the neck in patients with cancer of the oral cavity has gone through several cycles. Initially, it was thought that the removal of the primary cancer from the oral cavity without paying attention to the neck was sufficient. However, this policy of "waiting and watching the neck" resulted in approximately one-third of the patients developing recurrence in the neck; some of these recurrences were not operable, and therefore, the majority of these patients died of their cancer.

Neck dissection has evolved from radical neck dissection for patients with clinically detectable disease in the neck to selective neck dissection for patients who have N_0 or N+ neck and a "super"-selective neck dissection for patients who have persistent disease following chemoradiation. Although the use of the selective neck dissection in patients with an N_0 neck has not improved the cure rate, it has had a major positive impact on regional disease-free survival and has decreased the morbidity associated with surgical management of the neck.

The evolution of the neck dissection and its current use in the management of patients with cancer of the oral cavity are the subject of this chapter.

E.N. Myers (✉)
Department of Otolaryngology, University of Pittsburgh Medical Center,
Pittsburgh, PA, 15213, USA
e-mail: myersen@upmc.edu

J. Myers (ed.), *Oral Cancer Metastasis*,
DOI 10.1007/978-1-4419-0775-2_1, © Springer Science+Business Media, LLC 2010

Introduction

Squamous cell carcinoma of the oral cavity has a propensity to metastasize to the
cervical lymph nodes even in the early stages. The presence of lymph node metastasis is the most significant independent prognostic variable in determining survival
of patients with cancer of the head and neck (Fig. 1.1) (Hollenbeak et al. 2001).
Therefore, the diagnosis and treatment of cervical lymph node metastasis are the
most important responsibilities of the head and neck oncologist.

There are several important demographic factors that also appear to impact survival. According to the surveillance epidemiology and end results (SEER) data for
cancer of the oral cavity, the 5-year relative survival rate for the group of older
patients was lower than the corresponding value for the younger group (Fig. 1.2)
(Funk et al. 2002).

The 5-year relative survival rates for males was significantly lower than that for
females (Fig. 1.3) (Funk et al. 2002). The 5-year relative survival rate for African-
Americans is significantly worse than that whites (Fig. 1.4) (Funk et al. 2002).

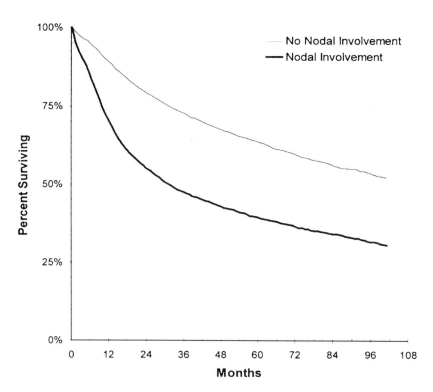

Fig. 1.1 Survival for patients with (n=9,938) lymph node involvement from the SEER database,
computed based on the Kaplan–Meier method ($P < 0.0001$). Reprinted with permission of Wiley-
Liss Inc., a subsidiary of John Wiley & Sons, Inc. (Hollenbeak et al. 2001)

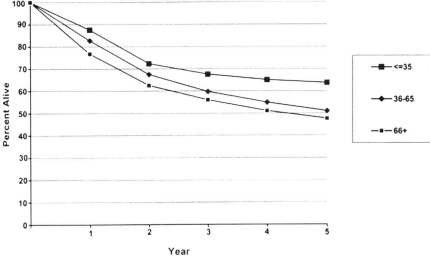

AGE	1	2	3	4	5	95% CIs	CASES
35 or younger	87.5	72.3	67.5	65.0	63.7	59.1 / 68.2	520
36-65	82.7	67.4	59.7	54.9	51.0	50.1 / 52.0	14215
66 or older	76.7	62.5	56.0	51.1	47.6	46.3 / 48.8	12846

Fig. 1.2 Five-year relative survival by age for oral SCC cases, 1985–1991. Five-year survival rates for all age groups were significantly different (95% confidence level) (95% CI: 95% confidence interval for 5-year relative survival). Reprinted with permission of John Wiley & Sons., Inc. (Funk et al. 2002)

A recent study of patients with cancer of the head and neck disclosed that there was a definite decrement in survival for individuals who did not have health care insurance, a difference presumably due to lack of access to health care (Chen et al. 2007). Goodwin et al. in a recent provocative article concluded that "Black Americans clearly bear a greater burden of head and neck cancer. The underlying causes are largely unknown but are most likely due to a complex interplay of differences in access to health care, quality of medical care, biologic/genetic factors, incidence of comorbid conditions, exposure to carcinogens, diet and cultural beliefs" (Goodwin et al. 2008).

Squamous cell carcinoma of the oral cavity is the most frequently encountered malignant tumor of the upper aerodigestive tract and accounts for 3% of all cancers in the United States (Greenlee et al. 2000). Throughout the world, cancer of the oral cavity is more frequent in regions where the use of tobacco and alcohol is high. The highest worldwide standardized incidence rate of cancer of the oral cavity is in France and the lowest rate is in Japan. It is estimated that 5,700 people die from cancer of the oral cavity in the United States each year (Chen and Myers 2001).

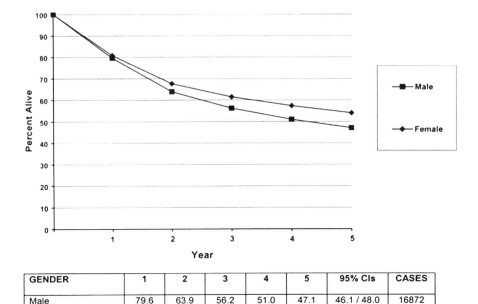

Fig. 1.3 Five-year relative survival by sex for oral SCC cases, 1985–1991. Five-year relative survival rate for males was significantly lower than for females (95% confidence level). (95% CI: 95% confidence interval for 5-year relative survival). Reprinted with permission of John Wiley & Sons., Inc. (Funk et al. 2002)

In Western countries, most of the tobacco-related cancers in the aerodigestive tract are related to cigarette smoking, whereas in Southeast Asia, a significant number of cases of squamous cell cancer of the oral cavity result from the use of betel nuts and pan, a mixture of betel nuts, tobacco, and slaked lime wrapped in a leaf.

Cancer of the head and neck was not a very common problem prior to the latter half of the nineteenth century. The increased incidence of these cancers is linked to the development of the mechanized production of cigarettes in factories. These factories made cigarettes readily available at a low price, which led to widespread addiction and the subsequent increased incidence of cancer of the head and neck (Klein 1996) (Fig. 1.5).

Diagnosis

The diagnostic approach to the mass in the neck depends on a variety of factors including the age of the patient, the time of appearance and the topographic location of the mass, and any associated symptoms. Hayes Martin, the "Father of

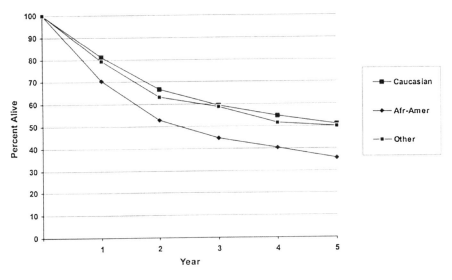

RACE	1	2	3	4	5	95% CIs	CASES
Caucasians	81	66.6	59.5	54.8	51.1	50.3 / 51.9	24111
African-American	70.5	62.9	44.7	40.1	35.5	33.2 / 37.8	2522
Other	79.4	63.2	58.9	51.5	50.1	44.3 / 56.0	442

Fig. 1.4 Five-year relative survival by race for oral SCC cases, 1985–1991. African-Americans demonstrated significantly lower 5-year relative survival than the other two groups (95% confidence level). (95% CI: 95% confidence interval for 5-year relative survival). Reprinted with permission of John Wiley & Sons., Inc. (Funk et al. 2002)

Modern Head and Neck Surgery" and Chief of the Division of Head and Neck Surgery at the Memorial Sloan-Kettering Cancer Center in New York City stated that in adult patients, the majority of the unilateral masses in the neck are malignant (Martin et al. 1951). By means of a thorough history and physical examination, and with the judicious use of laboratory studies and imaging, an accurate diagnosis can be made in the vast majority of these patients.

History and Physical Examination

Cancer of the oral cavity does not usually present much of a diagnostic dilemma. It is very important, however, to include the patient's past medical history in order to identify any comorbidities, which might play an important role in determining the management program. The social history is also quite important, because most of the patients with cancer of the oral cavity have been, or currently are, smoking cigarettes and consuming alcohol.

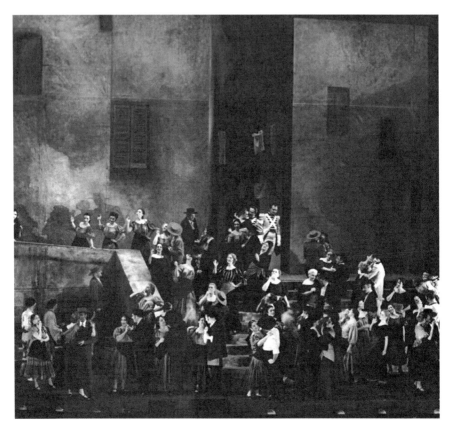

Fig. 1.5 The smoking chorus of cigarette makers, in the 1952 production of Carmen at the Metropolitan Opera, New York (Klein 1996). Reprinted with permission from the University of Nebraska Press

Since surgery is usually the key to successful management of cancer of the oral cavity, it is important for the surgeon to know what quantity of alcohol is being consumed because acute alcohol withdrawal following surgery often leads to delirium tremens. Prior to the availability of intravenous fluid administration, reliable and easily titrated sedation, and ventilatory support, this condition was often fatal. In the modern era, it is almost always managed successfully but at a very high cost since the patients usually spend 7–10 days on the ventilator in the Intensive Care Unit under sedation until the event has been adequately treated. The dollar cost for such treatment, added onto the costs of the actual surgery and reconstruction, amounts to resources that could have been conserved had the patient undergone a systematic, carefully monitored program of alcohol/withdrawal preoperatively. A subset of patients will develop a similar problem with acute nicotine withdrawal, which is also preventable.

The physical examination remains an important aspect of the initial evaluation. A complete inspection of the oral cavity with palpation of the lesion and surrounding tissues is important and provides a great deal of information as to the surface dimensions of the lesion and the depth of invasion. A tumor map should be created documenting the size and location of the tumor. Examination of the upper aerodigestive tract is vital in determining whether any other primary cancers are present. Palpation of the neck is of vital importance and is fundamental in determining whether the patient's tumor is operable. Fixation of cervical lymph node metastases is a sign of inoperability. Measuring the metastatic lymph nodes is essential for accurate staging. The measurements and location of metastatic nodes should also be documented on the tumor map. It is also very helpful as a baseline in the event the patient is treated nonsurgically in order to measure the progress of the treatment program.

Imaging

Imaging plays a vital role in the diagnosis and staging of metastatic cancer in the neck, and this will be covered in a comprehensive fashion in Chap. 2, "The Role of Diagnostic Imaging in Identifying Cervical Metastases in Oral Cavity Cancer." The most commonly used imaging studies have been computed tomography (CT), magnetic resonance imaging (MRI), and ultrasound (US). A newer modality, positron emission tomography (PET)–CT, has an expanded role in the evaluation of the patients with cancer of the head and neck, particularly in identifying cancer elsewhere, both related and unrelated to the cancer of the oral cavity. The role of sentinel node biopsy (SNB), using radioactive imaging techniques, has received a great deal of attention in recent years, and its utility is being evaluated. This topic will be covered in Chap. 3, "Sentinel Node Biopsy in Oral Cancer."

CT scanning is the imaging modality most frequently used in the evaluation of the cervical lymph nodes. It has been shown to be more sensitive and more specific than physical examination alone (Gavilan et al. 2003). MRI is used somewhat less but remains valuable because it is the best method for evaluation of perineural invasion associated with the primary cancer and gives very good definition to study the extent of cancer invasion into the tongue musculature. Squamous cell carcinoma metastatic in the lymph nodes tends to undergo necrosis, leading to filling defects within otherwise enhancing lymph nodes. Necrosis is more often evaluated with CT rather than MR and should be considered a suspicious finding for metastatic cancer even when the node is smaller than 10 mm (Bennett et al. 2007). Extracapsular spread (ECS) of cancer may be appreciated on CT scan as a blurring of the margin of the lymph node. Infiltration of the surrounding tissues may also be identified.

Ultrasound is a fast, safe, and inexpensive study that helps in the differentiation of benign from malignant tumors. This is highly operator dependent, but combined with fine-needle aspiration biopsy, the sensitivity and specificity of this test are increased (Gavilan et al. 2003).

Another interesting but not commonly used technique for indications for surgery of the neck is the measurement of tumor thickness of carcinoma of the oral tongue. Yuen et al. concluded that oral sonography has a satisfactory accuracy in the measurement of tumor thickness and is a useful adjunct in assisting pretreatment staging for prognosis and evaluation of carcinoma of the oral tongue (Yuen et al. 2008). Many studies have demonstrated that tumor thickness, rather than the surface diameter, is a more significant factor in predicting subclinical nodal metastatis, local recurrence, and survival in carcinoma of the oral tongue (Yuen et al. 2000, 2002; Kurokawa et al. 2002; Ocharoenrat et al. 2003; Lim et al. 2004; Sparano et al. 2004).

The role of SNB for oral and oral pharyngeal squamous cell carcinoma of the head and neck is still being defined Hart et al. 2007 (Rigual et al. 2005). Stoeckli (2007) studied 79 patients and concluded that SNB is technically feasible and reproducible with the highest sentinel node detection rate. Validation against selective neck dissection revealed a negative predictive value of 100%. Application of the SNB concept in clinical practice was very successful; the recurrence rate within the neck was very low, and the morbidity caused by elective neck dissection could be spared in 60% of the patients.

Ross et al. (2004) also concluded that SNB can be successfully applied to T1 and T2 cancers of the oral cavity and oral pharynx in a standardized fashion by centers worldwide. For the majority of these tumors, SNB technique can be used as a staging tool. At the Second International Conference on the Sentinel Node Biopsy for the Head and Neck Cancer, the delegates from 20 countries discussed technical and clinical aspects and clinical results. Their report confirmed the high accuracy and reliability of SNB for early oral and oral pharyngeal squamous cell carcinoma (Stoeckli et al. 2005).

Staging

Pretreatment staging constitutes the basis for an adequate selection of therapy in patients with cancer of the oral cavity. The clinical evaluation should be followed by a biopsy to stage the primary cancer and imaging of the regional lymph nodes and distant sites, particularly the lungs. Proper staging can then be carried out in accord with the following table (Gavilan et al. 2003) (Fig. 1.6).

The American Academy of Otolaryngology Head and Neck Surgery Foundation has adapted the Memorial Sloan Kettering Zone System to define the six levels of the neck (Werning and Mendenhall 2007; Robbins 2001, Robbins et al. 2008b) (Figs. 1.7 and 1.8).

Surgical Management of the Neck

The tongue is the most common site in the oral cavity for the development of squamous cell carcinoma (Chen and Myers 2001). In a review of 3,308 cases treated at The University of Texas M. D. Anderson Cancer Center between 1970 and 1999, 30% of all oral cancers were located on the tongue; the next most common

Regional Lymph Nodes (N)

NX Regional lymph nodes cannot be assessed

N0 No regional lymph node metastasis

°N1   Metastasis in a single ipsilateral lymph node, 3 cm or less in greatest
       dimension

°N2   Metastasis in a single ipsilateral lymph node, more than 3 cm but
       not more than 6 cm in greatest dimension, or in multiple
       ipsilateral lymph nodes, none more than 6 cm in greatest
       dimensions, or in bilateral or contralateral lymph nodes,
       none more than 6 cm in greatest dimension

°N2a   Metastasis in single ipsilateral lymph node more than 3 cm but not
       more than 6 cm in greatest dimension

°N2b   Metastasis in multiple ipsilateral lymph nodes, none more than
       6 cm in greatest dimension

°N2c   Metastasis in bilateral or contralateral lymph nodes, none more
       than 6 cm in gretest dimension

°N3   Metastasis in a lymph node more than 6 cm in greatest dimension

°*Note* a designation of "U" or "L" may be used to indicate metastasis above
        the lower border of the cricoid (U) or below the lower border of the
        cricoid (L).

Fig. 1.6 UICC and AJCC definitions of the nodal categories for all head and neck sites (except thyroid). Reprinted with permission from Elsevier (Gavilan et al. 2003). Used with the permission of the American Joint Committee on Cancer (AJCC), Chicago, Illinois. The original source for this material is the AJCC Cancer Staging Manual, Sixth Edition (2002) published by Springer-Verlag, New York, http://www.springer-ny.com

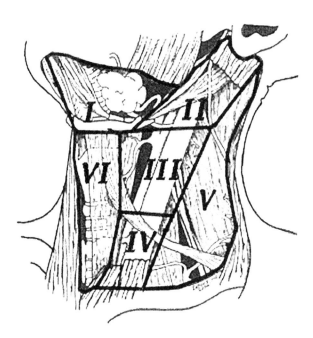

Fig. 1.7 The six levels of the neck. From Robbins (2001), with permission

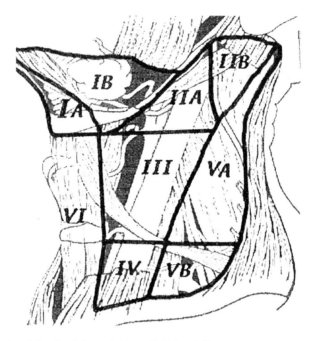

Fig. 1.8 The six sub levels of the neck. From Robbins (2001), with permission

sites in descending order include the floor of the mouth; retromolar trigone, alveolar ridge, hard palate, and buccal mucosa.

The treatment of early-stage cancer (T1–T2) is usually surgery alone. Later-stage lesions (T3–T4), patients who have perineural involvement in the primary cancer or metastasis to multiple cervical lymph nodes or ECS, are usually treated with a combination of surgery and postoperative radiation or chemoradiation. Good local control can be achieved by surgery alone, but the overall successful treatment of cancer of the oral cavity depends upon the appropriate treatment of the cervical lymph nodes.

The surgical anatomy of the lymphatics of the head and neck has been well researched. The publications of Trotter in 1930 on the surgery of the lymphatics of the head and neck is a classic (Trotter 1930). The definitive modern work on the human lymphatic system was published in 1932 by Rouviere (1932). Rouviere's work led to the development of a classification of the cervical lymph nodes according to their topography.

Before the early nineteenth century, there is no mention of a surgical procedure capable of controlling metastatic cancer to the cervical lymph nodes. The importance of cervical lymph node metastasis and the management of cancer of the head and neck was first reported in 1847 by Chelius (1847) in Ferlito et al. (2007). The development of ether anesthesia in the mid nineteenth century and the development of increased numbers of patients with of head and neck cancer coincided and made head and neck surgery possible.

Kocher (1880) recommended that positive lymph nodes be removed with a more ample resection margin and introduced what has come to be known as the Kocher incision, which provides better exposure. In 1881, Packard supported the recommendation that the submandibular and sublingual glands should be removed in the management of cancer of the tongue (Packard 1881).

Jawdynski, a Polish surgeon, performed the first lymph node dissection for metastatic cancer in 1888 (Jawdynski 1888; Ferlito et al. 2007). Jawdynski's work was not recognized until recently because it had been published in an obscure Polish medical journal.

We think of the systematic use of the selective neck dissection as being a rather recent development, but in fact, Butlin introduced this concept 123 years ago (Ferlito and Rinaldo 2005) (Fig. 1.9).

Sir Henry T. Butlin in London in 1885 noted that "every patient with cancer of the tongue must be regarded as having metastasis to the neck" and he advised the routine use of the elective dissection of the cervical lymphatics in the treatment of cancer of the tongue "because, if not, within 8 months after the operation on the tongue, cervical metastasis will become apparent" (Butlin 1885).

Butlin mentioned two alternative forms of management: "removal of the lymph nodes, though not enlarged, which correspond with the affected portion of the tongue, just as the axillary glands are excised as part of the routine operation for cancer of the breast or remove the glands as soon as the slightest enlargement of them is apparent." In his experience with 197 patients with cancer of the tongue, Butlin always excised the primary cancer 2 weeks before the operation, which would today might be described as a modified radical neck dissection. He compared the results of the 78 patients submitted to neck dissection with those of 44 patients treated with excision of the primary only. The 3-year survival rate was 42% in the neck dissection group, compared with 29% in those having excision of the primary. He also observed that 59% of patients who had no palpable lymph nodes at the time of initial visit survived 3 years in contrast to the 32% of patients who had palpable adenopathy. Thus, the concept of elective neck dissection was born.

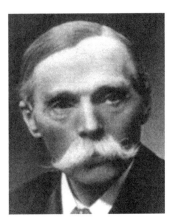

Fig. 1.9 Henry T. Butlin (1845–1912). From Ferlito and Rinaldo (2005)

Fig. 1.10 George W. Crile (1864–1943). From Ferlito and Rinaldo (2005)

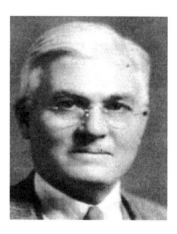

Butlin advised the "removal of ipsilateral nodes in all cases until ways of telling 'dangerous from less dangerous forms' of tongue cancer were available." More than a century later, we are still looking for a means of diagnosing occult metastasis to the neck to fulfill Butlin's prophecy.

George Crile of the Cleveland Clinic was the first surgeon in the United States to actually publish a paper on the systematic approach to neck dissection (Ferlito and Rinaldo 2005) (Fig. 1.10). His work entitled "On the Surgical Treatment of Cancer of the Head and Neck" in 1905 summarized his experience with 121 operations performed on 105 patients (Crile 1905). In 1906, he published a similar paper in the Journal of the American Medical Association, reporting on 132 cases of cancer of the head and neck (Crile 1906). The paper is richly illustrated with clear drawings and his personal experience with this surgical procedure. While similar to the paper published in 1905, it appeared in a high profile journal with a large readership; it is the paper most frequently cited and identified Crile as the leader in the field. It should be said that, although Dr. Crile's name is indelibly linked with the radical neck dissection, careful examination of the illustrations and discussion in his papers indicates that he also advocated supra-omohyoid neck dissection in patients with cancer of the tongue. Although Crile is often referred to as the "grandfather of radical neck dissection," he is actually the grandfather of neck dissection in its various modified forms (Crile 1905, 1906).

Radium and radon seed implants were commonly used to treat metastasis to the neck because external beam radiation therapy was in a very primitive state and was not used very often because of severe side effects. Despite Crile's contribution, radical surgery of the head and neck was also not frequently used because it was quite dangerous. After World War II, improved anesthesia techniques, the availability of antibiotics, and blood banking permitted advances in radical resections of cancer of the head and neck.

Dr. Hayes Martin (Fig. 1.11) became the Chief of the Head and Neck Service at Memorial-Sloan Kettering Hospital in 1934 and popularized the radical neck dissection (Martin et al. 1951). By 1950, 190 neck dissections had been performed at Memorial Hospital (Martin et al. 1951). Dr. Martin advocated exclusively the

Fig. 1.11 Dr. Hayes Martin (1892–1977). From Ferlito and Rinaldo (2005)

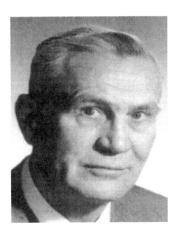

Fig. 1.12 Dr. John Conley (1912–1999)

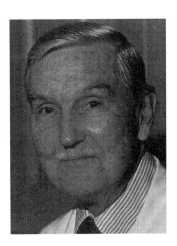

classical radical neck dissection, which included removal of the contents of the neck, including the spinal accessory nerve, the internal jugular vein, and the sternocleidomastoid muscle.

Dr. John Conley also strongly advocated radical neck dissection and said that "the radical neck dissection is the key to controlling metastatic cancer in the neck" (Conley 1967; Ferlito and Rinaldo 2005) (Fig. 1.12). Unfortunately, despite the radical procedure, there was a high recurrence rate in advanced-stage metastatic cancer. There was also a marked downgrading in the cosmetic appearance of the patient and a decreased functionality of the shoulder and arm. Bilateral radical neck dissection (RND) caused disfigurement because of severe facial edema and occasional blindness and/or death.

In 1952, Dr. Osvaldo Suarez, an otolaryngologist and anatomist from Argentina, developed the "functional neck dissection" (Ferlito and Rinaldo 2004). He recognized

Fig. 1.13 Dr. Ettore Bocca (1914–2003). From Ferlito and Rinaldo (2005)

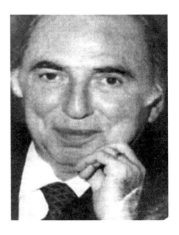

that the lymph nodes were enclosed in the fascial planes of the neck and observed that by respecting these fascial planes, the lymph nodes in the neck could be removed while preserving the very important structures such as the spinal accessory nerve, the internal jugular vein, and the sternocleidomastoid. This was a considerable improvement because the sternocleidomastoid muscle, which provides a major component of the contour of the neck, and the function of the spinal accessory function are preserved. In the 1960s, Dr. Ettore Bocca (Fig. 1.13) (Ferlito and Rinaldo 2005) and Cesar Gavilan popularized the functional neck dissection in Europe (Ferlito and Rinaldo 2004).

Byers, in 1985, reported that during the 1960s Ballantyne and others at the M. D. Anderson Cancer Center had begun to explore the possibilities of a less than radical neck dissection in which the lymph nodes with the highest potential for metastatic involvement were removed and the surrounding anatomic structures not grossly invaded with tumor were preserved (Byers 1985). When multiple positive nodes, unilateral or bilateral, were discovered on pathologic examination or if ECS was identified, postoperative radiation therapy was added to the treatment of the neck. This improvement in regional control set the stage for a conceptual revolution in the surgical treatment of cervical metastasis from squamous cell carcinoma of the head and neck.

The classic work of Shah was extraordinarily important in identifying the orderly progression of metastatic disease in the neck. He reported, in 1990, a series of 1,081 patients who had undergone radical neck dissection and pointed out that cancer of the oral cavity is most likely to metastasize to levels I, II, and III, and oral tongue cancers to level I to IV (Shah 1990). This information has led the way to a more coherent approach to the neck, and, in fact, the lymph node groups removed by the selective neck dissections are based on Shah's findings.

The Committee for Head and Neck Surgery and Oncology of the American Academy of Otolaryngology – Head and Neck Surgery, which was chaired by Dr. K. Thomas Robbins, published a pamphlet on standardized neck dissection

CONCEPTUAL GUIDELINES FOR NECK DISSECTION CLASSIFICATION

1. **Radical neck dissection** is considered to be the standard basic procedure for cervical lymphadenopathy. All other procedures represent one or more alterations of this procedure.

2. When the alteration involves *preservation of one or more nonlymphatic structures* routinely removed in the radical neck dissection, the procedure is termed **modified radical neck dissection.**

3. When the alteration involves *preservation of one or more lymph node groups* routinely removed in the radical neck dissection, the procedure is termed **selective neck dissection.**

4. When the alteration involves removal of *additional lymph node groups or nonlymphatic structures* not typically removed in the radical neck dissection, the procedure is termed an **extended radical neck dissection.**

From: Robbins, K T. 2001. *Pocket Guide to Neck Disection Classification and TNM Staging o Head and Neck Cancer*. 2nd ed. Alexandria: American Academy of Otolaryngology-Head and Neck Surgery Foundation. (Robbins 2001)

Reprinted with permission from American Academy of Otolaryngology – Head and Neck Surgery Foundation, Inc.

Fig. 1.14 Conceptual guidelines for neck dissection classification. From Robbins (2001) Robbins et al. (2008b). Reprinted with permission from American Academy of Otolaryngology – Head and Neck Surgery Foundation, Inc.

terminology in 1991 (Fig. 1.14) (Werning and Mendenhall 2007). The various types of neck dissections were described based on the different lymph nodes levels, and some of the levels were subdivided into several compartments.

The use of the elective neck dissection can be thought of as a continuing evolutionary cycle which, in contrast to other evolutionary cycles such as the dinosaur, does not necessarily mean that the RND or modified radical neck dissection (MRND) is no longer in use. Quite the contrary, for patients with advanced-stage cervical lymph node metastases, the RND or MRND remains the mainstay of treatment. However, throughout the world, the selective neck dissection (SND) appears to be more consistently accepted for use in patients with the N_0 neck and in selected cases of N_1–N_2 neck metastasis.

In the 1970s, in our Department at the University of Pittsburgh the approach for most patients with squamous cell carcinoma of the head and neck was to do an RND on patients with an N+ neck and "observation" for patients with an N_0 neck, with salvage surgery (RND) in patients who developed metastatic cancer to the neck (Schramm et al. 1980). Over the ensuing decades, with the trends toward more limited surgery in other tumor systems such as breast cancer and osteogenic sarcoma, we increasingly used more limited neck dissections because the morbidity associated with RND, both in terms of cosmesis and functionality, is significant (Myers and Gastman 2003) (Fig. 1.15). As we studied several series of patients, it also became clear that some of the patients in the observation group had presented late with inoperable cancer in the neck. Therefore, we continued with RND as a treatment of choice because of our concern over the poor prognosis associated with ECS in cervical lymph nodes.

Fig. 1.15 Patient with classic radical neck dissection demonstrating cosmetic deformity of the neck associated with dropped shoulder and a concave appearance. Reprinted with permission of the American Medical Association (Myers and Gastman 2003)

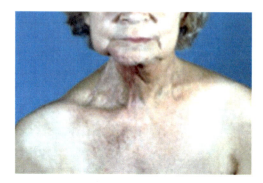

Extracapsular Spread

Professor Gordon Snow from Amsterdam, in 1979, presented a very important paper at the American Society of Head and Neck Surgeons (Snow et al. 1982). He reported that ECS in cervical lymph nodes carried a very poor prognosis based on both regional recurrence and development of distant metastasis. In his publication in 1982, the term "extracapsular spread" was introduced into the United States for the first time. Before that time, the term "soft tissue invasion" was associated with advanced lymph node metastasis, fixed deeply because of the invasion of the adjacent soft tissue. Snow's publication was also extremely important because he stated that 75% of patients with lymph nodes measuring more than 3 cm in diameter (N_1) would be found to harbor ECS. This meant that by the time that the patient or physician could palpate a mass in the neck, there was already a 75% chance that ECS would be present, providing a high degree of correlation with the poor prognosis. Even more frightening was the observation that ECS could be found in lymph nodes less than 1 cm; in such cases, ECS is usually undetectable by physical examination or imaging. Dr. Snow was stimulated by the work of Professor Yves Cachin, the Chief of Head and Neck Service at the Institute Gustave Roussy in France, who pointed out the same poor prognosis in what he referred to as "capsular rupture" (Cachin 1977).

Energized by Professor Snow's presentation, we carried out a study entitled "The ECS of tumor in cervical node metastasis" to validate these very important observations (Johnson et al. 1981). We examined specimens from 177 RNDs and surprisingly found no substantial difference in survivorship between patients who had no metastatsis in the cervical lymph nodes and another group of patients who had metastasis confined to the lymph nodes. However, the 2-year survivorship in patients with ECS was dramatically lower than in either of the above groups. This study was the first in the United States to systematically study this problem and call attention to the poor prognosis associated with ECS.

In a subsequent study published in 1985, we examined the records of an additional 349 patients who had undergone 371 RNDs and again demonstrated the dramatic reduction in survival with the finding of ECS when compared with a cohort of patients with similar-staged disease who had metastasis confined to the lymph nodes or to those patients who had no cervical lymph node metastasis (Johnson et al. 1985). The mean disease-free interval between surgical therapy and the development of recurrent disease was less than 18 months, and the patients with ECS had a higher incidence of regional recurrence and distant metastasis and a reduced disease-free survival. This study supported the original observation that ECS was an indicator of poor prognosis. These findings made our surgical group reluctant to do less than an RND because of the high rate of regional recurrence. Since the publication of our observations, the presence of ECS has become well recognized and has become an important feature in the management of squamous cell carcinoma of the head and neck. ECS is also now mentioned in articles on other types of tumors in the head and neck, such as melanoma, and thyroid and salivary gland tumors; although intuitively this finding cannot be good, it has not been systematically studied in the other tumor types.

The prognostic importance of ECS is illustrated by two recent retrospective studies at M. D. Anderson Cancer Center where the treatment records of 266 patients with cancer of the oral tongue were reviewed (Myers et al. 2001; Greenberg et al. 2003). In this series, the 5-year DSSS was 88% for pN_0 patients and 59% for pN+ patients. The risk of dying from cancer of the oral tongue was at least twice as great in patients with pN+ disease, with or without ECS, compared with patients with pN_0 disease. Five-year DSS was 66% in patients without ECS and 48% in patients with ECS.

With our own similar experience in the early 1980s, we treated all patients with ECS with postoperative radiation therapy as suggested by Professor Snow. However, we found that, although patients with ECS treated with surgery and radiation therapy had an improved regional control rate, they still had a poor survival rate. As a result of these observations, we instituted a program of adjuvant chemotherapy for those who would accept it. We published the results of a prospective nonrandomized study in which patients with ECS who had been treated with surgery and postoperative radiation were offered outpatient chemotherapy consisting of 18 courses of methotrexate and 5-fluorouracil. We were encouraged by the fact that the determinant 5-year disease-free survival rate was 54% for the patients treated with chemotherapy compared with the 17% for those who did not have chemotherapy. Each group was comparable in terms of cancer stage and Karnofsky's score (Johnson et al. 1987). With these improved results and with the development of better forms of chemotherapy, we have continued our program of treating these high-risk patients with ECS with concomitant postoperative chemoradiation using carboplatinum. These promising results were reported in Cancer (Johnson et al. 1996). While not generally accepted, this work has, in a way, been validated in a prospective randomized study of surgery, radiation, and chemotherapy by Bernier et al. (2004). The best survivorship results were achieved in patients who had surgery followed by adjuvant chemoradiotherapy as compared with those who had surgery alone or radiation therapy alone (Ambrosch and Brinck 1996; Enepekides et al. 1999).

In a review of 35 years experience with postoperative radiation for squamous cell carcinoma of the oral cavity, Hinerman et al. from the University of Florida reported that the local control rate in patients with ECS was 31% at 3 years after surgery alone versus 66% at 3 years after surgery followed by radiation therapy. Disease-free survival at 3 years was 25% with surgery alone and 45% after combined modality treatment (Hinerman et al. 2004).

Since it has been demonstrated in multiple publications that ECS portends a poor prognosis and that many patients having ECS benefit from postoperative radiation therapy, there should be a hightened vigilance in terms of determining the exact incidence of micrometastasis. The implication of this is that patients found to have pN_0 disease would not ordinarily be treated; but these patients may develop recurrence in the neck in cases in which the actual pathologic N status is pN+, as may be revealed on more thorough examination. Ambrosch et al. (1995) and Ambrosch and Brinck (1996) investigated the incidence of micrometastasis from squamous cell carcinoma of the head and neck in neck dissection specimens from patients originally staged as pN_0 relying upon serial microscopic sectioning and immunostaining with an antibody to pancytokeratin. They examined 1,020 lymph nodes from 76 neck dissections. Examination of these specimens disclosed eight micrometastases (7.9%) in six specimens from six patients with oral and pharyngeal cancers, which resulted in upstaging of disease in these patients. The micrometastases were detected in lymph nodes that were no more than 3–6 mm in diameter. All eight micrometastasis were located in the subcapsular sinus of the lymph node and all were found in nodes from Level II.

Enepekides found that of 40 patients with T1–T2 squamous cell carcinoma of the lip and oral cavity that had previously been pathologically staged as pN_0, 0.5% had micrometastasis as disclosed by immunoperoxidase staining of cervical lymph nodes with antibodies to cytokeratin (Enepekides et al. 1999). The study suggests that the true incidence of occult metastasis with squamous cell carcinoma of the oral cavity (stage I and II) is higher than previously documented.

Hamakawa et al. reviewed 544 cervical lymph nodes obtained from 73 patients with squamous cell cancer ; the specimens were sectioned at 200-μm intervals (Hamakawa et al. 2000). One series was used for hematoxylin-eosin (H&E) staining and the other for keratin immunostaining. In total, micrometastasis measuring less than 3 mm was detected in 29 sites in 23 lymph nodes in 16 patients, corresponding to 4.2% of the lymph nodes examined and 21.9% of the patients. These data indicate that immunohistochemical assessment and molecular analysis of cervical lymph nodes can be useful in refining the staging system and that a significant number of cases are found to have micrometastasis and the neck can be upstaged.

Functional Neck Dissection

As more information about functional neck dissection became available from Europe in the 1980s, there was a transition from the RND, which included the removal of the spinal accessory nerve as mandated by Dr. Hayes Martin, to an era of the MRND sparing the nerve. Shah et al. observed that in cases in which the spinal accessory nerve was spared, the patients had fewer problems with pain and decreased functionality, while the oncologic outcome was not changed from the classical RND (Shah 1990). Lingeman et al. (1977) reported on a series of 98 patients with cN_0 disease who underwent MRND, none of whom had regional recurrence. In 1980, Molinari also indicated low regional recurrence rate in patients with cancer of the larynx who underwent MRND (Molinari et al. 1980).

We began to use the MRND in the elective neck during the 1980s for patients with N_0 neck. In cases in which more than two lymph nodes were identified by pathology reports, the patients were treated with postoperative radiation therapy, and in cases in which ECS was identified, the patients were offered chemoradiation therapy. This was very helpful in preventing recurrence and improving survival in the ECS group of patients.

Our transition into the era of the elective neck dissection was slow to come, primarily because of our preoccupation with ECS. When we think back on Butlin's pioneering work with elective neck dissections at the end of the nineteenth century, we are remorseful about not bringing this technique to our patients earlier. We did, however, begin to use the SND for cN_0 neck in 1990. The evolution of our surgical approach was largely stimulated by the work of Bocca and Pignatoro, who in 1967 described the use of functional neck dissection, including dissection of the fascial spaces and removal of the lymph nodes without removal of nonlymphoid structures (Bocca and Pignataro 1967; Bocca 1975). The work was based on the surgical anatomical description of the fascial compartments of the neck by Professor Osvaldo Suarez , an otolaryngologist and anatomist from Argentina (Myers and Gastman 2003; Ferlito and Rinaldo 2005) (Fig. 1.16).

Dr. Bocca apparently had the opportunity to see Professor Suarez operate and later attended a course that he presented with Dr. Cesar Gavilan at the La Paz Hospital in Madrid .

Spiro and colleagues from Memorial Sloan-Kettering Cancer Center in New York in a landmark article found that the supra-omohyoid neck dissection (SOHND) (levels I, II, and III), which had been used with increasing frequency in their hospital since 1980 for patients with cancer of the oral cavity, accounted for about 25% of the neck dissections carried out at the time of their research (Spiro et al. 1988). They performed SOHND on 115 patients with cancer of the oral cavity. They found that metastasis to the cervical lymph nodes was present in 31% of the necks and that three of these specimens demonstrated ECS. Twenty of the patients were treated with postoperative radiation therapy and an 86% control rate of the neck through postoperative radiation therapy was achieved. Byers (1985) reported 100% control of the neck in patients with pathologically confirmed TN_1 disease who had undergone a SOHND and post-operative radiation therapy. Byers' conclusions were somewhat different in that he advocated SOHND alone as adequate treatment for PN_1 disease that did not show any evidence of ECS. This conclusion of Byers proved to be sound, as we have shown in our own work.

Fig. 1.16 Osvaldo Suarez (1912–1972)

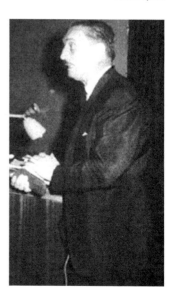

The Brazilian Head and Neck Cancer Study Group (1999) in a prospective trial compared the results of lateral neck dissection, an SND of levels II–IV of the neck, with that of MRND in 132 patients with cancer of the larynx. They concluded that the rate of recurrence in the neck in a 5-year overall survival were similar in both groups, confirming the efficacy of the more limited neck dissection in elective treatment of N_0 neck. (Group 1999)

We began to use SND in our department in 1990, and in 1997, Pitman et al. compared SND with RND for effective management in the clinically negative neck (Pitman et al. 1997). This study included 280 patients treated with 322 RNDs between 1974 and 1989 and 114 patients treated with 168 SNDs between January 1990 and March 1994. The overall regional recurrence rate for RND was 5.8%, which is not significantly different from the regional recurrence rate for SND of 3.5%, indicating that the SND is as effective as RND for treating the N_0 neck. In another study from our department, none of the patients with occult ECS positive nodes treated with SND had a recurrence. A trend towards decreased survival was seen in those with pN + ECS + nodes compared with patients with pN + lymph nodes. (Alvi and Johnson 1996). ECS was present in at least 19% of nodes with occult metastasis in the M. D. Anderson series (Myers et al. 2000).

J. Myers et al. at M. D Anderson Cancer Center analyzed a group of 64 patients with squamous cell carcinoma of the tongue in an age group younger than 39 years. The patients who were initially treated elsewhere or at M. D. Anderson who had a neck dissection as part of their initial treatment had a better outcome than those without neck dissection. Three and 5-year survival rates were 81% and 72%, respectively, in patients who had a neck dissection, and 44% and 22%, respectively, in patients whose necks were not dissected.

Kowalski in a series of 513 consecutive patients with squamous cell carcinoma of the oral cavity demonstrated a poor prognosis associated with patients who were managed with "watchful waiting" compared with those who had an END (Kowalski et al. 2000). The most important observation was that the 50% of the patients with metastasis in the neck discovered at follow-up were not candidates for surgical salvage and died of this cancer.

Kligerman et al. examined a cohort of 67 patients with T_1–T_2 squamous cell carcinoma of the tongue and floor of the mouth (Kligerman et al. 1994). The patients treated with SOHND at the time of the resection of the primary cancer had fewer recurrences in the neck and a better survival rate than did those who underwent resection of the primary cancer alone. Most importantly, the authors found a poor salvage rate among patients who did not undergo SOHND and who developed cervical metastasis under "observation."

The Head and Neck Group of the Swiss Society of Otolaryngology – Head and Neck Surgery, reported their results in patients with early (T1–T2) carcinoma of the oral cavity adequately treated by resection of the primary cancer and a neck dissection, at least levels I–III (Wolfensberger et al. 2001). One of the specific aims of the study was to achieve tumor-free margins by the use of intraoperative frozen section. The results in this study were somewhat equivocal since the tumor survival probability of 91% after 4 years confirmed the hypothesis that early oral cancer is adequately treated by resection alone without need for radiation therapy. Unfortunately, 16% of the patients had to be referred for additional therapy because of recurrence in the neck. The authors, for some reason, stated that 71% survival was very good so that no drawback resulted for the patient from the "wait and see" approach. These results stand in stark contrast to all the articles described above. The authors state that under no circumstances would they dispense with neck dissection in patients for whom reliable after care could not be guaranteed.

Akhtar et al. evaluated 94 patients with T_1–T_2 N_0 squamous cell carcinoma of the tongue treated with partial glossectomy and elective MRND and concluded that the occult micrometastasis rate of 32% in their patients warrants elective neck dissection. In early cases, the incidence of metastasis to levels IV and V in these cases is low, so these lymph nodes should be removed only when there is an intraoperative finding suspicious of extensive metastasis in levels I, II, or III. Otherwise, SOHND is sufficient (Akhtar et al. 2007). In this series, two patients had "skip metastasis" in levels III and IV and two patients had involvement of level V.

Hao et al. analyzed a series of 140 consecutive patients with squamous cell carcinoma of the oral cavity with an N_0 neck who underwent SOHND at Chang Gung Memorial Hospital in Taiwan (Hao and Tsang 2002). The patients were followed for at least 2 years. Thirty-seven patients had postoperative radiation therapy because of an advanced primary cancer, close margins or pN+. Twenty-four percent of the patients had occult cervical metastasis, and a control rate by SOHND of 91.4% was achieved. One of 21 patients who underwent postoperative radiation therapy had neck recurrence. Four of 13 patients who did not undergo postoperative radiation therapy had recurrence in the neck.

Hosal at the University of Pittsburgh studied the results of 300 neck dissections performed on 210 patients to study the efficacy of SND in the management of the clinically N_0 neck. He concluded that SND is effective for controlling metastases to the neck. In this group, 33% of the patients were pN+, and of those with positive nodes, 24% had ECS. Importantly, the patients who have more than two metastatic nodes when untreated had a higher incidence of recurrence than the patients with cancer limited to one or two lymph nodes. As a result of this study, we now systematically include radiation therapy as part of our program in patients who have more than two positive lymph nodes without ECS. All patients with ECS are treated with chemoradiation (Hosal et al. 2000).

Pitman compared the results of SND with MRND in a review of 556 patients with previously untreated N_0–N_2 squamous cell carcinoma of the oral cavity, oral pharynx, hypopharynx, and larynx. Among the 222 patients who had SND, the surgical specimens contained metastasis in 22%. One or more lymph nodes with ECS were detected in 24% of the node-positive specimens. Postoperative radiation therapy was given to 62% of patients with pN+. In this study, SND was indicated both as an elective and therapeutic procedure. For the pN_0 neck, the recurrence rate was 4.7%, in accordance with other reports showing the incidence of neck recurrence of 3–7% in the pN_0 neck (Pellitteri et al. 1997; Spiro et al. 1996; Pitman et al. 1997; Byers et al. 1988; Medina and Byers 1989; Spiro et al. 1993; Henick et al. 1995).

Use of the Selective Neck Dissection in the Management of the N+ Neck

We began to use the selective neck dissection as a staging procedure in patients with an N_0 neck in 1990. As we gained more experience with this procedure, we found that it was an operation that was soundly based in anatomical study and that understanding the fascial compartments allowed removal of the lymph nodes that were most likely to be involved by metastatic cancer from different primary sites in the head and neck, based on the observations of Shah (1990). This could be done without removing adjacent structures such as had been the case with RND and MRND. As we studied the results in elective neck dissections, it appeared that approximately one-third of the patients with cN_0 neck had, in fact, a pN+ neck. We found that if there were no more than two positive lymph nodes without ECS, and that the patients did not require adjunctive radiation therapy or a therapeutic neck and did well without recurrence.

The realization that we were in fact operating successfully on the cN_0 but pN+ neck one-third of the time with minimal recurrence led to the intentional use of the SND as a therapeutic procedure in patients who had cN_1 and selected cN_2 disease. Our indications presently are patients who have lymph nodes up to 6 cm (N_1–N_2a), which are mobile. We occasionally found intraoperatively some fixation to the sternocleidomastoid muscle and the jugular vein, in which case an adequate cuff of normal tissue from these structures was removed without any functional or cosmetic problems. The patients who had multiple positive nodes (N_2b) could also be treated with selective neck dissection as could patients with bilateral neck metastasis N_2c, as long as the nodes were in N_1–N_2 category. We considered these patients to be candidates for SND, understanding that most of the patients with cN+ will receive radiation therapy or chemoradiation in the event of ECS. If the node had decreased mobility, it was not deemed appropriate for the SND, and an MRND was employed. In some cases, the spinal accessory nerve could not be saved due to extensive tumor, so an RND was carried out. Fixed nodes were not treated primarily with surgery.

We reported the results of the use of SND for cN+ as a therapeutic option in 2006 in 65 patients (Simental et al. 2006). There was a recurrence rate of 6.1%, including inside and outside the dissected field This is similar to the recurrence rate reported by Chepeha et al. on 52 patients who underwent 58 SNDs for cN+ (Chepeha et al. 2002). They treated patients with cervical metastasis less than 3 cm. Postoperative radiation therapy was used for patients with more than two positive lymph nodes, ECS and T3–T4. The regional control rate was comparable to control rates obtained with MRND combined with similar indications for postoperative radiation therapy.

Anderson et al., in 2002, used SND on 170 patients with cN+ and reported regional recurrence rates in 8.4% of the patients who underwent SND and postoperative radiation therapy (Andersen et al. 2002). Byers et al. reported the use of SND in the management of cN+ (Byers et al. 1999). There was a regional recurrence rate of 35% in 517 SNDs in patients with pathologically positive nodes. However, when postoperative radiation therapy was given in the patients with pN+, the recurrence rate decreased to 5.6%. Thus, the authors recommended the use of postoperative radiation therapy for patients with pN+, a practice that is currently widely followed.

In another large series, Ambrosch et al. used postoperative radiation therapy in order to improve the regional control rate in patients with pN+ (Ambrosch et al. 2001). This was especially true for patients with ECS or multiple metastatic nodes. Lohuis et al. (2004) reported the effectiveness of the therapeutic SND in patients with laryngeal and hypopharygeal squamous cell carcinoma (N_1, N_2). They started performing SNDs (Level II–V) in patients with laryngeal and hypopharyngeal cancer and clinically proven N+ disease in the 1990s. This group had an experience similar to ours in that they found that one-third of the SNDs in the N_0 neck proved to be pN+. However, the authors state that the use of SND for the cN+ neck is much more controversial. Surgeons have reported results of therapeutic SND in N_1–N_2 in cancer of the larynx and hypopharynx, all of whom received postoperative radiation therapy with regional recurrence rates ranging from 0 to 33% (Spiro et al. 1993; Byers et al. 1999; Pellitteri et al. 1997; Traynor et al. 1996). The authors state that in the case of N3 disease, RND or MRND should remain the standard.

Pellitteri et al. stated that SND represents an accepted modality for the management of N_0 and selected N_1 necks in the treatment of squamous cell carcinoma of the upper aerodigestive tract (Pellitteri et al. 1997). Application of SND in the management of more advanced lymph node metastasis (N_{2a}, N_{2b}, and N_3) had not been advocated. The reluctance to apply this modality may be due to the belief that the predictability of cervical node metastasis can be altered following involvement of the first eschelon lymph node groups. They voiced additional concerns in this more advanced group, particularly with the incidence of ECS and with multiple nodal involvement that may not be addressed adequately by SND. Despite their concerns, they reported a regional recurrence rate of 10% for the group of patients with N_2–N_3 disease following SND and felt that this was not appreciably different from the entire study population.

Muzaffar (2003) reported a series of 359 consecutive patients. Of these, 269 patients had a pN+ neck on histological examination and 90 had a pN_0 neck. pN+ patients were treated with radiation therapy of 50 Gy on average. A total of eight patients (5%) had recurrence in the neck, and two of these had ECS. The overall mean time of recurrence was 19.5 months. Salvage surgery was attempted in five of the eight patients but was successful in only one. Indications for radiation therapy included the presence of two or more positive lymph nodes, nodes involved in multiple levels, evidence of ECS, positive surgical margins, or tumor size T3–T4. Disease-free survival 2 years after the end of this study was tabulated, and 80% of the SND group were either alive disease free or had died free of disease. The survival rates for the MRND and RND groups are similar at 29/45, 64% and 37/58, 64%, respectively, and a 14% incidence of distant metastasis.

Clark et al. raised the question of outcome of treatment for advanced cervical metastatic squamous cell carcinoma (Clark et al. 2005). The authors state that, in many centers, patients with advanced but resectable cancer of the head and neck (N2 and N3) are managed primarily with surgery and postoperative radiotherapy. The effectiveness of this strategy has been well established; however, a high rate of tumor response in the neck can also be achieved when primary chemoradiation protocols are used. The purpose of their study was to evaluate the outcomes of patients N2 or N3 metastatic squamous cell carcinoma managed with a consistent policy of surgery and postoperative RT in an attempt to identify subgroups for whom this combination therapy may be inadequate and for whom alternative treatment strategies could be investigated. The series included 181 patients, 70 of whom were treated with SND. Control in the treated neck was achieved in 86% of the patients. DSS was only 39% at 5 years. The authors state that the use of SND should be guided by the extent and distribution of nodal metastasis in addition to the characteristics of the primary tumor. These may be suitable when metastatic disease is limited, but in general, patients with advanced neck disease require a comprehensive dissection, including extended RND. Microscopic ECS remained a significant risk factor for regional failure, and the authors suggest the use of chemoradiation therapy since reports from prospective randomized trials show the beneficial effects from this therapy (Cooper et al. 2004; Bernier et al. 2001).

Verrucous Carcinoma

A subset of patients have verrucous carcinoma of the oral cavity. In a recent review of 2,350 cases of verrucous cancer of the head and neck in the National Cancer Database, the most frequent site of involvement was the oral cavity (55.9%) (Koch et al. 2001). Patients with pure verrucous carcinoma do not require neck dissection since this variation of squamous carcinoma does not metastasize. Treatment of such cases usually consists of local excision of the primary cancer. However, there is a hybrid form of verrucous carcinoma that coexists with the more typical invasive squamous cell carcinoma which does have the potential to metastasize. Patients who have verrucous carcinoma should be counseled that if a primary squamous cell carcinoma component is identified in the final pathology report after resection of the intraoral tumor, the patient should then be readmitted for an SND (Myers and Simental 2003).

Treatment Strategies

In the cN_0 neck, single modality therapy should be used whenever possible to manage squamous cell carcinoma of the upper aerodigestive tract since there is a high possibility of developing second primary cancers for which radiation therapy might be of importance. Since surgical resection of the primary cancer of the oral cavity is the method of choice, the neck at risk for metastasis to the lymph nodes is electively dissected (Werning and Mendenhall 2007). Many of the surgeons who advocate the elective management of the cN_0 neck in squamous cell carcinoma believe that treatment is warranted when the probability of metastasis exceeds 15–20%. This treatment threshold originally evolved from largely empirical recommendations that attempted to achieve a balance between the presumed improvement in survival provided by elective treatment and the calculated risk of morbidity and mortality. Decision analysis has been applied to the outcomes of treatment that were published for the N_0 neck between 1971 and 1991, leading to the conclusion that the probability of metastatic disease of more than 20% should be considered the appropriate threshold for elective management of the neck. A recent survey of board-certified otolaryngologists who treat patients with head and neck cancer, however, found that only 50% of the respondents treat the patients when the risk of metastasis exceeds 15–20% (Werning et al. 2003).

Cervical metastasis does not always correlate with T classification since patients with T1 cancer of the tongue and floor of the mouth have a significant risk of occult metastatic disease (Cunningham et al. 1986). Approximately, 21% of T1 cancers and 43% of T2 cancers and 56–70% of T3 cancers have pathologically positive lymph nodes revealed by SND. Elective or therapeutic treatment of the cervical lymphatics is recommended for virtually all patients with cancer of the oral tongue (Myers and Simental 2003). This is predicated on the notion that earlier treatment of cancer should result in improved outcomes. While the overall survival benefit of elective neck treatment may be small, there is a definite benefit in disease-free survival (Myers and Simental 2003). In addition, many patients who are simply observed are eventually discovered to have cervical lymph node metastasis that is unresectable (Cunningham et al. 1986).

Surgical Techniques

Since many excellent descriptions of techniques for neck dissections are available (Operative Otolaryngology-Head and Neck Surgery, Myers, 2nd ed, Saunders 2008), we have not included any detailed description of these procedures. However, there are two areas of controversy as to what levels should be included in the selective neck dissection. These include the dissection of sublevel IIB (submuscular recess) and the dissection of level IV (Fig. 1.8). Paleri et al. studied a series of 903 patients identified in 14 articles with 903 necks suitable for inclusion (Paleri et al. 2008). The overall incidence of metastatic disease at sublevel IIB in patients with cancer of the oral cavity is 3.9% (11 of 279). Contralateral positive nodes and isolated metastasis to this level were rare. Their conclusion was that there was no advantage in performing submuscular dissection (of sublevel IIB) in the contralateral neck or in cancer of the larynx. The primary concern in dissecting sublevel IIB is the potential for injury to the spinal accessory nerve, with associated pain, and shoulder dysfunction. Since oral cavity and oropharyngeal primary cancers have an incidence rate of metastasis to sublevel IIB of 4–5%, Paleri's recommendation is that this sublevel should be dissected in the setting of oral cavity and oropharyngeal primaries. An alternative suggestion based on the observation that "if it is evident that the patient will need postoperative radiation on the basis of the primary cancer, dissection of sublevel IIB can be avoided and subclinical metastasis can be treated adequately with radiation therapy."

Another controversial site is level IV. Byers, in 1997, reported finding "skip metastasis" to lymph nodes in level III and or level IV in 15.8% of the patients with cancer of the oral tongue (Byers et al. 1997). As a result of this study, the authors recommended removal of the lymph nodes of level IV whenever an SND is performed on any patient with cancer of the oral tongue. Medina (Khafif et al. 2001), however, recently published the results of a study undertaken to determine the incidence of occult metastasis to lymph nodes in level IV in patients with cancer of the oral tongue with N_0 neck to determine the efficacy of a clinical practice in which these lymph nodes were not routinely removed during elective dissection for cancer of the tongue. The authors concluded that occult nodal metastasis to level IV for patients T1–T3 N_0 cancer of the oral tongue was 4%. Dissection of these nodes only when there is intraoperative suspicion of metastasis to level II or III does not increase the risk of recurrent tumor in the neck.

Shah et al. studied RND specimens performed electively for cancer of the oral cavity and found metastasis in level IV lymph nodes in 3% of the patients (Shah 1990). Medina argued that extending a supra-omohyoid neck dissection to include the lymph nodes at level IV is a relatively simple maneuver that prolongs the operation by only a short period of time. However, exposure to that region through a high cervical incision, which they use for their SNDs, is awkward and increases the risk of a chylous fistula.

We favor elective neck dissection rather than the wait-and-see policy by observation. This should include levels I, II, III, and IV in all cases of oral cavity cancer, particularly with cancer of the oral tongue. The idea of only doing a neck dissection in cases with 15–20% possibility of metastasis is a form of gambling with the patient by playing the odds. After all, for the surgeon, the percentage of positive nodes may be small, but for the patient who is one of Medina's, 4% is actually 100%.

We know that because there is an incidence of metastasis to level IIb and IV, albeit a small one, not removing the lymph nodes in that area is similar to the obsolete method of "watch and wait," which we have cited over and over again in this chapter, being inadequate treatment instead of doing an elective neck dissection. In my philosophy, as long as there is any incidence of metastasis to the subsite, the subsite should be dissected carefully and the potential lymph node metastasis removed , particularly since so little extra time and effort is necessary. Naturally, caution must be exercised to avoid injury to the spinal accessory nerve and thoracic duct.

Conclusion

- Metastasis to the neck from squamous cell carcinoma of the oral cavity is a negative predictor of survival.
- Diagnostic modalities such as CT scan, MRI, PET-CT, ultrasound, FNAB, and sentinel lymph node biopsy should be used in an effort to stage the neck as accurately as possible since understaging leads to under treatment of the neck.
- A "watch and wait" approach to the N_0 neck, even for early stage primary squamous cell carcinoma of the oral cavity, is dangerous and not in the patient's best interest.
- The selective neck dissection is based on sound anatomic principles and in practice has proved to be as effective in the management of both the N_0 and selected N+ necks as the radical or modified radical neck dissection and should be practiced by all head and neck surgeons.
- There remains a role for RND/MRND in patients with advanced lymph node metastasis.

In the future, we are certain to improve the cure rate of cancer of the oral cavity not with more or better surgery, but based upon a better understanding of the biology of lymph node metastasis and development of effective interventions at a molecular level.

References

Akhtar S, Ikram M, Ghaffar S (2007) Neck involvement in early carcinoma of tongue. Is elective neck dissection warranted? J Pak Med Assoc 57:305–307

Alvi A, Johnson JT (1996) Extracapsular spread in the clinically negative neck (N0): implications and outcome. Otolaryngol Head Neck Surg 114:65–70

Ambrosch P, Brinck U (1996) Detection of nodal micrometastases in head and neck cancer by serial sectioning and immunostaining. Oncology (Williston Park) 10:1221–1226 discussion 1226, 1229

Ambrosch P, Kron M, Fischer G, Brinck U (1995) Micrometastases in carcinoma of the upper aerodigestive tract: detection, risk of metastasizing, and prognostic value of depth of invasion. Head Neck 17:473–479

Ambrosch P, Kron M, Pradier O, Steiner W (2001) Efficacy of selective neck dissection: a review of 503 cases of elective and therapeutic treatment of the neck in squamous cell carcinoma of the upper aerodigestive tract. Otolaryngol Head Neck Surg 124:180–187

Andersen PE, Warren F, Spiro J, Burningham A, Wong R, Wax MK, Shah JP, Cohen JI (2002) Results of selective neck dissection in management of the node-positive neck. Arch Otolaryngol Head Neck Surg 128:1180–1184

Bennett JA, Deol P, Abrahams JJ (2007) Imaging of patients with oral cancer. In: Werning JW (ed) Oral Cancer. Diagnosis, Management, and Rehabilitation. Thieme Medical Publishers, New York

Bernier J, Ozsahin M, Greiner R et al (2001) Results of EORTC Phase III Trial 22931 comparing, in post-operative setting, radiotherapy and radiotherapy combined to cisplatin in locally advanced head and neck squamous cell carcinoma (abstract). Int J Radiat Oncol Biol Phys 51(Suppl 1):3

Bernier J, Domenge C, Ozsahin M, Matuszewska K, Lefebvre JL, Greiner RH, Giralt J, Maingon P, Rolland F, Bolla M, Cognetti F, Bourhis J, Kirkpatrick A, van Glabbeke M (2004) Postoperative irradiation with or without concomitant chemotherapy for locally advanced head and neck cancer. N Engl J Med 350:1945–1952

Bocca E (1975) Conservative neck dissection. Laryngoscope 85(9):1511–1515

Bocca E, Pignataro O (1967) A conservation technique in radical neck dissection. Ann Otol Rhinol Laryngol 76(5):975–987

Butlin HT (1885) Diseases of the Tongue. Cassell and Company, London

Byers RM (1985) Modified neck dissection. A study of 967 cases from 1970 to 1980. Am J Surg 150(4):414–421

Byers RM, Clayman GL, McGill D, Andrews T, Kare RP, Roberts DB, Goepfert H (1999) Selective neck dissections for squamous carcinoma of the upper aerodigestive tract: patterns of regional failure. Head Neck 21(6):499–505

Byers RM, Weber RS, Andrews T, McGill D, Kare R, Wolf P (1997) Frequency and therapeutic implications of "skip metastases" in the neck from squamous carcinoma of the oral tongue. Head Neck 19(1):14–19

Byers RM, Wolf PF, Ballantyne AJ (1988) Rationale for elective modified neck dissection. Head Neck Surg 10(3):160–167

Cachin Y (1977) Treatment of cervical lymph node metastases from carcinomas of the upper respiratory and digestive tracts. Recent Results Cancer Res 62:215–219

Chelius JM (1847) A System of Surgery. Lea and Blanchard, Philadelphia

Chen AY, Myers JN (2001) Cancer of the oral cavity. Dis Mon 47(7):275–361

Chen AY, Schrag NM, Halpern M, Stewart A, Ward EM (2007) Health insurance and stage at diagnosis of laryngeal cancer: does insurance type predict stage at diagnosis? Arch Otolaryngol Head Neck Surg 133(8):784–790

Chepeha DB, Hoff PT, Taylor RJ, Bradford CR, Teknos TN, Esclamado RM (2002) Selective neck dissection for the treatment of neck metastasis from squamous cell carcinoma of the head and neck. Laryngoscope 112(3):434–438

Clark J, Li W, Smith G, Shannon K, Clifford A, McNeil E, Gao K, Jackson M, Mo Tin M, O'Brien C (2005) Outcome of treatment for advanced cervical metastatic squamous cell carcinoma. Head Neck 27(2):87–94

Conley J (1967) Cancer of the Head and Neck. Proceedings of the International Workshop on CANCER of the HEAD and NECK. Butterworths, Washington

Cooper JS, Pajak TF, Forastiere AA, Jacobs J, Campbell BH, Saxman SB, Kish JA, Kim HE, Cmelak AJ, Rotman M, Machtay M, Ensley JF, Chao KS, Schultz CJ, Lee N, Fu KK (2004) Postoperative concurrent radiotherapy and chemotherapy for high-risk squamous-cell carcinoma of the head and neck. N Engl J Med 350(19):1937–1944

Crile GW (1905) On the surgical treatment of cancer of the head and neck. With a summary of one hundred and twenty-one operations performed upon one hundred and five patients. Trans South Surg Gynecol Assoc 18:108–127

Crile GW (1906) Excision of cancer of the head and neck. With special reference to the plan of dissection based on one hundred and thirty-two operations. JAMA 47:1780–1786

Cunningham MJ, Johnson JT, Myers EN, Schramm VL Jr, Thearle PB (1986) Cervical lymph node metastasis after local excision of early squamous cell carcinoma of the oral cavity. Am J Surg 152(4):361–366

Enepekides DJ, Sultanem K, Nguyen C, Shenouda G, Black MJ, Rochon L (1999) Occult cervical metastases: immunoperoxidase analysis of the pathologically negative neck. Otolaryngol Head Neck Surg 120(5):713–717

Ferlito A, Rinaldo A (2005) Neck dissection: historical and current concepts. Am J Otolaryngology – Head and Neck Medicine and Surgery 26:289–295

Ferlito A, Johnson JT, Rinaldo A, Pratt LW, Fagan JJ, Weir N, Suarez C, Folz BJ, Bien S, Towpik E, Leemans CR, Bradley PJ, Kowalski LP, Herranz J, Gavilan J, Olofsson J (2007) European surgeons were the first to perform neck dissection. Laryngoscope 117(5):797–802

Ferlito A, Rinaldo A (2004) Osvaldo Suarez: often-forgotten father of functional neck dissection. Laryngoscope 114(7):1177–1178

Funk GF, Karnell LH, Robinson RA, Zhen WK, Trask DK, Hoffman HT (2002) Presentation, treatment, and outcome of oral cavity cancer: a National Cancer Data Base report. Head Neck 24(2):165–180

Gavilan J, Herranz-Gonzalez JJ, Lentsch EJ (2003) Cancer of the Neck. In: Myers EN, Suen JY, Myers JN, Hanna EYN (eds) Cancer of the Head and Neck. Saunders, Philadelphia

Goodwin WJ, Thomas GR, Parker DF, Joseph D, Levis S, Franzmann E, Anello C, Hu JJ (2008) Unequal burden of head and neck cancer in the United States. Head Neck 30(3):358–371

Greenberg JS, Fowler R, Gomez J, Mo V, Roberts D, El Naggar AK, Myers JN (2003) Extent of extracapsular spread: a critical prognosticator in oral tongue cancer. Cancer 97(6): 1464–1470

Greenlee RT, Murray T, Bolden S, Wingo PA (2000) Cancer statistics. CA Cancer J Clin 50:7–33

Group, Brazilian Head and Neck Cancer Study (1999) End results of a prospective trial on elective lateral neck dissection vs. type III modified radical neck dissection in the management of supraglottic and transglottic carcinomas. Head Neck 21(8):694–702

Hamakawa H, Takemura K, Sumida T, Kayahara H, Tanioka H, Sogawa K (2000) Histological study on pN upgrading of oral cancer. Virchows Arch 437:116–121

Hao SP, Tsang NM (2002) The role of supraomohyoid neck dissection in patients with oral cavity carcinoma. Oral Oncol 38(3):309–312

Hart RD, Henry E, Nasser JG, Trites JR, Taylor SM, Bullock M, Barnes D (2007) Sentinel node biopsy in N0 squamous cell carcinoma of the oral cavity and oropharynx in patients previously treated with surgery or radiation therapy: a pilot study. Arch Otolaryngol Head Neck Surg 133(8):806–809

Henick DH, Silver CE, Heller KS, Shaha AR, El GH, Wolk DP (1995) Supraomohyoid neck dissection as a staging procedure for squamous cell carcinomas of the oral cavity and oropharynx. Head Neck 17(2):119–123

Hinerman RW, Mendenhall WM, Morris CG, Amdur RJ, Werning JW, Villaret DB (2004) Postoperative irradiation for squamous cell carcinoma of the oral cavity: 35-year experience. Head Neck 26(11):984–994

Hollenbeak CS, Lowe VJ, Stack BC Jr (2001) The cost-effectiveness of fluorodeoxyglucose 18-F positron emission tomography in the N0 neck. Cancer 92(9):2341–2348

Hosal AS, Carrau RL, Johnson JT, Myers EN (2000) Selective neck dissection in the management of the clinically node-negative neck. Laryngoscope 110(12):2037–2040

Jawdynski F (1888) Przypadek raka pierwotnego szyi. t.z. raka skrzelowego Volkmann'a. Wyciecie nowotworu wraz z rezekcyja tetnicy szyjowej wspolney i zyly szyjowej wewnctrznej. Wyzdrowienie Gaz Lek 8:530–537

Johnson JT, Barnes EL, Myers EN, Schramm VL Jr, Borochovitz D, Sigler BA (1981) The extracapsular spread of tumors in cervical node metastasis. Arch Otolaryngol 107(12):725–729

Johnson JT, Myers EN, Bedetti CD, Barnes EL, Schramm VL Jr, Thearle PB (1985) Cervical lymph node metastases. Incidence and implications of extracapsular carcinoma. Arch Otolaryngol 111(8):534–537

Johnson JT, Myers EN, Schramm VL Jr, Mayernik DG, Nolan TA, Sigler BA, Wagner RL (1987) Adjuvant chemotherapy for high-risk squamous-cell carcinoma of the head and neck. J Clin Oncol 5(3):456–458

Johnson JT, Wagner RL, Myers EN (1996) A long-term assessment of adjuvant chemotherapy on outcome of patients with extracapsular spread of cervical metastases from squamous carcinoma of the head and neck. Cancer 77(1):181–185

Khafif A, Lopez-Garza JR, Medina JE (2001) Is dissection of level IV necessary in patients with T1–T3 N$_0$ tongue cancer? Laryngoscope 111(6):1088–1090

Klein R (1996) Where there's smoke, there's.. In: Hutcheon L, Hutcheon M (eds) Opera. Desire. Disease. Death. University of Nebraska Press, Lincoln & London

Kligerman J, Lima RA, Soares JR, Prado L, Dias FL, Freitas EQ, Olivatto LO (1994) Supraomohyoid neck dissection in the treatment of T1/T2 squamous cell carcinoma of oral cavity. Am J Surg 168(5):391–394

Koch BB, Trask DK, Hoffman HT, Karnell LH, Robinson RA, Zhen W, Menck HR (2001) National survey of head and neck verrucous carcinoma: patterns of presentation, care, and outcome. Cancer 92(1):110–120

Kocher T (1880) Radicalheilung des Krebses. Dtsch Z Chir 13:134–166

Kowalski LP, Bagietto R, Lara JR, Santos RL, Silva JF Jr, Magrin J (2000) Prognostic significance of the distribution of neck node metastasis from oral carcinoma. Head Neck 22(3):207–214

Kurokawa H, Yamashita Y, Takeda S, Zhang M, Fukuyama H, Takahashi T (2002) Risk factors for late cervical lymph node metastases in patients with stage I or II carcinoma of the tongue. Head Neck 24(8):731–736

Lim SC, Zhang S, Ishii G, Endoh Y, Kodama K, Miyamoto S, Hayashi R, Ebihara S, Cho JS, Ochiai A (2004) Predictive markers for late cervical metastasis in stage I and II invasive squamous cell carcinoma of the oral tongue. Clin Cancer Res 10(1 Pt 1):166–172

Lingeman RE, Helmus C, Stephens R, Ulm J (1977) Neck dissection: radical or conservative. Ann Otol Rhinol Laryngol 86(6 Pt 1):737–744

Lohuis PJ, Klop WM, Tan IB, van Den Brekel MW, Hilgers FJ, Balm AJ (2004) Effectiveness of therapeutic (N1, N2) selective neck dissection (levels II to V) in patients with laryngeal and hypopharyngeal squamous cell carcinoma. Am J Surg 187(2):295–299

Martin HE, Del Valle B, Ehrlich H et al (1951) Neck dissection. Cancer 4:441–499

Medina JE, Byers RM (1989) Supraomohyoid neck dissection: rationale, indications, and surgical technique. Head Neck 11(2):111–122

Molinari R, Cantu G, Chiesa F, Grandi C (1980) Retrospective comparison of conservative and radical neck dissection in laryngeal cancer. Ann Otol Rhinol Laryngol 89:578–581

Muzaffar K (2003) Therapeutic selective neck dissection: a 25-year review. Laryngoscope 113(9):1460–1465

Myers EN (2008) Operative Otolaryngology-Head and Neck Surgery. 2nd Ed., Saunders, Philadelphia

Myers EN, Simental AA (2003) Cancer of the Oral Cavity. In: Myers EN, Suen JY, Myers JN, Hanna EYN (eds) Cancer of the Head and Neck. Saunders, Philadelphia

Myers EN, Gastman BR (2003) Neck dissection: an operation in evolution. Arch Otolaryngol Head Neck Surg 129(1):14–25

Myers JN, Elkins T, Roberts D, Byers RM (2000) Squamous cell carcinoma of the tongue in young adults: increasing incidence and factors that predict treatment outcomes. Otolaryngol Head Neck Surg 122(1):44–51

Myers JN, Greenberg JS, Mo V, Roberts D (2001) Extracapsular spread. A significant predictor of treatment failure in patients with squamous cell carcinoma of the tongue. Cancer 92(12):3030–3036

Ocharoenrat P, Pillai G, Patel S, Fisher C, Archer D, Eccles S, RhysEvans P (2003) Tumour thickness predicts cervical nodal metastases and survival in early oral tongue cancer. Oral Oncol 39:386–390

Packard JH (1881) A system of surgery, theoretical and practical. In: Holmes ET (ed) In treatises by various authors. 1st American, from the 2d English ed. thoroughly revised and much enlarged. H C Lea's Son & Co, Philadelphia

Paleri V, Kumar Subramaniam S, Oozeer N, Rees G, Krishnan S (2008) Dissection of the submuscular recess (sublevel IIb) in squamous cell cancer of the upper aerodigestive tract: Prospective study and systematic review of the literature. Head Neck 30(2):194–200

Pellitteri PK, Robbins KT, Neuman T (1997) Expanded application of selective neck dissection with regard to nodal status. Head Neck 19(4):260–265

Pitman KT, Johnson JT, Myers EN (1997) Effectiveness of selective neck dissection for management of the clinically negative neck. Arch Otolaryngol Head Neck Surg 123(9):917–922

Rigual N, Douglas W, Lamonica D, Wiseman S, Cheney R, Hicks W Jr, Loree T (2005) Sentinel lymph node biopsy: a rational approach for staging T2N0 oral cancer. Laryngoscope 115(12):2217–2220

Robbins KT (2001) Pocket Guide to Neck Disection Classification and TNM Staging o Head and Neck Cancer, 2nd edn. American Academy of Otolaryngology-Head and Neck Surgery Foundation, Alexandria, VA

Robbins KT, Doweck I, Samant S, Vieira F (2008a) Effectiveness of superselective and selective neck dissection for advanced nodal metastases after chemoradiation. Arch Otolaryngol Head Neck Surg 131:965–969

Robbins KT, Shaha AR, Medina JE, Califano JA, Wolf GT, Ferlito A, Som PM, Day TA, Committee for Neck Dissection Classification, American Head and Neck Society (2008b) Consensus statement on the classification and terminology of neck dissection. Arch Otolaryngol Head Neck Surg 134(5):536–538

Ross GL, Soutar DS, Gordon MacDonald D, Shoaib T, Camilleri I, Roberton AG, Sorensen JA, Thomsen J, Grupe P, Alvarez J, Barbier L, Santamaria J, Poli T, Massarelli O, Sesenna E, Kovacs AF, Grunwald F, Barzan L, Sulfaro S, Alberti F (2004) Sentinel node biopsy in head and neck cancer: preliminary results of a multicenter trial. Ann Surg Oncol 11(7):690–696

Rouviere H (1932) Anatomie des lymphatiques de l'homme. Mason et cie, Paris

Schramm VL Jr, Myers EN, Sigler BA (1980) Surgical management of early epidermoid carcinoma of the anterior floor of the mouth. Laryngoscope 90(2):207–215

Shah JP (1990) Patterns of cervical lymph node metastasis from squamous carcinomas of the upper aerodigestive tract. Am J Surg 160:405–409

Simental AA Jr, Duvvuri U, Johnson JT, Myers EN (2006) Selective neck dissection in patients with upper aerodigestive tract cancer with clinically positive nodal disease. Ann Otol Rhinol Laryngol 115(11):846–849

Snow GB, Annyas AA, van Slooten EA, Bartelink H, Hart AA (1982) Prognostic factors of neck node metastasis. Clin Otolaryngol Allied Sci 7(3):185–192

Sparano A, Weinstein G, Chalian A, Yodul M, Weber R (2004) Multivariate predictors of occult neck metastasis in early oral tongue cancer. Otolaryngol Head Neck Surg 131(4):472–476

Spiro JD, Spiro RH, Shah JP, Sessions RB, Strong EW (1988) Critical assessment of supraomohyoid neck dissection. Am J Surg 156(4):286–289

Spiro RH, Gallo O, Shah JP (1993) Selective jugular node dissection in patients with squamous carcinoma of the larynx or pharynx. Am J Surg 166(4):399–402

Spiro RH, Morgan GJ, Strong EW, Shah JP (1996) Supraomohyoid neck dissection. Am J Surg 172(6):650–653

Stoeckli SJ (2007) Sentinel node biopsy for oral and oropharyngeal squamous cell carcinoma of the head and neck. Laryngoscope 117(9):1539–1551

Stoeckli SJ, Pfaltz M, Ross GL, Steinert HC, MacDonald DG, Wittekind C, Soutar DS (2005) The second international conference on sentinel node biopsy in mucosal head and neck cancer. Ann Surg Oncol 12(11):919–924

Traynor SJ, Cohen JI, Gray J, Andersen PE, Everts EC (1996) Selective neck dissection and the management of the node-positive neck. Am J Surg 172(6):654–657

Trotter HA (1930) The surgical anatomy of the lymphatics of the head and neck. Ann Otol Rhinol Laryngol 39:384–397

Werning JW, Mendenhall WM (2007) Management of the neck. In: Werning JW (ed) Oral cancer. Diagnosis, management, and rehabilitation. Thieme Medical Publishers, New York

Werning JW, Heard D, Pagano C, Khuder S (2003) Elective management of the clinically negative neck by otolaryngologists in patients with oral tongue cancer. Arch Otolaryngol Head Neck Surg 129(1):83–88

Wolfensberger M, Zbaeren P, Dulguerov P, Müller W, Ornoux A, Schmid, S (2001) Surgical treatment of early oral carcinoma–Results of a prospective controlled multi center study. Head and Neck 23:525–530

Yuen AP, Lam KY, Lam LK, Ho CM, Wong A, Chow TL, Yuen WF, Wei WI (2002) Prognostic factors of clinically stage I and II oral tongue carcinoma. A comparative study of stage, thickness, shape, growth pattern, invasive front malignancy grading, Martinez-Gimeno score, and pathologic features. Head Neck 24:513–520

Yuen AP, Lam KY, Wei WI, Lam KY, Ho CM, Chow TL, Yuen WF (2000) A comparison of the prognostic significance of tumor diameter, length, width, thickness, area, volume, and clinico-pathological features of oral tongue carcinoma. Am J Surg 180(2):139–143

Yuen AP, Ng RW, Lam PK, Ho A (2008) Preoperative measurement of tumor thickness of oral tongue carcinoma with intraoral ultrasonography. Head Neck 30(2):230–234

Chapter 2
The Role of Diagnostic Imaging in Identifying Cervical Metastases in Oral Cavity Cancer

Lawrence E. Ginsberg

Abstract Radiologic imaging is an integral part of the diagnostic evaluation of the newly diagnosed or suspected head and neck cancer patient. At the M.D. Anderson Cancer Center, for most head and neck malignancies we prefer CT for evaluation of the neck. Small nodes, or those that are nonpalpable because of location (e.g., lateral retropharyngeal or deep to the sternocleidomastoid muscle) but are nevertheless abnormal based on necrosis, shape, clustering, or other criteria, can be diagnosed with CT. This diagnosis, important for its treatment and prognostic implications, requires knowledge not only of the known or suspected primary cancer, its location, and expected sites of nodal drainage, but also of the proper imaging technique and appearance of nodal metastases. This chapter will familiarize the reader with imaging strategies, radiographic appearance, and other findings that may diagnose or suggest a likehood of nodal metastasis.

Introduction

Nodal metastasis in oral cavity cancer has a profound effect not only on prognosis but also on therapeutic approach. Primary tumors arising from certain sites, including the oral tongue, are far more likely to be associated with nodal spread than are tumors arising from the buccal mucosa, with the likelihood of nodal metastasis increasing with T stage. Because physical examination is relatively insensitive to the detection of nodal metastases, the role of imaging becomes important. When nodal metastases are clinically or radiologically evident in an oral cavity malignancy, neck dissection and adjuvant therapy are often indicated. In cases in which routine cross-sectional imaging (magnetic resonance imaging [MRI] or computed tomography [CT]) is equivocal for nodal metastases, further imaging may be

L.E. Ginsberg (✉)
Departments of Diagnostic Radiology and Head and Neck Surgery, Department of Diagnostic Radiology Unit 370, The University of Texas M. D. Anderson Cancer Center, 1515 Holcombe Blvd, Houston, TX, 77030, USA
e-mail: lginsberg@di.mdacc.tmc.edu

J. Myers (ed.), *Oral Cancer Metastasis*,
DOI 10.1007/978-1-4419-0775-2_2, © Springer Science+Business Media, LLC 2010

33

warranted. This can include ultrasound and ultrasound-guided fine-needle aspiration (USG-FNA) or positron emission tomography (PET)/CT imaging. In patients for which imaging cannot firmly establish the presence of nodal disease, the treating physician is faced with the difficult issue of whether or not to dissect the neck at the time of resection of the primary cancer. Among the issues to be considered in this determination is tumor thickness, to which imaging may contribute (Fukano et al. 1997; Asakage et al. 1998; Okura et al. 2008; Kane et al. 2006).

In this chapter, we review the imaging strategies and findings relevant to the staging evaluation in patients with oral cavity carcinoma. The histologic subtype in the majority of cases is squamous cell carcinoma, but it should be remembered that minor salivary cancers may occur in any location of the upper aerodigestive tract mucosa, and these tumors have imaging findings indistinguishable from squamous cell carcinoma. Choice of imaging modality is still somewhat controversial. However, at The University of Texas M. D. Anderson Cancer Center, CT remains the imaging modality of choice for known or suspected cancers of the upper aerodigestive tract except nasopharyngeal carcinoma, for which MRI is the preferred modality. The basis of this choice is that while some small or superficial cancers may not be visible on CT, most are CT is chosen because, with the exception of some small or superficial cancers, most are visible on CT, and CT is excellent for detecting bony invasion, a finding that influences surgical approach and prognosis. In addition, it is our feeling that nodal disease, and particularly necrosis within small metastatic nodes, can generally be better seen on CT than MRI. This does not, however, address the issue of metastatic disease within nodes lacking the CT characteristics suggestive of malignancy. Philosophical issues arise as to how aggressive pretreatment imaging should be in unearthing the smallest of nodal metastases, and which imaging modality is best. In truth, no available imaging modality can detect the smallest of micrometastases.

While statistics can be presented based on the best objective imaging data for each modality, one immeasurable factor is experience. Experience of the radiologist comes into play in every case he or she reads, and lack of experience can result in the failure to detect radiologically evident lesions, whether primary or metastatic. Another factor in imaging worth mentioning is that shortcomings of imaging technique can result in lesions being inconspicuous when they might otherwise be more readily seen. There is no way to measure experience or the importance of good imaging technique.

Nodal Classification

For the purpose of this chapter, and in common clinical parlance, the nodal usage terminology will conform to that published in 2000 by Som et al. (1999, 2000) (Fig. 2.1). This work sought to match the imaging description of lymph node metastases to the most commonly used clinical descriptions, in order to improve communication between radiologists and clinicians.

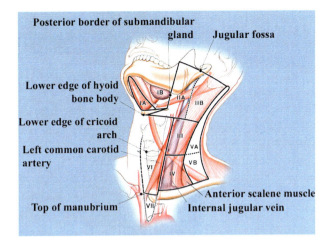

Fig. 2.1 Nodal classification Reprinted with permission from Som and Brandwein (2003)

Nodal Staging

The most commonly accepted nodal staging classification for squamous cell carcinoma of the oral cavity is as follows:

Nx: nodes cannot be assessed
N0: no lymph nodes with evidence of metastasis
N1: a single ipsilateral node with evidence of metastasis 3 cm or less
N2:
> N2a- a single ipsilateral lymph node with evidence of metastasis greater than 3 cm, but not greater than 6 cm in greatest dimension.
> N2b- multiple ipsilateral lymph nodes with evidence of metastasis, none greater than 6 cm in greatest dimension.
> N2c- bilateral or contralateral lymph nodes with evidence of metastasis, none greater than 6 cm in greatest dimension.
N3- a lymph node with evidence of metastasis greater than 6 cm in greatest dimension.

Nodal Drainage Patterns

The vast majority of nodal metastases in oral cavity cancer involve levels I, II, and III. For oral tongue cancer, the likelihood of nodal disease is the highest among the oral cavity primary sites. Cancers of the oral tongue that are anteriorly situated tend to spread to nodes in levels I or II. Tumors more laterally or posteriorly situated tend to spread to nodes in levels II and III. Nodal disease from other oral cavity primary sites is less common than from tongue carcinoma but follows a similar pattern (Som and Brandwein 2003). Primary sites that are more anteriorly situated, such as anterior floor of mouth or gingiva, tend to spread to level I or II; primary cancers more posteriorly located tend to spread to levels II and III. In general, there is an orderly downhill, superior-to-inferior spread, whereby once levels I and II are involved, the tendency to spread then occurs more inferiorly into level IV and so forth. The posterior triangle or level V of the neck is relatively uninvolved in the nodal spread of oral cavity malignancy (Shah et al. 1990). Primary lesions that involve or approach the midline (e.g., floor of mouth or oral tongue) are more likely to access the lymphatics bilaterally (Fig. 2.2). While larger lesions and higher N status are generally associated with a greater likelihood and degree of adenopathy, some early-stage, small primary cancers may give rise to a fairly extensive degree of nodal disease (Fig. 2.2).

Imaging Criteria for Nodal Metastasis by Imaging

CT and MRI

If a lymph node has internal heterogeneity or necrosis by imaging, there is a very high likelihood that it harbors tumor, regardless of size (Som and Brandwein 2003; Glastonbury 2004; Wiggins 2004) (Figs. 2.2–2.5). On CT, this can be seen as an area of low density ("attenuation" in CT terminology), which may be subtle or quite obvious. In the extreme, necrosis can result in a nearly cystic or cyst-like appearance (Fig. 2.3), though this is far more common in oropharyngeal carcinomas than in carcinomas of oral cavity origin (Asakage et al. 1998; Okura et al. 2008; Kane et al. 2006). Central necrosis may be observed in nodes that are quite small and nonpalpable, thus justifying imaging in the clinically N0 neck (Fig. 2.4). On MRI, internal necrosis can be harder to appreciate in smaller nodes, but in larger nodes, it can be seen as internal "high signal" or "hyperintensity" on T2-weighted images, and nonenhancement of the necrotic area on post-contrast, T1-weighted images (Fig. 2.5). Although figures vary by study design (for instance, use of a cutoff based on lymph node size, with a 1-cm size cutoff or the presence of internal necrosis), CT has a negative predictive value (NPV) of 84% and a positive predictive value (PPV) of 50% (Curtin et al. 1998).

On MRI, the differentiation between metastatic and benign or reactive nodes can be challenging. If a node is nonnecrotic or not clearly enlarged, the differentiation is difficult because metastatic and benign nodes have similar imaging characteristics, being isointense on T1-weighted images, hyperintense on T2-weighted images, and enhancing following intravenous administration of Gadolinium-based contrast agents (Som and Brandwein 2003; Glastonbury 2004; Wiggins 2004; Som 1992). With MRI, the NPV and PPV are on the order of 79% and 52%, respectively (Curtin et al. 1998).

If internal necrosis is not radiographically evident, other imaging criteria must be employed. Historically, size has been long-used as a determinant of malignancy but is highly unreliable. The generally accepted size cutoff is 1.5 cm for the subdigas-

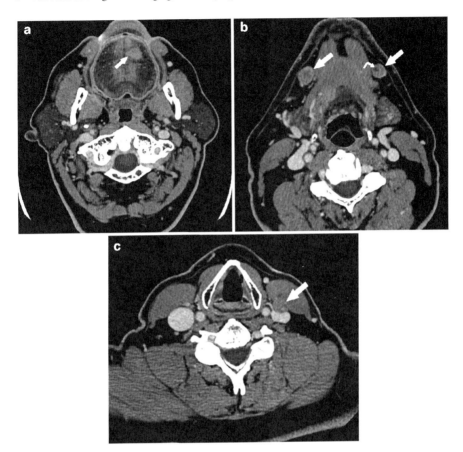

Fig. 2.2 Early-stage oral tongue carcinoma that approaches the midline, with bilateral nodal metastases. (**a**) Axial CT images shows fairly small left anterior oral tongue primary that reaches the midline (*arrow*). (**b**) Bilateral level 1b nodal metastases (*straight arrows*), each with internal areas of necrosis, perhaps more obvious on the left side (*curved arrow*). (**c**) Level 3 nodal metastasis (*arrow*), somewhat inapparent due to similar density compared with adjacent sternocleidomastoid muscle. The node is compressing the anterior surface of the internal jugular vein. Necrosis in this node is difficult to discern

tric node (the upper internal jugular nodes, or in the current classification scheme, level IIA), and 1 cm for other cervical lymph nodes. The lateral retropharyngeal nodes of Rouviere, which generally have a smaller size cutoff (perhaps 6–8 mm) are seldom involved by metastases in patients with oral cavity primary tumors. One exception to this is primary cancers of the maxillary alveolar ridge, which can metastasize to the lateral retropharyngeal nodes (Kimura et al. 1998) (Fig. 2.6). The smaller the size used for cutoff, the greater the sensitivity (fewer metastases missed), but also the greater the number of nonmetastatic nodes included (lower specificity) (Curtin et al. 1998). This is the trade-off when size alone is used. Thus, it is important to look at other features of lymph nodes in addition to size. The shape of a node has diagnostic value, benign nodes tending to be more oval or bean-shaped, and metastatic

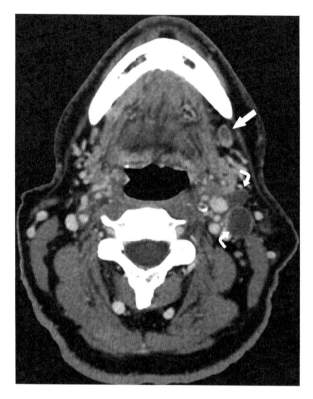

Fig. 2.3 Maxillary alveolar ridge carcinoma (not shown) with cystic nodal metastases. Level 1b node (*straight arrow*) has internal necrosis but some solid enhancement posteriorly. Level 2 nodes are so necrotic as to be essentially cystic, without any solid enhancement (*curved arrows*)

nodes tending to be round. The location of a node is important, specifically its location with respect to the known or suspected primary cancer and the expected lymphatic drainage of that site. For instance, a right-sided anterior oral tongue carcinoma, lacking ipsilateral nodal metastases, would be very unlikely to have a nodal metastasis in the left level IV; a borderline-sized node in such a location would be relatively discounted in terms of its likelihood of being metastatic in this scenario. Were a borderline-sized, non-necrotic node to be seen precisely in the location of drainage (and obviously ipsilateral) to a primary cancer, it would not as readily be dismissed. Put another way, the "oncology" of a node should reasonably enter into the interpretation of its imaging. Clustering, or the tendency of nodal metastases to congregate, should also be taken into consideration; a group of 3–5 nodes in a single location on a single image should arouse suspicion even if none of the nodes is individually abnormal based on size or morphology (Som and Brandwein 2003).

Special mention should be made of the imaging findings that suggest extracapsular extension (ECE), a known predictor of local recurrence and decreased survival (Woolgar et al. 2003; Myers et al. 2001). Imaging findings that suggest ECE include irregular spiculated margins and indistinct borders between the nodal

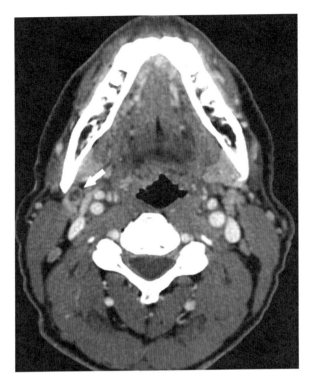

Fig. 2.4 Patient with clinically N0 neck. Small but clearly necrotic right level 2a node (*arrow*)

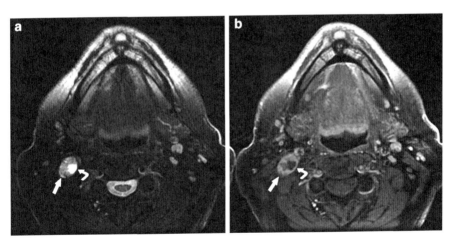

Fig. 2.5 MR images of necrotic nodal metastasis. (**a**, **b**) T2-wighted and post-contrast T1-weighted MR images, respectively, show a right upper internal jugular nodal metastasis (*straight arrow*). As with reactive and benign nodes, T2 hyperintensity is typical, but this metastatic node is enlarged, and there is a medially situated focus of internal necrosis that is seen as even greater signal hyperintensity on T2, and nonenhancement on the post-contrast image (*curved arrows* in **a** and **b**, respectively)

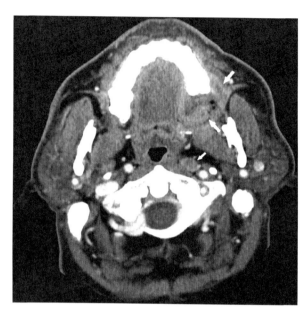

Fig. 2.6 Metastatic lateral retropharyngeal node of Rouviere in maxillary alveolar ridge carcinoma. Axial CT image shows the obvious primary along the posterior maxilla (*large arrows*) and an enlarged, perhaps subtly necrotic left-sided lateral retropharyngeal lymph node (*small arrow*)

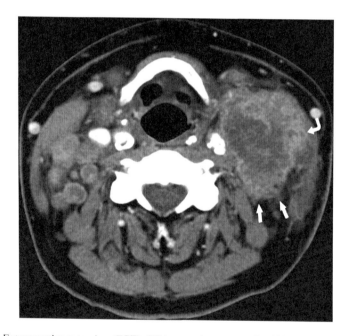

Fig. 2.7 Extracapsular extension (ECE). CT image shows extensive bilateral nodal disease, but the large left-sided node has very irregular margins, especially posteriorly (*straight arrows*), and very blurred margins between the node and the medial surface of the sternocleidomastoid muscle (*curved arrow*)

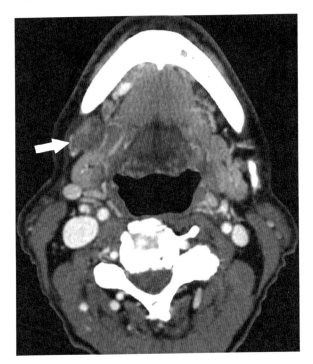

Fig. 2.8 Extracapsular extension (ECE) undetectable on imaging. Axial CT image of a patient with mandibular alveolar ridge carcinoma. There is an obviously enlarged, necrotic right-sided level 1b nodal metastasis (*arrow*), with none of the signs that would suggest ECE, but which was evident histologically

metastasis and adjacent structures such as the inner surface of the sternocleidomastoid muscle (Som 1992) (Fig. 2.7). Unfortunately, imaging is not able to detect every case of ECE, which may be only visible histologically (Fig. 2.8).

If, then, a node is not frankly pathologic at initial staging by CT or MRI because of grossly abnormal size or the presence of necrosis, how does one deal with the borderline node (for example, a node that is 1.6 cm in the subdigastric region, or 1.2 cm in level III with no other tell-tale sign of cancer)? Such cases may require further attention, depending on whether or not there is other indication for neck dissection. If, in the case of a thick oral tongue cancer, surgery is planned, then a borderline node will be addressed at the time of neck dissection. If surgery is not otherwise indicated, then further imaging may be used to assess the borderline or questionable lymph node. Ultrasound (US), with fine-needle aspiration (FNA), may be performed to determine if a node is truly metastatic. In experienced hands, US is very useful and highly accurate in predicting the presence or absence of metastatic disease within a lymph node and in identifying those cases that would benefit from confirmatory FNA. Unfortunately, US-guided FNA can be subject to sampling error, and false negative results may occur (Fig. 2.9). In our institution, US is often used as an adjunct test in staging the neck. The sonographic features of nodal metastases are described in this chapter.

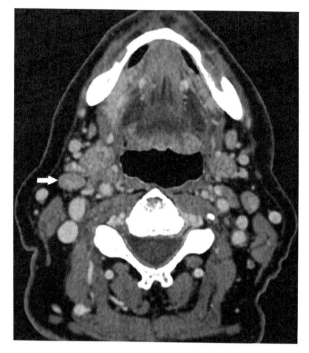

Fig. 2.9 Clinically T2 possible N1 right-sided oral tongue carcinoma. CT image shows a prominent but not frankly abnormal right subdigastric node (1.2 cm, *arrow*). Ultrasound was considered worrisome, but FNA revealed only reactive lymphocytes. Neck dissection was performed because of thickness of the primary (~1.5 cm), and histologically this node contained small foci of metastatic carcinoma that were simply nondefinitive on CT and that were apparently missed at USG-FNA due to sampling error

Generally, imaging serves to upstage, by demonstrating nodal metastases that are not evident clinically. Occasionally, particularly in the case of floor of mouth cancer, imaging can downstage. This can occur if the floor of mouth cancer obstructs the submandibular duct, causing the gland to obstruct and enlarge; in such cases, the resulting enlarged gland may be clinically interpreted (palpated) as nodal disease. Imaging can reliably differentiate an obstructed submandibular gland from a nodal metastasis (Fig. 2.10).

One additional matter is false positive imaging results. If a node is observed to be asymmetrically enlarged and within the drainage basin of a known malignancy, then one may be tempted to call it metastatic radiographically. This can be compounded if the presumably reactive node is palpable (Fig. 2.11); however, such a node may be merely reactive. Another pitfall in nodal imaging is the pseudonecrosis that may result from partial volume averaging of a normal fatty hilum. Specifically,

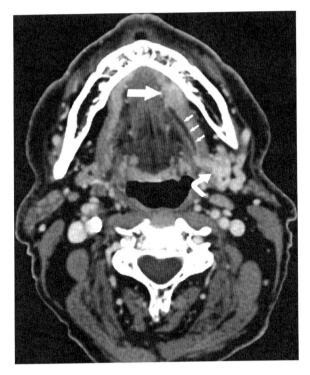

Fig. 2.10 Floor of mouth carcinoma, clinically N1. Axial CT image shows the enhancing floor of mouth primary (*large straight arrow*). Note the obstructed, dilated submandibular duct (*small arrows*) and an enlarged, enhancing left submandibular gland (*curved arrow*). This gland was palpable and presumed to be a nodal metastasis. In this case, imaging served to downstage the neck. There were no nodal metastases detectable elsewhere in the neck

when a CT slice overlaps a portion of normally low-density fat within the hilum of a lymph node and also includes a portion of normal lymphoid tissue, the "averaged" tissue may be misinterpreted as necrosis (Fig. 2.12).

Ultrasound

Ultrasound has long been used to evaluate lymph nodes, in the neck and elsewhere. Criteria for metastatic disease in a node include a rounded (abnormal) vs. oval or fusiform (normal) shape, increased size (unreliable as in cross-sectional), or an abnormal internal echo pattern. The abnormal internal echo pattern can take the form of a diffusely hypoechoic appearance or diffusely increased echogenicity – this often coincides with loss or disordering of the expected central hilar echo pattern (Evans 2003; van den Brekel and Castelijns 2005) (Fig. 2.13). Though much

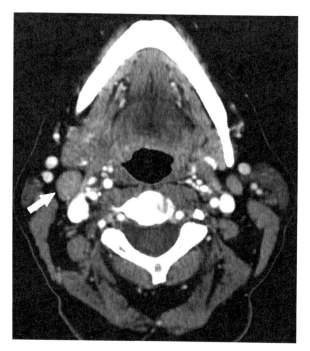

Fig. 2.11 Right-sided retromolar trigone carcinoma with clinically N1 neck. Axial CT image shows a borderline enlarged (1.5 cm) right subdigastric node (*arrow*), which was presumed metastatic because of its location relative to the primary lesion as well as the clinical impression. At neck dissection, no tumor was found in this or any other neck node

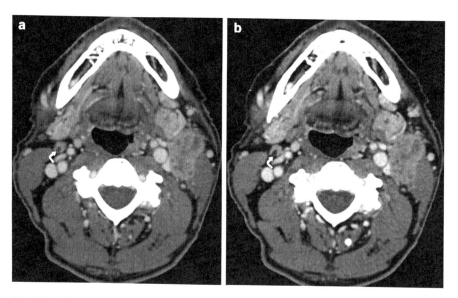

Fig. 2.12 Metastatic carcinoma to the left neck. (**a**) Axial CT image, in addition to obvious left-sided nodal disease, suggests the possibility of necrosis within a contralateral node (*curved arrow*). (**b**) The image at a slightly lower level shows that, rather than necrosis, this is a normal fatty hilum (hypodense area, *curved arrow*). The image more superiorly represents partial volume averaging and thus the illusion of necrosis that does not exist

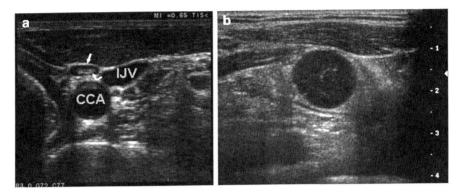

Fig. 2.13 Sonographic findings in normal and metastatic nodes. (**a**) Axial ultrasound image shows normal oval node (*straight arrow*), with organized central internal echoes (*curved arrow*). The common carotid artery (CCA) and internal jugular vein (IJV) are labeled. (**b**) Nodal metastasis with round shape, internal hypoechoic appearance, and absence of the normal central echoes seen in (**a**). (Images courtesy of Beth S. Edeiken, M.D.)

more common in thyroid cancer metastases, the presence of calcification in a lymph node suggests malignancy. Another sign of malignancy in a node is abnormal vascularity by color Doppler determination. Normal flow should be primarily central in location; color flow Doppler findings of malignancy include displacement of normal hilar flow, aberrant or extra vessels, focal absence of expected normal areas of perfusion, and abnormally increased peripheral, subcapsular vessels (Fig. 2.14) (Evans 2003; van den Brekel and Castelijns 2005). Internal necrosis may take the appearance of cystic degeneration (Evans 2003). One benefit of ultrasound is the ability to perform USG-FNA on any suspicious lymph node, with essentially immediate cytologic results.

PET/CT

Recent advances in F[18]-labeled fluorodeoxyglucose (FDG) PET technology have made widely available the fusion of PET and CT in a single machine (PET/CT). The presence of correlative CT images allows far more accurate spatial and anatomic localization of abnormalities seen on the PET images. In numerous studies, PET/CT has proven to be more sensitive than MR/CT in the detection of nodal metastases from a variety of head and neck malignancies, including the oral cavity (Ng et al. 2006) (Fig. 2.15). Unfortunately, PET/CT is so sensitive that it can lead to false positives. As an example, reactive nodes may be associated with abnormally elevated FDG activity, and thus mistakenly characterized as metastatic (Schoder et al. 2006). Furthermore, PET/CT remains unable to detect micrometastases, and as such, does not have high enough NPV to prevent elective neck dissection in every case (Schoder et al. 2006). On PET/CT, nodal metastases (and potentially negative, reactive or inflammatory nodes) are seen as "hot" areas of increased FDG activity, yellow in color as presented in most systems (Fig. 2.15).

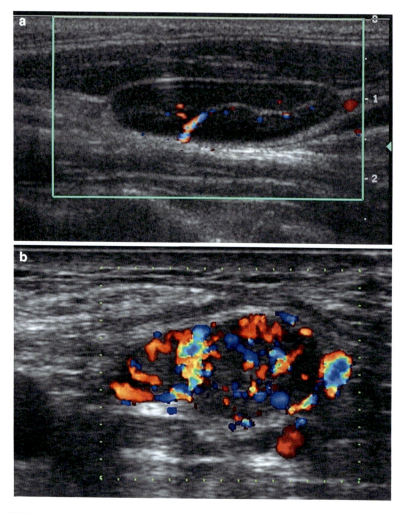

Fig. 2.14 Normal and abnormal color flow Doppler. (**a**) Normal centrally located internal Doppler signal. (**b**) Grossly abnormal increased internal vascular flow typical of metastasis. (Images courtesy of Beth S. Edeiken, M.D.)

Sentinel Lymph Node Biopsy

Recent investigations have begun examining the feasibility and efficacy of sentinel node biopsy, which is based on the concept that if one can identify the first echelon nodal drainage from a given primary cancer, then that node can be sampled even if normal by other modalities of imaging (Hart et al. 2005). Such sampling is accomplished through intratumoral or peritumoral injection of a radioisotope and then performing imaging with scintigraphy and subsequent biopsy of the sentinel

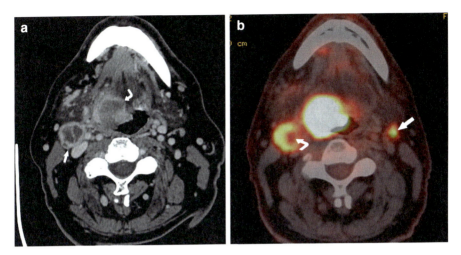

Fig. 2.15 Base of tongue carcinoma. (**a**) Axial CT image shows the obvious right-sided tongue base primary (*curved arrow*) and necrotic ipsilateral adenopathy (*straight arrow*), but contralateral nodal disease cannot be called. (**b**) Fused PET/CT image shows a small but striking area of increased metabolic activity in the left neck (*straight arrow*). This represents a nodal metastasis not detectable by any other means and illustrates the utility of PET/CT. Note that some of the internal necrosis of the right-sided nodal metastasis is not associated with abnormal metabolic activity (*curved arrow*); this is expected and a potential source of false-negative PET scan in the case of purely cystic/necrotic nodal metastases

node, either surgically or by USG-FNA. Sentinel lymph node mapping appears to have a very high NPV and thus may prove to be very useful in patients with N0 necks. While currently used primarily in cutaneous malignancies, it holds promise for mucosal tumors as well and will be discussed elsewhere in this text.

Conclusion

Imaging has much to offer in the staging evaluation of patients with oral cavity cancer. At M. D. Anderson Cancer Center, disease in most patients is staged with contrast-enhanced CT. While there are guidelines on how to approach and diagnose metastatic lymph nodes radiologically, experience is important for the evaluation of nodes that are borderline, those which cannot obviously be called metastatic. Identification of such nodes requires a high level of vigilance, an understanding of the behavior of the malignancy, attention to imaging technique, and knowledge of which adjunct tests would increase diagnostic sensitivity and avoid false negative results. Unfortunately, however, at this time there is no single imaging test that is 100% sensitive and specific and that has a 100% negative predictive value. Until there is such a test, surgeons will need to rely on other features of a primary cancer to determine who would most benefit from elective neck dissection.

References

Fukano H, Matsuura H, Hasegawa Y, Nakamura S (1997) Depth of invasion as a predictive factor for cervical lymph node metastasis in tongue carcinoma. Head Neck 19:205–210

Asakage T, Yokose T, Mukai K et al (1998) Tumor thickness predicts cervical metastasis in patients with stage I/II carcinoma of the tongue. Cancer 82:1443–1448

Okura M, Iida S, Aikawa T et al (2008) Tumor Thickness and Paralingual Distance of Coronal MR Imaging Predicts Cervical Node Metastases in Oral Tongue Carcinoma. AJNR Am J Neuroradiol 29:45–50

Kane SV, Gupta M, Kakade AC, D'Cruz A (2006) Depth of invasion is the most significant histological predictor of subclinical cervical lymph node metastasis in early squamous carcinomas of the oral cavity. Eur J Surg Oncol 32:795–803

Som PM, Curtin HD, Mancuso AA (2000) Imaging-based nodal classification for evaluation of neck metastatic adenopathy. Am J Roentgenol 174:837–844

Som PM, Curtin HD, Mancuso AA (1999) An imaging-based classification for the cervical nodes designed as an adjunct to recent clinically based nodal classifications. Arch Otolaryngol Head Neck Surg 125:388–396

Som PM, Brandwein MS (2003) Lymph Nodes. In: Som PM, Curtin HD (eds) Head and neck imaging. Mosby, St. Louis, pp 1865–1934

Shah JP, Candela FC, Poddar AK (1990) The patterns of cervical lymph node metastases from squamous carcinoma of the oral cavity. Cancer 66:109–113

Glastonbury CM (2004) Squamous cell carcinoma nodes. In: Harnsberger HR, Wiggins RH, Hudgins PA, Michel MA, Swartz J, Davidson HC, et al. (eds) Diagnostic imaging: Head and neck, vol III. Amirsys, Salt Lake City, UT, pp. 2–28; 22–31

Wiggins RH (2004) Nodal metastases, SCCa (SMS). In: Harnsberger HR, Wiggins RH, Hudgins PA, Michel MA, Swartz J, Davidson HC, et al. (eds) Diagnostic imaging: Head and neck, vol III. Amirsys, Salt Lake City, UT, pp. 4–46; 44–47

Curtin HD, Ishwaran H, Mancuso AA, Dalley RW, Caudry DJ, McNeil BJ (1998) Comparison of CT and MR imaging in staging of neck metastases. Radiology 207:123–130

Som PM (1992) Detection of metastasis in cervical lymph nodes: CT and MR criteria and differential diagnosis. Am J Roentgenol 158:961–969

Kimura Y, Hanazawa T, Sano T, Okano T (1998) Lateral retropharyngeal node metastasis from carcinoma of the upper gingiva and maxillary sinus. AJNR Am J Neuroradiol 19:1221–1224

Woolgar JA, Rogers SN, Lowe D, Brown JS, Vaughan ED (2003) Cervical lymph node metastasis in oral cancer: the importance of even microscopic extracapsular spread. Oral Oncol 39:130–137

Myers JN, Greenberg JS, Mo V, Roberts D (2001) Extracapsular spread a significant predictor of treatment failure in patients with squamous cell carcinoma of the tongue. Cancer 92:3030–3036

Evans RM (2003) Ultrasound of cervical lymph nodes. Imaging 15:101–108

van den Brekel MW, Castelijns JA (2005) What the clinician wants to know: surgical perspective and ultrasound for lymph node imaging of the neck. Cancer Imaging 5 Spec No A:S41–S49.

Ng S-H, Yen T-C, Chang JT-C et al (2006) Prospective study of [18F]fluorodeoxyglucose positron emission tomography and computed tomography and magnetic resonance imaging in oral cavity squamous cell carcinoma with palpably negative neck. J Clin Oncol 24:4371–4376

Schoder H, Carlson DL, Kraus DH et al (2006) 18F-FDG PET/CT for detecting nodal metastases in patients with oral cancer staged n0 by clinical examination and CT/MRI. J Nucl Med 47:755–762

Hart RD, Nasser JG, Trites JR, Taylor SM, Bullock M, Barnes D (2005) Sentinel lymph node biopsy in N0 squamous cell carcinoma of the oral cavity and oropharynx. Arch Otolaryngol Head Neck Surg 131:34–38

Chapter 3
Sentinel Node Biopsy in Oral Cancer

L.W.T. Alkureishi, G.L. Ross, and S.J. Stoeckli

Abstract In patients with cT1-T2 oral/oropharyngeal squamous cell cancer, involvement of the cervical lymph nodes is associated with a 50% decrease in 5-year survival and represents the most important prognostic factor in this patient group. Precise staging of the cervical nodes is therefore of utmost importance, to ensure an accurate prognosis and provision of the most appropriate treatment.

The gold standard for staging the cervical nodes is elective neck dissection, providing both diagnostic and therapeutic measures. However, only one-fourth of cT1-T2 patients are found to harbor occult nodal disease, and the remainder of patients may be unnecessarily exposed to the considerable morbidity associated with neck dissection.

The sentinel node biopsy procedure provides a means of obtaining tissue for pathological staging of the cervical lymph node basin, while potentially avoiding the morbidity of an elective neck dissection. This chapter describes the technique, its accuracy and current applications, and its potential role in the management of patients with early oral/oropharyngeal squamous cell cancer.

Introduction: Difficulties in Managing the N0 Neck

Lymph Node Metastases and Survival

Oral cancer and oropharyngeal squamous cell carcinoma (OSCC) are relatively common, with a U.S. prevalence of approximately 240,000. The estimated annual incidence is 10.4/100,000, with an annual mortality rate of 2.5/100,000. Incidence is greatest in high-risk groups, including older males and tobacco and alcohol users, and both incidence and mortality are higher in African-Americans. The overall 5-year survival is approximately 60% (Ries et al. 2008).

G.L. Ross(✉)
Plastic Surgery department, Christie Hospital, Wilmslow, M20 4BX, UK
e-mail: Gary.Ross@christie.nhs.uk

J. Myers (ed.), *Oral Cancer Metastasis*,
DOI 10.1007/978-1-4419-0775-2_3, © Springer Science+Business Media, LLC 2010

As with many cancers, prognosis in OSCC is closely related to staging. Regional and distant metastases are associated with reduced overall survival rates, and may require significantly different treatment goals and modalities. The primary route of spread of OSCC is via the lymphatics, draining to the cervical lymph node basin, and the presence or absence of disease in the cervical lymph nodes is the single most important prognostic factor in this patient group (Alvi and Johnson 1996). The National Cancer Institute reports that the overall 5-year survival drops from 82% to 53% as a result of regional lymphatic involvement, and is reduced to 28% for patients with distant metastases (Ries et al. 2008).

Only approximately 10% of patients are found to have distant metastases at presentation, with the remainder of patients having stage I/II (33%) or stage III (50%) disease. The marked difference in outcome between the latter two patient groups serves to highlight the importance of detecting lymphatic involvement, both for prognostic and treatment purposes (Ferlito et al. 2003).

Detection of Occult Lymph Node Involvement

Determining the extent of disease begins with clinical evaluation, and palpation of the neck. Palpation has previously demonstrated a poor sensitivity of approximately 70% (O'Brien et al. 2000; Woolgar et al. 1995), preventing its use as a sole staging tool in this patient group. This has led several groups to investigate the utility of clinical imaging tools such as ultrasound, CT, MRI, and even positron emission tomography (PET)/CT (Stoeckli et al. 2002a, b). However, there are ongoing concerns regarding the true sensitivities of all currently available imaging modalities, and it is generally held that none are sufficiently accurate to permit their use as a sole staging tool (O'Brien et al. 2000; Yuen et al. 1999; Persky and Lagmay 1999). There is currently no consensus regarding the optimal criteria for detection of diseased nodes by imaging. The most commonly used criteria are related to nodal size. However, recommended threshold values between "high-risk" and "low-risk" vary widely among groups, and nodal size as a sole criterion has been demonstrated to have poor sensitivity and specificity at all available size thresholds (Alkureishi et al. 2007). Combining size, central necrosis, peripheral contrast enhancement, and clustering of nodes in CT raises the sensitivity considerably, but still leaves a low specificity and negative predictive value. The most accurate staging modality for the neck has been shown to be ultrasound with fine-needle aspiration cytology (FNAC). However, even in the most expert hands, only 80–85% of negative necks on imaging will remain negative after neck dissection (Stoeckli et al. in press) or wait-and-scan (Nieuwenhuis et al. 2002) .Overall, 20–30% of patients with clinically negative (N0) necks, determined using currently available clinical staging tools, will subsequently be found to harbor occult disease within the cervical lymph nodes (van den Brekel et al. 1990; Ross et al. 2004a, b).

Elective Neck Dissection

Currently, the decision to electively treat the cN0 neck is made on the basis of primary tumor characteristics, including primary site and T classification. Patients whose tumor has a greater than 20% risk of subclinical lymph metastases are recommended to undergo elective neck dissection (END) (Yuen et al. 1999).

The current gold standard for both staging and treatment of the cN0 neck remains END. This provides material for histopathologic analysis and also removes the lymph nodes at risk for involvement (Pitman et al. 1997). This reduces the risk of subsequent nodal involvement, and has been shown by some groups to prolong disease-free survival (Kligerman et al. 1994). However, neck dissection is not without considerable morbidity and would represent overtreatment for approximately three-fourths of all cN0 patients. Historically, neck dissection involved a radical approach, with removal of lymph nodes from all neck levels, sternocleidomastoid and omohyoid muscles, internal and external jugular veins, and the spinal portion of the accessory nerve. The morbidity from this procedure was considerable, and included pain, shoulder stiffness, muscle atrophy, facial swelling, and poor cosmesis. Mortality rates in patients undergoing bilateral radical neck dissections were as high as 10% (Razack et al. 1981). This led to the use of various modified radical neck dissections (MRNDs), designated MRND I-III depending on the structures preserved (accessory nerve, sternocleidomastoid and/or internal jugular vein). Several groups reported that the MRND could be performed without compromising the oncologic safety of the procedure, and the radical neck dissection fell out of favor (Bocca et al. 1984).

Since the introduction of the MRND, investigators have continued to develop more conservative surgical management techniques for the cervical lymph nodes, particularly for patients with cN0 necks. Improved understanding of the patterns of lymphatic metastasis has allowed surgeons to tailor the neck dissection to a smaller group of lymph nodes, a procedure named selective neck dissection (SND) (Fisch and Sigel 1964; Shah and Andersen 1994; Werner et al. 2003). In the setting of stage I/II oral cavity SCC, the SND most commonly performed is the level I–III neck dissection, while a level II–IV dissection is preferred for oropharyngeal tumors. The major benefit of SND over MRND is a further reduction in the associated morbidity of the procedure (Chepeha et al. 2002).

Despite these advances in surgical selection and technique, SND remains an invasive procedure and may ultimately be unnecessary for majority of patients. The most frequently encountered postoperative complication is shoulder dysfunction, which occurs in up to 22% of patients despite preservation of the spinal accessory nerve (Sobol et al. 1985).

Wait-and-See Policy

Conversely, a "wait-and-see" policy avoids the initial morbidity of neck dissection, but approximately one-fourth of patients will subsequently develop cervical disease. While salvage surgery is often technically possible in these patients, it usually means a more extensive dissection and postoperative radiotherapy. Nieuwenhuis et al. (2002) reported on the series of 161 N0 patients who were evaluated with ultrasound-guided FNAC (USgFNAC). Thirty-four patients (21%) went on to develop nodal recurrence during follow-up, and salvage treatment required therapeutic neck dissection and radiotherapy. Seven of the 34 patients (21%) presented with advanced disease that was not amenable to salvage.

Rationale for Sentinel Node Biopsy

Sentinel node biopsy (SNB) continues the trend of minimizing the invasiveness of the staging procedure, utilizing lymphatic mapping to selectively target the small group of lymph nodes most likely to harbor metastases.

The sentinel node concept states that spread from the primary tumor will follow a predictable pattern, with involvement of the sentinel node(s) before progression to the remainder of the lymph node basin (Fig. 3.1). Identification, surgical excision, and histopathological evaluation of the sentinel nodes should therefore provide an accurate prediction of the disease status of the rest of the basin (Morton et al. 1992). Patients with OSCC who have a positive sentinel node biopsy can then proceed to definitive treatment of the involved neck, while sentinel node–negative patients may avoid the need for further surgery. The minimally invasive nature of the SNB procedure may potentially avoid some of the complications associated with neck dissection (Wrightson et al. 2003).

Sentinel node biopsy also offers some additional advantages over neck dissection. Among these, the per-patient cost of performing the procedure is reported to be less than the cost of a comprehensive neck dissection (Kosuda et al. 2003; Brobeil et al. 1999), and the small number of harvested lymph nodes allows for a more detailed histopathological evaluation. The comparatively large number of nodes harvested during a standard neck dissection represents a significant burden of work for the pathologist and effectively restricts evaluation of each node to standard hematoxylin-eosin (H&E) staining. In-depth examination of the small number of sentinel nodes can include additional techniques such as step-serial sectioning and immunohistochemistry (van den Brekel et al. 1992). These additional pathological techniques, and their role in the detection of micrometastases, will be discussed later in this chapter.

The SNB technique is not without disadvantages, however. The technique can be technically challenging (Morton et al. 1992), and has been demonstrated to have a steep learning curve (van der Veen et al. 1994). As a result, it is recommended that investigators wishing to begin using the technique should do so within the context of SNB-assisted END (Ross et al. 2004a, b). There is also the potential for false-negative results, and the sensitivity of the procedure appears to be between 90% and 95% (Ross et al. 2004a, b; Stoeckli 2007; Civantos et al. 2005). Finally, SNB should not be applied to patients with clinically positive (cN+) nodal disease or T3/T4 primary tumors, in whom there is an increased likelihood of extensive

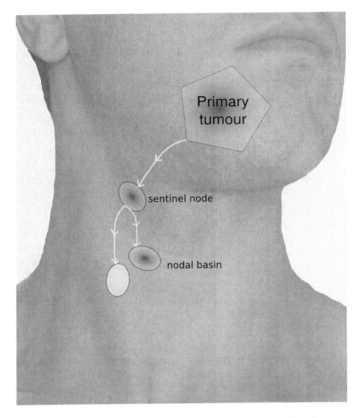

Fig. 3.1 The sentinel node concept. Lymphatic drainage passes from the primary tumor to the first-echelon lymph node (the "sentinel node") before draining to the remaining lymphatic basin

tumor involvement. This can potentially distort the normal lymphatic architecture, blocking the usual drainage pathways and leading to aberrant drainage patterns (Fig. 3.2). Biopsy of these uninvolved second-tier lymph nodes can lead to false-negative results (Dünne et al. 2001).

Early Applications: Melanoma and Other Cancers

The concept of a "sentinel" lymph node is not new, with the first description dating back to 1960. Gould et al. (1960) reported on a total parotidectomy, during which intraoperative frozen section examination of a single facial lymph node was used to guide the decision to proceed to radical neck dissection. Cabanas (1977) subsequently described "sentinel node biopsy" in 46 patients with penile squamous cell cancer. However, the authors erroneously believed the sentinel node to be in a fixed

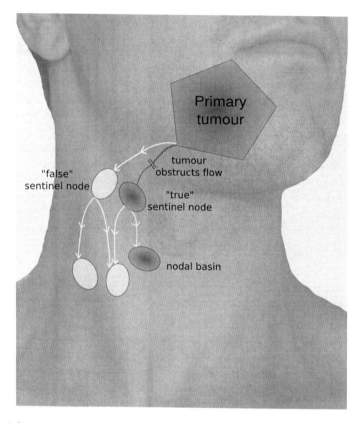

Fig. 3.2 Advanced primary tumor. Extensive infiltration of lymphatic channels by tumor blocks free passage of lymph and radiotracer to the true sentinel node. Redirection of lymph/radiotracer results in biopsy of a different node ("false sentinel node"), which may not accurately reflect the disease status of the remaining nodal basin

location in all patients. Nevertheless, they reported 90% 5-year survival for sentinel node-negative patients. Similarly, Weissbach and Boedefeld proposed a limited retroperitoneal lymph node dissection as a means of "…prevention of long-term damage without compromising diagnostic accuracy" in patients with testicular cancer (Weissbach and Boedefeld 1987).

In parallel with the work by Cabanas (1977), Holmes et al. reported in 1977 on the use of radioactive colloidal gold injection to determine which lymph node basin was draining melanomas in ambiguous areas such as the midline (Holmes et al. 1977). Fifteen years later, the same group described a novel technique for intraoperative identification of the sentinel lymph node (SLN) using injection of vital dye (Morton et al. 1992), a technique which closely resembles the SNB procedure used today for a variety of solid tumors, including melanoma (Morton et al. 1992) and breast cancer (Wilke and Giuliano 2003). The use of a handheld gamma camera was subsequently added in order to ease intraoperative identification and improve sentinel node identification rates (Alex and Krag 1993).

For many surgeons, sentinel node biopsy has become an increasingly important staging tool in patients with melanoma. However, its exact role has yet to be fully defined and is to a large degree dependent on the results of large-scale prospective multicenter trials such as MSLT-I and MSLT-II (Morton et al. 2006).

Interest in applying the SNB technique to patients with head and neck squamous cell cancer was relatively more recent, with a report of successful SNB in a patient with supraglottic cancer in 1996 (Alex and Krag 1996). The further development of SNB in OSCC will be described later in this chapter.

Peritumoral Injection and Lyphoscintigraphy

The sentinel node is defined as "...the first draining lymph node on the direct lymphatic pathway from the primary tumour site" (Morton and Bostick 1999)

Radiolocalization of the sentinel node begins with preoperative lymphoscintigraphy (LSG), a technique first applied to head and neck cancer by Koch et al. (1998). Injection of radiolabeled colloid solution around the primary tumor leads to drainage along the afferent lymphatics to the first-echelon, or sentinel, nodes. Here, the radiocolloid solution can accumulate and the resultant radioactivity may be visualized using a gamma camera.

The lymphatic anatomy of the head and neck region has been extensively studied, and patterns of drainage from the oral cavity and oropharynx are thought to be relatively predictable. However, aberrant lymph drainage can occur, and in these cases, this may lead to inappropriate placement of initial incisions or failure to correctly identify a true sentinel node (Werner et al. 2003). Preoperative LSG is particularly useful in guiding the surgeon for placement of the initial access incision.

Radioisotopes and Optimal Radiation Dose

The choice of radiopharmaceutical is dependent on a number of factors. The agent should have a short half-life, limiting the radiation dose to the injection site. It should emit only gamma rays, with a suitable energy to allow detection, and should be cleared rapidly from the injection site, allowing early visualization of the lymphatics. The particle size should be uniform, to allow reproducible results, and should allow the agent to accumulate and persist in the lymph node until imaging can be performed (Cody 1999; Ross et al. 2002a). The best currently available radiopharmaceutical is radiolabeled technetium (^{99m}Tc), which was first used in 1965 (Garzom et al. 1965).

A variety of ^{99m}Tc-labeled colloids are commercially available. However, licensing varies between regions, and this frequently restricts the available choices. In Europe and parts of the United States, there are two colloids available: Albures™ and Nanocoll™ (Nycomed Amersham, Buckinghamshire, UK). Albures™ has a larger particle size (500 nm), is slower moving, and tends to remain in the first echelon lymph nodes. The large size limits its use to primary tumor sites with a high density of terminal lymphatic vessels, and it is commonly used in the anterior tongue and floor of the mouth. Nanocoll™ is a smaller colloid, with a mean particle size of 50 nm. This theoretically allows its use in sites with lower densities of terminal lymphatics, such as the remainder of the oral cavity and oropharynx. However, its small particle size also potentially allows it to pass more readily from the sentinel node to the second-echelon lymph nodes (Ross et al. 2002a; Ross et al. 2004a, b). In some regions, including parts of the United States, colloids based on human serum albumin have not been approved, and therefore, the most commonly used colloid in these areas is sulfur colloid. Sulfur colloid preparations are available in both unfiltered (particle size 300–340 nm) and filtered (particle size <200 nm) forms (Tafra et al. 1999).

Injection Technique

Patients undergo LSG up to 1 day prior to surgery. Depending on the timing of surgery, up to 80 MBq ^{99m}Tc radiolabeled colloid is injected throughout the normal mucosa surrounding the tumor edge and submucosa on the deep and lateral aspect of the tumor. A volume of approximately 0.2–1.0 ml is used to completely encircle the tumor (Ross et al. 2002a, b). At the end of injection, the tumor should be completely surrounded by colloid. A permanently secured needle should be used to prevent inadvertent spillage into the mouth. Immediately following injection of the radiopharmaceutical, a mouthwash should be used to prevent sumping or swallowing of residual radioactivity. Care should be taken in patients with ulcerated lesions to minimize leakage from tumor edge to the ulcer and thereby into the general oral cavity (Shoaib et al. 1999).

Lymphoscintigraphy

Lymphoscintigraphy imaging may be either static or dynamic. There is currently no evidence favoring either technique. Static LSG is performed at predefined intervals, until the appearance of radioactive nodes. The exact timing of static imaging varies widely between centers. All areas of focal increased uptake visualized on LSG, outside of the primary injection site, should be considered sentinel nodes regardless of the sequence in which they arise. It is usual to see focal increased activity within the first 15 min before injection. One hour before injection, if there has been no visualization of lymph nodes, they may be located in close proximity to the primary injection site. Leakage of radiocolloid from the injection site into the oral cavity may also prevent visualization of the sentinel nodes. At each time point, images should be acquired in two planes: anterior, and lateral or lateral-oblique.

A radiolabeled Cobalt (^{57}Co) marker may be employed to trace the patient's outline, or a flood source of ^{57}Co or ^{99m}Tc can be placed behind the patient to produce a silhouette of the patient's outline. A gamma camera fitted with a low energy, high-resolution (LEHR) collimator is used to image the patient.

It is recommended that the skin overlying any localized SLNs should be marked with indelible marker pen. However, the final decision as to whether the skin should be marked at the site of SLN should be made locally following discussion with the surgical team. If skin marking is performed, it should be confirmed in two planes. The SLN may be located using a handheld gamma probe, or by moving a radioactive marker source over the patient's skin during imaging until its position coincides with the surface projection of the SLN. A lead plate of an appropriate thickness (e.g., 3 mm) may be used to shield the injection site, reducing the high signal detected from the primary tumor (Shoaib et al. 1999; Ross et al. 2002a, 2004a, b).

Planar Lymphoscintigraphy vs. Single Photon Emission CT with CT

Planar lymphoscintigraphy in two projections, with the addition of an anterior oblique view if necessary, allows for safe and reliable SLN detection with a previously published SLN detection rate of 96% (Stoeckli 2007). In the meantime, technology has evolved, and single photon emission computed tomography with CT (SPECT/CT) has become available in some centers (Fig. 3.3). Preliminary reports suggested a benefit of SPECT/CT over dynamic planar lymphoscintigraphy alone, especially for carcinomas of the floor of mouth with close proximity to sentinel nodes in level I.

There is no doubt that SPECT/CT allows the surgeon better topographical orientation and delineation of SLNs against surrounding structures (e.g., muscles, vessels, and bones), but this subjective impression and benefit of SPECT/CT do not influence the final success of the procedure. In a recent study, SPECT/CT was not superior to planar LSG alone with respect to number and localization of hot spots and ultimately excised SLNs (Haerle et al. in press).

The data of this study are in contrast with the results of Bilde et al. (2006), who have identified 47% more SLNs by SPECT/CT than on planar LSG, but in agreement with those of Keski et al., who found no additional value from SPECT/CT over planar LSG alone (Keski-Säntti et al. 2006). In summary, planar LSG seems sufficient for successful lymphatic mapping, but SPECT/CT may help the surgeon with three-dimensional orientation.

Operative Technique

Patients should undergo SNB within 24 h of the injection of radiocolloid, in order to ensure detectable radioactivity levels. The patient should be anaesthetized, prepared, and draped as for a standard excision and neck dissection.

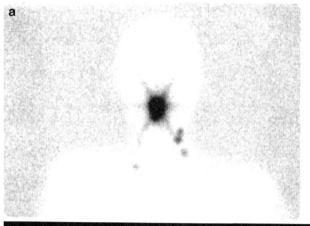

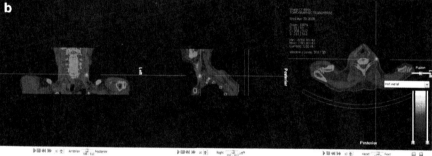

Fig. 3.3 Lymphoscintigraphy and single photon emission CT (SPECT)/CT images: (**a**) Anterior projection static lymphoscintigraphy, (**b**) anteroposterior, lateral, and axial SPECT/CT views in the same patient

Use of Blue Dye

In many centers, the SNB procedure begins with injection of blue dye around the primary tumor. The dye enters the local lymphatics, staining them a vivid blue color and aiding visualization of both the draining channels and the sentinel nodes themselves (Morton et al. 1992). However, this technique is not universally accepted, and many investigators feel that its disadvantages outweigh its perceived benefits. Principally, there is a concern that the injection of blue dye at the tumor edge can obscure the true surgical margins, making adequate resection more difficult to ensure. Additionally, it has been reported that blue dye is unnecessary in order to ensure excellent sentinel node identification rates (Dünne et al. 2001). Proponents of the technique report that injection of blue dye is a useful adjunct that serves to facilitate easier – and faster – identification of the draining lymphatics (Shoaib et al. 1999, 2001; Ross et al. 2002b). The combination of preoperative lymphoscintigraphy, intraoperative injection of blue dye, and use of the handheld gamma probe has been termed the *triple-diagnostic technique*.

If blue dye is to be used, it should be injected by the same operator as the injection of radiocolloid, in order to ensure uniform and consistent administration. Every effort should be made to ensure that the same injection points are used. Up to 2 ml of dye is injected throughout the mucosa and submucosa, surrounding the tumor on its lateral and deep aspects. The brand of dye used is dependent on the geographical region, with Patent Blue V Dye (Laboratoire Guerbet, Aulnay-Sous-Bois, France) employed in Europe, and Lymphazurin™ (Tyco Healthcare Group LP, Norwalk, CT, USA) in the United States.

Risk of Anaphylaxis

There is a small but appreciable risk of anaphylactic reaction associated with the use of blue dyes injected during SNB. A number of reports have described cases of anaphylaxis following administration of isosulphan blue and Patent Blue, and there have also been reports of cross-reactivity between the dyes (Scherer et al. 2006). In a recent large series of over 3,300 patients, the authors reported their first anaphylactic complication after 12 years of experience with the technique (Kaufman et al. 2008); however, other investigators have reported incidences of up to 2.7% (Scherer et al. 2006).

Management of anaphylaxis in this patient group should follow the management of any patient with anaphylaxis; close monitoring and hemodynamic support are critical. However, a recent report has highlighted that a biphasic response to the allergen may be seen, with anaphylactic episodes at 15 min and 2-h postinjection, and this should be borne in mind when managing these patients (Liang and Carson 2008).

Skin Incision

Following injection, the neck incision is made. Placement of this incision should be guided by the preoperative LSG images and skin markings made by the nuclear medicine physician. The placement and orientation of the incision should also facilitate excision of the scar in the event of a subsequent neck dissection. For patients undergoing SNB-assisted ENB, the neck dissection skin flaps may be elevated after injection of blue dye, facilitating surgical access for the remaining procedure.

Use of the Handheld Gamma-Probe

Surgical dissection is guided by the preoperative LSG images, which should be made available in the operating room, and by a handheld gamma probe fitted with a 14-mm diameter straight collimated probe. The pulse height analysis window should be set just to include the ^{99m}Tc photopeak with a cut-off on the low energy side at about 130 keV. The handheld probe can be directed toward areas of high signal, providing more immediate guidance regarding the direction of dissection. A series of 1-mm-thick, malleable sterilized lead plates may be used to mask the primary tumor, reducing detection of "shine-through" radioactivity from the injection site and aiding intraoperative identification of radioactive nodes. If blue dye was previously injected, visualized lymphatic channels should be followed to the first-echelon lymph nodes. All "hot" (radioactive) nodes, and all blue nodes, are regarded as sentinel nodes and should be excised. Radioactivity should be confirmed ex vivo before sending the nodes for pathological evaluation. All harvested nodes should be labeled according to neck level, radioactivity, and color. Patients undergoing SNB-assisted END may then proceed to completion of the neck dissection. At the end of the procedure, the handheld gamma camera should be used to detect any residual radioactivity in the surgical bed and in the neck dissection specimen. When no radioactivity is present in the neck, closure can then be undertaken (Shoaib et al. 1999; Ross et al. 2002b).

In some centers, lymph nodes that exhibit radioactivity less than 10% of the "hottest" node are not routinely removed. The rationale for this is based on the results of the large Sunbelt Melanoma Trial (McMasters et al. 2004), which determined that removing only those nodes with a radioactivity count greater than 10% of the hottest node is associated with a failure rate of approximately 2%. To date, no similar data have been reported for squamous cell carcinoma.

Pathologic Evaluation of Harvested Lymph Nodes

Histopathologic Work-Up

SNB is mainly a minimally invasive staging procedure with implications on further patient management. Earlier work has shown that increasing the number of lymph node sections taken from neck dissection specimens also increases the detection of occult disease (Ambrosch and Brinck 1996). In SNB, the number of lymph nodes to be investigated is considerably reduced in comparison with END. This reduction in workload for the pathologist allows for more extensive work-up of the SLN. Thorough histopathologic examination of the SLNs is most crucial for the accuracy of this technique.

There is still some debate on how best to section SLNs. The goal should be to detect most of the occult metastases in order to correctly stage the neck. The current recommendation, formulated at the Second International Conference on Sentinel Node Biopsy in Mucosal Head and Neck Cancer in 2003, is step serial sectioning of the entire SLNs at intervals of 150 μm (Stoeckli et al. 2005). Conventional staining with H&E and immunohistochemistry with cytokeratin staining must be available. SLNs that appear negative on H&E have to be stained with cytokeratin, as immunohistochemistry facilitates the detection and increases the rate of micrometastatic deposits.

The presence of occult metastases is assessed and their size measured with standardized ocular measurement devices. If there is no evidence of disease on H&E and cytokeratin staining, the node is declared tumor free. If cytokeratin deposits are detected, the positive section must be compared with the immediately adjacent serial section, previously stained with H&E, to determine whether the positivity was due to the presence of viable tumor cells. Artifacts, or inclusion of tissues other than SCC, present challenging pitfalls and warrant an experienced pathologist to avoid false positive reports.

Classification of Occult Metastases

Histologically detected lymph node metastases in clinically nodal negative necks are, by definition, occult metastases. Some authors erroneously use the term *micrometastasis* for any metastasis detected by histological work-up of a clinically N0 neck. Hermanek et al. proposed a classification of occult metastases according to well-defined histologic criteria, and this is shown in Table 3.1 (Hermanek et al. 1999).

Occult metastases are subdivided into isolated tumor cells (ITC; small clusters of tumor cells within the lymph node sinuses), micrometastases, and metastases. ITC have been defined in the sixth edition of the TNM classification of malignant tumors as "...single tumor cells or small clusters of cells not more than 0.2 mm in greatest dimension that are usually detected by immunohistochemistry or molecular methods, but which may be verified with H&E stains. ITC do not typically show evidence of metastatic activity (e.g., proliferation or stromal reaction) or penetration of vascular or lymphatic sinus walls" (Sobin and Wittekind 2006).

Micrometastases and metastases represent infiltrations of the lymph node parenchyma by tumor deposits smaller and larger than 2 mm, respectively. This classification has also been proposed for use in the context of SNB for oral and oropharyngeal SCC (Stoeckli et al. 2002a, b), and widely accepted as ITC, micrometastases and metastases may have different therapeutic and prognostic implications.

Table 3.1 Classification of isolated tumor cells (ITC) and micrometastasis (Hermanek et al. 1999)

	ITC	Micrometastasis
Size	Single tumor cells or small clusters	Smaller than 2 mm
Contact with lymph sinus wall	No	Yes
Invasion of lymph sinus wall	No	Yes
Extrasinusoidal stromal reaction	No	Usually yes
Extrasinusoidal tumor cell proliferation	No	Yes

Implications of SNB on the TNM Classification

The sixth edition of the TNM classification of malignant tumors, published in 2002, presents both a definition of the sentinel node and a proposed classification system for its use in oral/oropharyngeal SCC (Sobin and Wittekind 2002).

When SNB is attempted, this should be indicated by the addition of the designation (sn) after the N category. Cases with ITC are classified as pN0 (i+) (sn), while those with a micrometastasis designated pN1 (mi) (sn). The presence of micrometastases leads to upstaging of the N category, whereas *isolated tumor cells do not result in upstaging of the neck.* Classification according to these criteria is pivotal to avoid stage migration when comparing the results of treatment with historical cohorts.

Frozen Section

Traditionally, the detection of occult disease by SNB is followed by a therapeutic neck dissection. This represents a disadvantage for those patients who have to undergo a second surgical procedure. Intraoperative frozen section analysis of SLN was discouraged for a long period of time because of the disadvantages of freezing artefacts, loss of tissue, and high expenditures of labor and time. Several groups have investigated the accuracy of frozen sections for SLN in OSCC. In a study by Stoeckli et al. (2007), the negative predictive value of a negative SNB on frozen section achieved 83%. Only 17% of the patients had to undergo a second procedure because of false negative frozen sections of the SLNs, mostly due to ITC or tiny micrometastatic disease not revealed on frozen sections. Two other studies have reported equally encouraging results (Terada et al. 2005; Tschopp et al. 2005). Currently, novel intraoperative staging techniques such as imprint cytology (Asthana et al. 2003), and even intraoperative real-time genetic evaluation (Hamakawa et al. 2004), are under investigation and may change the protocols in the near future. For the time being, frozen section analysis can be considered as safe and accurate, sparing a second surgical procedure in the majority of patients with occult disease in the SLNs.

Management of SLN Positive Patients

Currently, the recommendation is to dissect all necks with tumor deposits in the SLNs, regardless of the type of occult disease. With more data and experience, this general recommendation may be modified.

Early Applications of Sentinel Node Biopsy in OSCC

Phase I Trials

The technique of sentinel node biopsy was first successfully applied to OSCC by Alex and Krag in 1996. The authors reported a patient with neck metastases from a supraglottic cancer, successfully identified by gamma-probe radiolocalization (Alex and Krag 1996). Interest in the technique mounted, but many of the initial reports were unfavorable. Pitman et al. (1998) described a series of 16 patients with HNSCC, in which identification of sentinel nodes was unsuccessful using injection of blue dye alone. Koch et al. (1998) reported unsuccessful gamma-probe SNB in three of five patients with cN0 OSCC, and suggested that while the technique appears feasible for selected patients, the problems they encountered may indicate that further study is not warranted. In a larger study of 20 patients, Shoaib et al. reported problems with the use of blue dye alone, and inaccuracy of SNB for patients with a clinically positive neck. However, as part of the same study, the authors reported that SNB with both blue dye and radiocolloid was successful in identifying subclinical metastases in seven of seven patients (Shoaib et al. 1999). The difficulties posed by the cN+ neck were previously noted in other cancers such as melanoma, and were subsequently highlighted in patients with HNSCC by Werner et al. (1999). These problems are thought to be due to the raised hydrostatic pressures and distorted architecture within grossly metastatic lymph nodes, preventing entry of radiocolloid or dye into the lymph node and diverting flow to a different, uninvolved, node (Werner et al. 1999; Dünne et al. 2001).

Most centers began to focus on patients with clinically negative necks, primarily with clinical stage T1 or T2 primary tumors in the oral cavity and oropharynx. Early reports took the form of validation studies, with patients undergoing sentinel node biopsy followed by immediate END and comparison of the pathology. As experience with the procedure increased, the reported identification rates for sentinel nodes improved and many authors began to describe successful SLN harvest in 90–100% of cases (Taylor et al. 2001; Stoeckli et al. 2001; Zitsch et al. 2000; Bilchik et al. 1998; Mozzillo et al. 2001; Dünne et al. 2001). Significantly, these early phase I validation studies were also beginning to demonstrate a very low false negative rate (0–6%) for the sentinel node procedure; that is, the immediate END did not appear to detect a significant number of cases in which nodal disease had been "missed" by the SNB (Table 3.2). This finding led to further interest in the procedure as a staging tool for early OSCC, and paved the way for subsequent stage II trials.

Learning Curve

Experience has shown that lymphatic mapping in the neck can be technically challenging (Morton et al. 1992), and there is a significant learning curve associated with

Table 3.2 Phase I studies: SNB in head and neck SCC

Author	Primary tumor	Clinical stage	Methods of SNB	n	Numbers of patients with occult metastasis	SN identified (%)	False negative (%)	Negative predictive value (%)
Shoaib et al. (2001)	Oral cavity	T1-T4, N0	Tc-99m-HSA+patent blue V dye	37	20 (54%)	6	90	95
Chiesa et al. (2000)	Oral cavity	T1-T2, N0, M0	Tc-99m-HSA	11	3 (27%)	0	73[a]	100
Alex and Krag (1996)	Oral cavity oropharynx larynx	T1-T4, N0, M0	Tc-99m-SC	8	1 (13%)	0	100	100
Werner et al. (1999)	Oropharynx hypopharynx larynx	T1-T3, N0, M0	Tc-99m-HSA	5	1 (20%)	0	100	100
Koch et al. (1998)	Oral cavity oropharynx	T1-T2, N0, M0	Tc-99m-SC	5	1 (20%)	0	40	100
Taylor et al. (2001)	Oral cavity oropharynx	T1-T2, N0, M0	Tc-99m-SC	9	4 (44%)	0	100	100
Stoeckli et al. (2001)	Oral cavity oropharynx	T1-T3, N0, M0	Tc-99m-SC+methyl blue dye	19	6 (32%)	0	100	100
Alex et al. (2000)	Supraglottic	T1, N0, M0	Tc-99m-SC	1	1 (100%)	0	100	100
Zitsch et al. (2000)	Oral cavity oropharynx	T1-T2, N0, M0	Tc-99m-SC	8	1 (20%)	0	100	100
Bilchik et al. (1998)	Oral cavity	T1, N0, M0	LSG+lymphazurin blue dye	4	1 (25%)	0	100	100
Mozzillo et al. (2001)	Oral cavity	T1-T2, N0, M0	Tc-99m-HSA+blue dye	41	4 (10%)	0	95	100
Dünne et al. (2001)	Oropharynx hypopharynx larynx	T1-T2, N0, M0	Tc-99m-HSA	38	6 (16%)	0	100	100
Stoeckli et al. (2002a, b)	Oral cavity oropharynx	T1-T3, N0, M0	Tc-99m-HSA	19	6 (32%)	0	100	100
Kosuda et al. (2003)	Oral cavity oropharynx hypopharynx larynx	T2-T3, N0, M0	Tc-99m-tin colloid	11	4 (36%)	0	100	100
Höft et al. (2004)	Oral cavity oropharynx hypopharynx larynx	T1-T4, N0, M0	Tc-99m-HSA	50	12 (24%)	0	92	100
Werner et al. (2004)	Oral cavity oropharynx hypopharynx larynx	T1-T3, N0, M0	Tc-99m-HSA	90	23 (26%)	13	100	97

Nieuwenhuis et al. (2005)	Oral cavity oropharynx	T2–T4, N0, M0	Tc-99m-HSA	22	9 (45%)	11	91	92
Hart et al. (2005)	Oral cavity oropharynx	T1–T4, N0, M0	Tc-99m-SC	20	4 (20%)	0	100	100
Gallegos-Hernández et al. (2005)	Oral cavity	T1–T2, N0, M0	Tc-99m-SC+blue dye	48	13 (27%)	17	100	89
Payoux et al. (2005)	Oral cavity oropharynx	T1–T4, N0, M0	Tc-99m-SC	30 (38 necks)	6 (20%)	3	97	97
Thomsen et al. (2005)	Oral cavity	T1–T2, N0, M0	Tc-99m-SC+patent blue dye	40	14 (35%)	20	100	96
Rigual et al. (2005)	Oral cavity	T2, N0, M0	Tc-99m-SC+isosulfan blue dye	20	12 (60%)	14	100	80

SN sentinel node; LSG lymphoscintigraphy; HSA human serum albumin; SC sulfur colloid

[a]Injection of radioactive tracer and neck dissection performed 1 month after primary intraoral tumor resection

the procedure (van der Veen et al. 1994; Ross et al. 2004a, b; Haerle et al. in press). This learning curve, coupled with the still-evolving technique, may account for some of the early difficulties encountered in some reports. As such, it is recommended that all centers wishing to participate in a clinical trial should first validate the technique by performing SNB-assisted END, with comparison of the pathological results. An overall accuracy of 90% and an identification rate of 90% in ten consecutive cases should be demonstrated before patients may be entered into the trial.

Cost-Effectiveness of Sentinel Node Biopsy

Sentinel node biopsy may potentially also offer some financial advantages, compared to traditional management of the cN0 neck. Traditionally, patients with a greater than 20% chance of subclinical neck metastasis would be managed with an END (O'Brien et al. 2000). Each neck dissection specimen can potentially consists of 20 or more lymph nodes, each of which must be examined individually by the pathologist. While the evaluation of a sentinel node is generally more extensive in comparison with a routine neck dissection specimen, the nature of the procedure allows the pathologist to focus attention on just a few selected nodes. This can potentially lead to a significant reduction in the pathologist's workload by reducing the number of unnecessary neck dissections performed. The cost of analyzing a sentinel node specimen is estimated to be approximately half that of a modified radical neck dissection specimen (van Diest et al. 2001).

Although there are a few studies demonstrating these benefits in patients with OSCC, a number of reports have demonstrated tangible cost benefits for the management of melanoma (Genta et al. 2007). It is postulated that the use of SNB for melanoma reduces the operative morbidity seen with END due to the limited dissection required. Brobeil et al. (1999) estimated cost savings to the health care system of approximately $172 million per year for SNB in melanoma, where in SNB was used instead of END for staging regional disease. The cost analysis included total hospital charges and professional fees, and demonstrated that patients, providers, payers, employers, and industry are all beneficiaries of SNB technology. The long-term cost savings and benefit were found to far outweigh the initial investment of purchasing equipment and training personnel.

Current Status: Where Do We Stand?

Inclusion Criteria

During the last decade, SNB has been validated for feasibility and accuracy against the gold standard, END, in many studies from different centers throughout the world. These validation studies have been performed within the context of END

(Mamelle et al. 2006; Civantos et al. 2006; Shoaib et al. 1999; Stoeckli et al. 2001). Most of the studies were restricted to oral and oropharyngeal squamous cell carcinoma, with a strong preponderance of oral cavity cancers. Therefore, with respect to the anatomic site of the primary tumor, the SNB procedure can currently only be considered validated for tumors arising in the oral cavity and in accessible subsites of the oropharynx (i.e., soft palate, lateral wall). Several investigators have reported on successful SNB for other locations such as the hypopharynx and the supraglottic larynx (Werner et al. 2004). Due to the limited number of studies and patients included, these sites should still be considered investigational.

Tumors in hidden areas such as the hypopharynx, base of tongue, and supraglottic larynx cannot be reached with the patient awake for injection of the radiotracer. Therefore, preoperative evaluation with LSG is not possible, and the tracer must be injected under general anesthesia with endoscopic guidance. Whether lymphatic mapping based solely on the use of the intraoperative gamma probe gives equivalent results remains questionable, since the regional nodes along the jugular chain are located in close proximity to the injection site in the hypopharynx and larynx. Radioactive scatter from the primary site makes the detection of the sentinel nodes difficult. In addition, node-negative squamous cell carcinoma of the hypopharynx and supraglottic larynx are rather rare, as these tumors mainly present in advanced stages, and many of these tumors will be treated nonsurgically. Therefore, the main indication for SNB, to date, includes squamous cell carcinoma of the oral cavity and accessible oropharynx.

For successful SNB of squamous cell carcinomas of the oral cavity and the oropharynx, there are further limitations with respect to tumor size. Large tumors are difficult to completely surround with the tracer injection, they show a tendency to drain to multiple lymphatic basins, and in most patients, they require a neck dissection for either access to tumor resection or defect reconstruction. In the early phase I trials, large tumors (T3/4) were included in SNB protocols, leading to unreliable results for the reasons mentioned above (Ross et al. 2002a). As a result, there is a current consensus that SNB should be restricted to early tumors staged T1/2 (Ross et al. 2004a, b; Stoeckli et al. 2005).

There are three main clinical situations for which SNB in early oral and oropharyngeal squamous cell carcinoma is an accepted indication. The first and most frequent is to stage the ipsilateral cN0 neck in a unilateral primary tumor. The second indication is to assess the ipsilateral and contralateral cN0 necks in primary tumors close to or crossing the midline. The third indication is to assess the contralateral cN0 neck in primary tumors close to or crossing the midline with an ipsilateral cN+ neck, in order to decide whether these patients need bilateral neck dissections, or whether the morbidity can be reduced by performing an ipsilateral neck dissection and contralateral SNB alone.

A further potential indication has, to date, been largely unexplored and is more anecdotal, but nevertheless clinically highly attractive. Patients with previous treatment to the neck by either radiation or neck dissection are routinely excluded from SNB protocols. The strength of lymphatic mapping and SNB is the individual analysis of the lymphatic drainage of a specific tumor in a distinct individual. Prior radiation or surgery to the neck obviously distorts lymphatic drainage patterns, potentially giving rise to unexpected patterns of nodal metastases. In the case of a small recurrent or second primary tumor, lymphatic mapping can be used in these patients to analyze the lymphatic pathways directing surgical intervention to the region at risk.

Exclusion Criteria

Many patients undergoing SNB for early oral cancer are included in prospective trial protocols. Most protocols exclude children, pregnant women, and lactating women for safety reasons; most radiotracers are not approved for use in these patients. Off-label use should be considered with caution, and with respect to a risk-benefit analysis in each individual case.

Sentinel Node Biopsy as the Sole Staging Procedure

Some centers have subsequently abandoned END in the case of a negative SNB, largely as a result of the encouraging outcomes of validation studies. The reported high level of accuracy of the SNB procedure, with a false-negative rate of approximately 5%, has allowed some investigators to proceed with SNB as the sole staging tool in selected patients.

To date, two large prospective clinical observational trials have been published (Ross et al. 2004a, b; Stoeckli 2007). The first, a multicenter trial based at the Canniesburn plastic surgery department in Scotland, reported the results of SNB in 134 patients from 6 European centers. All patients had cT1/2 N0 disease and underwent either SNB-assisted END or SNB alone. The interim results were published at 2 years of follow-up in 2004, and reported a 93% SN identification rate and 93% sensitivity for the SNB procedure (Ross et al. 2004a, b). After a full 5 years of follow-up, one further patient developed nodal recurrent disease, bringing the overall sensitivity to 91% and negative predictive value to 95% at 5 years (Alkureishi et al. 2008). Of particular note in this patient series, both the SN identification rate and sensitivity were found to be significantly lower in patients whose tumors were located in the floor of the mouth. The authors attribute these discrepancies to the technical difficulties of accessing tumors in this location, and the close proximity of the primary tumor potentially masking the true location of the sentinel nodes. As a result, the authors concluded that SNB can be successfully applied as the sole staging tool for the majority of tumors in the oral cavity and oropharynx, but advise caution when applying the technique to floor-of-mouth tumors.

The second study represents the largest single-institution experience published to date (Stoeckli 2007). In this study, the total number of 51 consecutive patients with cT1/2, cN0 OSCC were prospectively enrolled in the observational part of the trial. The sentinel node detection rate was 98%. Forty percent of the patients were upstaged as a result of a positive SNB, and underwent neck dissection. Only two patients with negative SNB experienced a neck recurrence. The negative predictive value of SNB for the remaining neck was therefore 94%. All patients with positive SNB were treated with an END of levels I–III for oral cavity primaries, and levels II–IV for oropharyngeal SCC. No postoperative radiotherapy was employed. The authors conclude that SNB as the sole staging procedure is reliable and that patients with positive SNB can be safely treated with neck dissection.

The data from these observational trials have subsequently been merged with data from a number of experienced European centers to form the prospective European Sentinel Node Trial, known as SENT. The mean follow-up for this data-set is currently at 27 months, and the authors have reported on an interim analysis focusing on sentinel node–positive patients (Ross et al. 2008).

The authors report 72 patients (86 neck sides) who were found positive by sentinel node biopsy and who went on to receive therapeutic neck dissection as part of the sentinel node protocol. Thirty-six of the 86 neck sides (42%) were found to have additional disease in the neck dissection specimen. Of these additional positive lymph nodes, 52% were found in the same neck level as the positive SLN, while a further 44% were located in a level immediately adjacent (higher or lower) to the positive SLN. Only 4% of the positive nodes were located in a neck level other than that of the positive SLN or its immediate relations. Additionally, only one of the 86 neck sides (2%) was found to have positive disease beyond levels I–III. The authors conclude that based on these data, it may be feasible to limit the therapeutic neck dissection following SNB to three levels – one above and one below the positive SLN – as a means of further reducing the morbidity of the procedure without compromising the oncologic safety.

In the United States, the American College of Surgeons' Oncology Group (ACOSOG) Z0360 trial completed accrual in 2006. This prospective multicenter validation study involves 137 cT1/T2 patients from 25 institutions and is currently in the follow-up phase. The authors recently published an interim analysis of their data, with promising results (Civantos 2007). Based on preliminary pathology with H&E staining alone, the authors reported a negative predictive value of 94%, and this is expected to rise when the data from additional pathologic evaluation become available. Similar to the results of the Canniesburn multicenter trial, the authors found that the accuracy of sentinel node biopsy was significantly lower for tumors located in the floor of the mouth, with a negative predictive value of 88.5% compared with 95.8% for other sites, and concluded that while SNB is a promising technique, further advances in its application are required before it can be reliably applied to tumors in the floor of the mouth.

The Future of Sentinel Node Biopsy in OSCC

The sentinel node biopsy procedure currently provides an additional tool for the staging of patients with early oral/oropharyngeal squamous cell cancer. However, it is not without its limitations, and sound knowledge of these is essential for the physician wishing to employ it. Presently, the exact role of SNB in the management of squamous cell cancer remains largely undefined, and it is hoped that the results of upcoming large-scale prospective studies will go some way toward further elucidating this role. The SENT trial is ongoing, as is the ACOSOG Z0360 study (Civantos et al. 2005). The results of these studies may pave the way for true randomized phase III trials, comparing the outcomes of patients undergoing SNB alone (with therapeutic neck dissection for SNB-positive patients) with those of patients undergoing END, which remains the standard of care in most institutions.

References

Alex JC, Krag DN (1993) Gamma probe guided lymph node localization in malignant melanoma. Surg Oncol 2:137–143

Alex JC, Krag DN (1996) The gamma-probe-guided resection of radiolabeled primary lymph nodes. Surg Oncol Clin N Am 5(1):33–41 Review

Alex JC, Sasaki CT, Krag DN, Wenig B, Pyle PB (2000) Sentinel lymph node radiolocalization in head and neck squamous cell carcinoma. Laryngoscope 110:198–203

Alkureishi LW, Ross GL, MacDonald DG, Shoaib T, Gray H, Robertson G, Soutar DS (2007) Sentinel node in head and neck cancer: use of size criterion to upstage the N0 neck in head and neck squamous cell carcinoma. Head Neck 29(2):95–103

Alkureishi LWT, Ross GL, Shoaib T, Sorensen J, Alvarez J, Poli T, Kovacs A, Alberti F, Soutar DS (2008) Sentinel node biopsy in oral/oropharyngeal squamous cell cancer: five year follow-up. Presented at the Annual Meeting of the American Head and Neck Society (AHNS), San Francisco, July 2008

Alvi A, Johnson JT (1996) Extracapsular spread in the clinically negative neck (N0): implications and outcome. Otolaryngol Head Neck Surg 114:65–70

Ambrosch P, Brinck U (1996) Detection of nodal micrometastases in head and neck cancer by serial sectioning and immunostaining. Oncology 10:1221–1226

Asthana S, Deo SVS, Shukla NK, Jain P, Anand M, Kumar R (2003) Intraoperative neck staging using sentinel node biopsy and imprint cytology in oral cancer. Head Neck 25:368–372

Barzan L, Sulfaro S, Alberti F, Politi D, Pin M, Savignano MG, Marus W, Zarcone O, Spaziante R (2004) An extended use of the sentinel node in head and neck squamous cell carcinoma: results of a prospective study of 100 patients. Acta Otorhinolaryngol Ital 24(3):145–149

Bilchik AJ, Giuliano A, Essner R, Bostick P, Kelemen P, Foshag LJ, Sostrin S, Turner RR, Morton DL (1998) Universal application of intraoperative lymphatic mapping and sentinel lymphadenectomy in solid neoplasms. Cancer J Sci Am 4:351–358

Bilde A, Von Buchwald C, Mortensen J et al (2006) The role of SPECT-CT in the lymphoscintigraphic identification of sentinel nodes in patients with oral cancer. Acta Otolaryngol 126(10):1096–1103

Bocca E, Pignataro O, Oldini C, Cappa C (1984) Functional neck dissection: an evaluation and review of 843 cases. Laryngoscope 94(7):942–945

Brobeil A, Cruse CW, Messina JL, Glass LF, Haddad FF, Berman CG, Marshburn J, Reintgen DS (1999) Cost analysis of sentinel lymph node biopsy as an alternative to elective lymph node dissection in patients with malignant melanoma. Surg Oncol Clin N Am 8(3):435–445 viii

Cabanas RM (1977) An approach for the treatment of penile carcinoma. Cancer 39(2):456–466

Chepeha DB, Hoff PT, Taylor RJ, Bradford CR, Teknos TN, Esclamado RM (2002) Selective neck dissection for the treatment of neck metastasis from squamous cell carcinoma of the head and neck. Laryngoscope 112(3):434–438

Chiesa F, Mauri S, Grana C, Tradati N, Calabrese L, Ansarin M, Mazzarol G, Paganelli G (2000) Is there a role for sentinel node biopsy in early N0 tongue tumors? Surgery 128:16–21

Civantos FJ, Werner JA, Bared A (2005) Sentinel node biopsy in cancer of the oral cavity. Oper Tech Otolaryngol Head Neck Surg 16(4):275–285. American College of Surgeons Oncology Group trial Z0360, https://www.acosog.org

Cody HS III (1999) Sentinel lymph node mapping breast cancer. Oncology 13:25–34

Dünne AA, Külkens C, Ramaswamy A, Folz BJ, Brandt D, Lippert BM, Behr T, Moll R, Werner JA (2001) Value of sentinel lymphonodectomy in head and neck cancer patients without evidence of lymphogenic metastatic disease. Auris Nasus Larynx 28(4):339–344

Ferlito A, Rinaldo A, Robbins KT, Leemans CR, Shah JP, Shaha AR, Andersen PE, Kowalski LP, Pellitteri PK, Clayman GL, Rogers SN, Medina JE, Byers RM (2003) Changing concepts in the surgical management of the cervical node metastasis. Oral Oncol 39(5):429–435

Fisch UP, Sigel ME (1964) Cervical lymphatic system as visualized by lymphography. Ann Otol Rhinol Laryngol 73:870–882

Gallegos-Hernández JF, Hernández-Hernández DM, Flores-Díaz R, Sierra-Santiesteban I, Pichardo-Romero P, Arias-Ceballos H, Minauro-Muñoz G, Alvarado-Cabrero I (2005) The number of sentinel nodes identified as prognostic factor in oral epidermoid cancer. Oral Oncol 41(9):947–952

Garzom OL, Palcos MC, Radicella R (1965) Technetium-99 m labelled colloid. Int J Appl Radiat Isotopes 16:613

Genta F, Zanon E, Camanni M, Deltetto F, Drogo M, Gallo R, Gilardi C (2007) Cost/accuracy ratio analysis in breast cancer patients undergoing ultrasound-guided fine-needle aspiration cytology, sentinel node biopsy, and frozen section of node. World J Surg 31(6):1155–1163

Gould EA, Winship T, Philbin PH, Kerr HH (1960) Observations on a 'sentinel node' in cancer of the parotid. Cancer 13:77–78

Haerle SK, Hany TF, Strobel K, Sidler D, Stoeckli SJ (in press) Is there an additional value of SPECT/CT over lymphoscintigraphy for sentinel node mapping in oral/oropharyngeal squamous cell carcinoma? J Nucl Med

Hamakawa H, Onishi A, Sumida T, Terakado N, Hino S, Nakashiro KI, Shintani S (2004) Intraoperative real-time genetic diagnosis for sentinel node navigation surgery. Int J Oral Maxillofac Surg 33:670–675

Hart RD, Nasser JG, Trites JR, Taylor SM, Bullock M, Barnes D (2005) Sentinel lymph node biopsy in N0 squamous cell carcinoma of the oral cavity and oropharynx. Arch Otolaryngol Head Neck Surg 131(1):34–38

Hermanek P, Hutter RV, Sobin LH, Wittekind C (1999) International Union Against Cancer. Classification of isolated tumor cells and micrometastasis. Cancer 86(12):2668–2673

Höft S, Maune S, Muhle C, Brenner W, Czech N, Kampen WU, Jänig U, Laudien M, Gottschlich S, Ambrosch P (2004) Sentinel lymph-node biopsy in head and neck cancer. Br J Cancer 91(1):124–128

Holmes EC, Moseley HS, Morton DL, Clark W, Robinson D, Urist MM (1977) A rational approach to the surgical management of melanoma. Ann Surg 186(4):481–490

Kaufman G, Guth AA, Pachter HL, Roses DF (2008) A cautionary tale: anaphylaxis to isosulfan blue dye after 12 years and 3339 cases of lymphatic mapping. Am Surg 74(2):152–155 Review

Keski-Säntti H, Mätzke S, Kauppinen T, Törnwall J, Atula T (2006) Sentinel lymph node mapping using SPECT-CT fusion imaging in patients with oral cavity squamous cell carcinoma. Eur Arch Otorhinolaryngol 263(11):1008–1012

Kligerman J, Lima RA, Soares JR, Prado L, Dias FL, Freitas EQ, Olivatto LO (1994) Supraomohyoid neck dissection in the treatment of T1/T2 squamous cell carcinoma of oral cavity. Am J Surg 168(5):391–394

Koch WM, Choti MA, Civelek AC, Eisele DW, Saunders JR (1998) Gamma probe-directed biopsy of the sentinel node in oral squamous cell carcinoma. Arch Otolaryngol Head Neck Surg 124:455–459

Kosuda S, Kusano S, Kohno N, Ohno Y, Tanabe T, Kitahara S, Tamai S (2003) Feasibility and cost-effectiveness of sentinel lymph node radiolocalization in stage N0 head and neck cancer.

Arch Otolaryngol Head Neck Surg 129(10):1105–1109 Erratum in: Arch Otolaryngol Head Neck Surg 2003;129(11):1229

Liang MI, Carson WE III (2008) Biphasic anaphylactic reaction to blue dye during sentinel lymph node biopsy. World J Surg Oncol 6:79

Mamelle G, Temam S, Casiraghi O, Lumbroso J, Laplanche A, Bourhis J (2006) Role and perspectives of sentinel node biopsy in head and neck tumors. Cancer Radiother 10(6–7):349–353

McMasters KM, Noyes RD, Reintgen DS, Goydos JS, Beitsch PD, Davidson BS, Sussman JJ, Gershenwald JE, Ross MI, Sunbelt Melanoma Trial (2004) Lessons learned from the Sunbelt Melanoma Trial. J Surg Oncol 86(4):212–223

Morton DL, Bostick PJ (1999) Will the true sentinel node please stand? Ann Surg Oncol 6:12–14

Morton DL, Wen DR, Wong JH, Economou JS, Cagle LA, Storm FK, Foshag LJ, Cochran AJ (1992) Technical details of introperative lymphatic mapping for early stage melanoma. Arch Surg 127:392–399

Morton DL, Thompson JF, Cochran AJ, Mozzillo N, Elashoff R, Essner R, Nieweg OE, Roses DF, Hoekstra HJ, Karakousis CP, Reintgen DS, Coventry BJ, Glass EC, Wang HJ, MSLT Group (2006) Sentinel-node biopsy or nodal observation in melanoma. N Engl J Med 355(13):1307–1317 Erratum in: N Engl J Med 2006;355(18):1944

Mozzillo N, Chiesa F, Botti G, Caraco C, Lastoria S, Giugliano G, Mazzarol G, Paganelli G, Ionna F (2001) Sentinel node biopsy in head and neck cancer. Ann Surg Oncol 8:103S–105S

Nieuwenhuis EJ, Castelijns JA, Pijpers R, van den Brekel MW, Brakenhoff RH, van der Waal I, Snow GB, Leemans CR (2002) Wait-and-see policy for the N0 neck in early-stage oral and oropharyngeal squamous cell carcinoma using ultrasonography-guided cytology: is there a role for identification of the sentinel node? Head Neck 24(3):282–289

Nieuwenhuis EJ, van der Waal I, Leemans CR, Kummer A, Pijpers R, Castelijns JA, Brakenhoff RH, Snow GB (2005) Histopathologic validation of the sentinel node concept in oral and oropharyngeal squamous cell carcinoma. Head Neck 27(2):150–158

O'Brien CJ, Traynor SJ, McNeil E, McMahon JD, Chaplin JM (2000) The use of clinical criteria alone in the management of the clinically negative neck among patients with squamous cell carcinoma of the oral cavity and oropharynx. Arch Otolaryngol Head Neck Surg 126(3):360–365

Payoux P, Dekeister C, Lopez R, Lauwers F, Esquerré JP, Paoli JR (2005) Effectiveness of lymphoscintigraphic sentinel node detection for cervical staging of patients with squamous cell carcinoma of the head and neck. J Oral Maxillofac Surg 63(8):1091–1095

Persky MS, Lagmay VM (1999) Treatment of the clinically negative neck in oral squamous cell carcinoma. Laryngoscope 109(7 Pt 1):1160–1164

Pitman KT, Johnson JT, Myers EN (1997) Effectiveness of selective neck dissection for management of the clinically negative neck. Arch Otolaryngol Head Neck Surg 123(9):917–922

Pitman KT, Johnson JT, Edington H, Barnes EL, Day R, Wagner RL, Myers EN (1998) Lymphatic mapping with isosulfan blue dye in squamous cell carcinoma of the head and neck. Arch Otolaryngol Head Neck Surg 124(7):790–793

Razack MS, Baffi R, Sako K (1981) Bilateral radical neck dissection. Cancer 47(1):197–199

Ries LAG, Melbert D, Krapcho M, Stinchcomb DG, Howlader N, Horner MJ, Mariotto A, Miller BA, Feuer EJ, Altekruse SF, Lewis DR, Clegg L, Eisner MP, Reichman M, Edwards BK (eds) (2008) SEER Cancer Statistics Review, 1975–2005. National Cancer Institute, Bethesda, MD

Rigual N, Douglas W, Lamonica D, Wiseman S, Cheney R, Hicks W Jr, Loree T (2005) Sentinel lymph node biopsy: a rational approach for staging T2N0 oral cancer. Laryngoscope 115(12):2217–2220

Ross GL, Shoaib T, Soutar DS, MacDonald DG, Camilleri IG, Bessent RG, Gray HW (2002a) The first international conference on sentinel node biopsy in mucosal head and neck cancer and adoption of a multicenter trial protocol. Ann Surg Oncol 9(4):406–410

Ross GL, Soutar DS, Shoaib T, Camilleri IG, MacDonald DG, Robertson AG, Bessent RG, Gray HW (2002b) The ability of lymphoscintigraphy to direct sentinel node biopsy in the clinically N0 neck for patients with head and neck squamous cell carcinoma. Br J Radiol 75:950–958

Ross GL, Soutar DS, MacDonald DG, Shoaib T, Camilleri IG, Robertson AG (2004a) Improved staging of cervical metastases in clinically node-negative patients with head and neck squamous cell carcinoma. Ann Surg Oncol 11(2):213–218

Ross GL, Soutar DS, Gordon MacDonald D, Shoaib T, Camilleri I, Roberton AG, Sorensen JA, Thomsen J, Grupe P, Alvarez J, Barbier L, Santamaria J, Poli T, Massarelli O, Sesenna E, Kovács AF, Grünwald F, Barzan L, Sulfaro S, Alberti F (2004b) Sentinel node biopsy in head and neck cancer: preliminary results of a multicenter trial. Ann Surg Oncol 11(7):690–696

Ross GL, on behalf of the Sentinel European Node Trial (SENT) organising committee. Sentinel Node Biopsy for Squamous Cell Carcinoma of the Oral Cavity: Preliminary results of the SENT Trial. Presented at the Annual Meeting of the American Head and Neck Society (AHNS), San Francisco, July 2008

Scherer K, Studer W, Figueiredo V, Bircher AJ (2006) Anaphylaxis to isosulfan blue and cross-reactivity to patent blue V: case report and review of the nomenclature of vital blue dyes. Ann Allergy Asthma Immunol 96(3):497–500 Review

Shah JP, Andersen PE (1994) The impact of patterns of nodal metastasis on modifications of neck dissection. Ann Surg Oncol 1(6):521–532

Shoaib T, Soutar DS, Prosser JE et al (1999) A suggested method for sentinel node biopsy in squamous cell carcinoma of the head and neck. Head Neck 21(8):728–733

Shoaib T, Soutar DS, MacDonald DG, Camilleri IG, Dunaway DJ, Gray HW, McCurrach GM, Bessent RG, MacLeod TI, Robertson AG (2001) The accuracy of head and neck carcinoma sentinel lymph node biopsy in the clinically N0 neck. Cancer 91(11):2077–2083

Sobin LH, Wittekind Ch (eds) (2002) TNM classification of malignant tumors, 6th edn. Wiley, New York

Sobol S, Jensen C, Sawyer W II, Costiloe P, Thong N (1985) Objective comparison of physical dysfunction after neck dissection. Am J Surg 150(4):503–509

Stoeckli SJ (2007) Sentinel node biopsy for oral and orophayrngeal squamous cell carcinoma of the head and neck. Candidate's thesis. Laryngoscope 117:1539–1551

Stoeckli SJ, Schuknecht B, Strobel K (in press) Initial Staging of the Neck in HNSCC: Is PET/CT the best? Head Neck

Stoeckli SJ, Steinert H, Pfaltz M, Schmid S (2001) Sentinel lymph node evaluation in squamous cell carcinoma of the head and neck. Otolaryngol Head Neck Surg 125:221–226

Stoeckli SJ, Steinert H, Pfaltz M, Schmid S (2002a) Is there a role for positron emission tomography with 18F-Fluorodeoxyglucose in the initial staging of nodal negative oral and oropharyngeal squamous cell carcinoma. Head Neck 24:345–349

Stoeckli SJ, Pfaltz M, Steinert H, Schmid S (2002b) Histopathological features of occult metastasis detected by sentinel lymph node biopsy in oral and oropharyngeal squamous cell carcinoma. Laryngoscope 112(1):111–115

Stoeckli SJ, Pfaltz M, Ross GL, Steiner HC, MacDonald DG, Wittekind C, Soutar D (2005) The second international conference on sentinel node biopsy in mucosal head and neck cancer. Ann Surg Oncol 12:919–924

Tafra L, Chua AN, Ng PC, Aycock D, Swanson M, Lannin D (1999) Filtered versus unfiltered technetium sulfur colloid in lymphatic mapping: a significant variable in a pig model. Ann Surg Oncol 6(1):83–87

Taylor RJ, Wahl RL, Sharma PK, Bradford CR, Terrell JE, Teknos TN, Heard EM, Wolf GT, Chepeha DB (2001) Sentinel node localization in oral cavity and oropharynx squamous cell cancer. Arch Otolaryngol Head Neck Surg 127(8):970–974

Terada A, Hasegawa Y, Goto M, Sato E, Hyodo I, Ogawa T, Nakashima T, Yatabe Y (2005) Sentinel lymph node radiolocalization in clinically negative neck oral cancer. Head Neck 28:114–120

Thomsen JB, Sørensen JA, Grupe P, Karstoft J, Krogdahl A (2005) Staging N0 oral cancer: lymphoscintigraphy and conventional imaging. Acta Radiol 46(5):492–496

Tschopp L, Nuycns M, Stauffer E, Krause T, Zbären P (2005) The value of frozen section analysis of the sentinel lymph node in clinically N0 squamous cell carcinoma of the oral cavity and oropharynx. Otolaryngol Head Neck Surg 132:99–102

van den Brekel MW, Stel HV, Castelijns JA, Nauta JJ, van der Waal I, Valk J, Meyer CJ, Snow GB (1990) Cervical lymph node metastasis: assessment of radiologic criteria. Radiology 177(2):379–384

van den Brekel MW, Stel HV, van der Valk P, van der Waal I, Meyer CJ, Snow GB (1992) Micrometastases from squamous cell carcinoma in neck dissection specimens. Eur Arch Otorhinolaryngol 249(6):349–353

van der Veen H, Hoekstra OS, Paul MA, Cuesta MA, Meijer S (1994) Gamma probe-guided sentinel node biopsy to select patients with melanoma for lymphadenectomy. Br J Surg 81(12):1769–1770

van Diest PJ, Torrenga H, Meijer S, Meijer CJ (2001) Pathologic analysis of sentinel lymph nodes. Semin Surg Oncol 20(3):238–245

Weissbach L, Boedefeld EA (1987) Localization of solitary and multiple metastases in stage II nonseminomatous testis tumor as basis for a modified staging lymph node dissection in stage I. J Urol 138:77–82

Werner JA, Dunne AA, Brandt D, Ramaswamy A, Kulkens C, Lippert BM, Folz BJ, Joseph K, Moll R (1999) Studies on significance of sentinel lymphadenectomy in pharyngeal and laryngeal carcinoma. Laryngorhinootologie 78:663–670

Werner JA, Dünne AA, Myers JN (2003) Functional anatomy of the lymphatic drainage system of the upper aerodigestive tract and its role in metastasis of squamous cell carcinoma. Head Neck 25(4):322–332

Werner JA, Dünne AA, Ramaswamy A, Dalchow C, Behr T, Moll R, Folz BJ, Davis RK (2004) The sentinel node concept in head and neck cancer: solution for the controversies in the N0 neck? Head Neck 26(7):603–611

Wilke LG, Giuliano A (2003) Sentinel lymph node biopsy in patients with early-stage breast cancer: status of the National Clinical Trials. Surg Clin North Am 83(4):901–910

Woolgar JA, Beirne JC, Vaughan ED, Lewis-Jones HG, Scott J, Brown JS (1995) Correlation of histopathologic findings with clinical and radiological assessments of cervical lymph-node metastases in oral cancer. Int J Oral Maxillofac Surg 24(1 Pt 1):30–37

Wrightson WR, Wong SL, Edwards MJ, Chao C, Reintgen DS, Ross MI, Noyes RD, Viar V, Cerrito PB, McMasters KM, Sunbelt Melanoma Trial Study Group (2003) Complications associated with sentinel lymph node biopsy for melanoma. Ann Surg Oncol 10(6):676–680

Yuen AP, Lam KY, Chan AC, Wei WI, Lam LK, Ho WK, Ho CM (1999) Clinicopathological analysis of elective neck dissection for N0 neck of early oral tongue carcinoma. Am J Surg 177(1):90–92

Zitsch RP, Todd DW, Renner GJ, Singh A (2000) Intraoperative radiolymphoscintigraphy for detection of occult nodal metastasis in patients with head and neck squamous cell carcinoma. Otolaryngol Head Neck Surg 122:662–666

Chapter 4
Prediction of Nodal Metastases from Genomic Analyses of the Primary Tumor

Amy S. Whigham and Wendell G. Yarbrough

Abstract Due to the associated poor prognostic significance, the finding of nodal metastases during the evaluation and staging of patients with head and neck cancer drives therapeutic decisions. Advances in imaging have enabled the detection of smaller cervical metastases with more certainty; however, an unacceptable portion (a minority) of patients with negative clinical and radiographic evaluation for cervical disease actually has metastases upon pathologic evaluation of resected nodes. Clinicians are left in the uncomfortable position of treating cervical nodal basins in patients with greater than 20% risk of metastases based on historical data, despite the fact that, in the majority of patients, this intervention may not be beneficial. This treatment frequently results in patient morbidity and is a health care expenditure that could be redirected if physicians could better predict metastases. On the cellular level, metastasis is a rare event due to its complex nature requiring that the metastatic tumor cells acquire a number of disparate behaviors through gene alterations. Recent data suggest that gene expression profiling of the primary tumor can predict metastatic potential. Because primary tumor biopsies provide adequate material for gene expression profiling, one can imagine that data derived from a diagnostic biopsy could be used to direct therapeutic decisions.

Introduction

Head and neck squamous cell carcinoma (HNSCC) remains a significant source of morbidity in the United States and worldwide. Current treatment for head and neck cancer is based on relatively unsophisticated information, such as the site of origin, tumor size, and the presence of lymphatic or hematogenous metastases. Oral cavity squamous cell carcinoma (OSCC) displays a wide range of metastatic behavior that

W.G. Yarbrough (✉)
Department of Otolaryngology & Department of Cancer Biology, Vanderbilt-Ingram Cancer Center, Vanderbilt University School of Medicine, 2220 Pierce Avenue, 654 Preston Research Building, Nashville, TN, 37232, USA
e-mail: wendell.yarbrough@vanderbilt.edu

J. Myers (ed.), *Oral Cancer Metastasis*,
DOI 10.1007/978-1-4419-0775-2_4, © Springer Science+Business Media, LLC 2010

cannot be predicted by tumor size, standard histology, or even individual gene or protein expression/activity. The use of multimodality therapy in the treatment for HNSCC has rendered the American Joint Committee on Cancer (AJCC) staging system less adequate as a prognostic indicator (Salesiotis and Cullen 2000). Although the head and neck cancer staging system may be antiquated, the presence or absence of neck metastases consistently retains statistical correlation with survival (Spiro et al. 1974; Schuller et al. 1980; Anderson et al. 1994; Sessions et al. 2000, 2002, 2003). Molecular characteristics such as estrogen/progesterone receptor and HER2 status in breast cancer and chromosomal translocations in lymphomas are used clinically to subclassify these tumors and to guide therapy; however, no molecular characteristics are currently used in clinical decision making for HNSCC.

More recently, global gene expression techniques have been used to classify tumors and predict behavior with the goal of improving treatment strategies. Despite the clinically obvious heterogeneity of OSCC, there are currently no means of predicting individual tumor behavior. Treatment decisions are based on experience, including clinical trials designed to identify modalities with the greatest percentage of patient response. While this strategy maximizes overall response of the population of HNSCC cancer patients, it condemns those patients whose tumor may behave less aggressively to unnecessary morbidity. Based on clinical trials and personal experience, treatments that benefit only a minority of patients may be abandoned as noneffective. Microarray gene expression analyses provide semiquantitative detection of thousands of individual genes. Perhaps the most important application of this technique is to correlate changes in gene expression with changes in tumor behavior, such as proliferation, metastases, or response to drug therapy (He and Friend 2001). Accurate prediction of metastases in oral and HNSCC would have an immediate clinical impact through avoidance of unnecessary treatment of patients at low risk with appropriate direction of resources toward aggressive treatment of patients at high risk of having metastatic disease. Additionally, elucidation of key pathways involved in tumor metastasis may direct therapeutic investigation and intervention (Fidler 1990).

Oral Cavity Cancer

Head and neck cancer cases within the United States number more than 45,000 per year with oral cavity cancer accounting for approximately 20,000 cases annually (Jemal et al. 2007). Head and neck cancer is the fifth most common cancer and the sixth leading cause of cancer-related death in the United States (Kim et al. 2002). Histology of oral cavity cancers is relatively uniform, with squamous cell carcinomas comprising 80–90% of these tumors (Chung et al. 2006b). OSCC is strongly associated with tobacco and alcohol use, but recently human papillomavirus (HPV) has been etiologically implicated in HNSCC, including up to 50% of oropharyngeal tumors and potentially a portion of oral cavity cancers (Gillison et al. 2000; Mellin et al. 2000; Lindel et al. 2001; Schwartz et al. 2001;Ritchie et al. 2003).

The clinical behavior of HNSCC varies greatly from one tumor to another, but all are treated similarly based on tumor location, tumor size, and the presence of lymph node and distant metastases. The oral cavity includes the subsites of tongue, floor of mouth, lip, alveolar ridge, hard palate, and buccal mucosa (Fig. 4.1); carcinoma of the lip is most often etiologically linked to sun exposure and may consequently be viewed as a distinct clinical entity. The oral cavity is critical for alimentation and communication, and therapy for OSCC can have deleterious effects on swallowing and speech. Advanced tumors of the oral cavity are frequently treated with surgery followed by concurrent chemotherapy and radiation therapy. Even small primary tumors of the oral cavity have a propensity to metastasize to cervical nodes, mandating that the majority of patients, even those with no clinical or radiographic evidence of nodal metastases, undergo some form of neck treatment either for staging or therapeutic purposes (Kligerman et al. 1994). To minimize the adverse effects of neck dissection for staging, sentinel node techniques are now being evaluated for their ability to accurately predict the absence of cervical metastases (Taylor et al. 2001; Ross et al. 2004; Werner et al. 2004; Kovacs 2007). Unfortunately, sentinel node biopsies still require a neck procedure to remove one or more lymph nodes. Although techniques are being developed to rapidly analyze resected sentinel nodes, current practice requires a staging surgery followed by definitive neck dissection for histologically positive sentinel nodes (Ross et al. 2002; Becker et al. 2004; Ferris et al. 2005; Stoeckli 2007). Currently, there are no molecular characteristics of the primary tumor that are used clinically to predict the risk of cervical metastases.

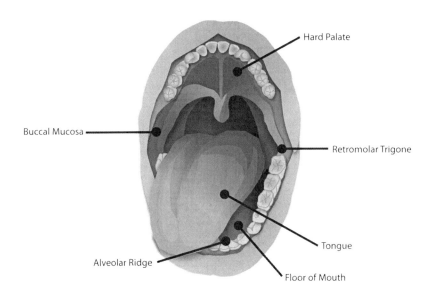

Fig. 4.1 Oral Cavity. The oral cavity and its subsites of tongue, hard palate, floor of mouth, alveolar ridge, buccal mucosa, and retromolar trigone

Microarray Analyses of Gene Expression

Technologies in functional genomics, such as microarray analysis, permit qualitative and quantitative biologic investigations on a genome-wide scale (Mohr et al. 2002). The basic technique requires extraction of DNA or RNA from biological samples, such as tumor biopsies or resection specimens. The nucleic acids can be amplified before labeling with a fluorescent marker. The labeled DNA/RNA is then hybridized to a microarray, a platform on which thousands of gene sequences are localized in specific and distinct locations (Warner et al. 2004). Because nucleic acid hybridization relies on complementary sequences, each deposited gene sequence will specifically bind homologous DNA or RNA derived from the original sample. Unbound DNA/RNA is washed away and the fluorescent intensities are measured (Butte 2002). The intensity of fluorescence at a particular location is a measure of the amount of a particular gene or RNA sequence in the original sample. If messenger RNA (mRNA) derived from a sample of interest (e.g., tumor) is used as the starting material, then the intensity of fluorescence corresponding to a particular gene will give an indication of the level of expression of that gene within the tumor. Microarrays containing all human gene sequences are readily available, allowing creation of gene expression profiles containing all known genes (Warner et al. 2004). Obviously, the amount of data created from a single microarray experiment is enormous. Comparisons of data from multiple samples or even from multiple different array platforms require sophisticated bioinformatics and biostatistical tools.

There are several roles for microarrays in oncologic research, with implications for clinical practice. Microarrays can be used to detect specific gene mutations with improved speed, accuracy, and sensitivity compared with classical sequencing or screening techniques. In cancer research, oligonucleotide arrays have been used to screen for mutations in oncogenes and tumor suppressors (Mohr et al. 2002). By combining oligonucleotide arrays with comparative genomic hybridization techniques, gene copy number changes can be detected. The screening of single nucleotide polymorphisms (SNPs) by oligonucleotide array can be used to determine or predict loss of heterozygosity, individual variability of drug metabolism or activity, and in particular individual disease susceptibility for conditions that rely on the interaction of multiple genes (e.g., hypertension, diabetes, cardiovascular disease, cancer) (Mohr et al. 2002). Microarrays can also augment investigation of gene function and have solidified connections between previously unrecognized signaling pathways. Arguably, the major use of microarrays for clinical applications in oncologic research has been to determine differences in gene expression between disparate tumors, between tumor and normal, or between tumors with similar clinical and histologic characteristics (Mohr et al. 2002). These comparisons are used to provide insight into differences that in some way correlate with tumor behavior, such as growth, metastases, or response to therapy, or with clinical course of disease, such as recurrence or survival.

Regardless of the molecular technique utilized, there are inherent limitations imposed by examination of RNA as a measure of gene expression. Since techniques, including expression microarrays, that measure mRNA do not directly detect proteins, they may not accurately predict expression or activity of the encoded protein. Proteins are the effectors that guide cellular behavior; consequently, it would be ideal to measure protein levels or activity within biological samples. For example, transcription of some genes, such as p53, remains relatively constant despite the wide variation in its protein levels, which are regulated primarily by protein stabilization. Additionally, some proteins, such as signaling molecules, are not primarily regulated by either transcription or protein stability. Activity of these critical proteins is frequently regulated by posttranscriptional modifications, including phosphorylation, acetylation, and ubiquitination. Despite these limitations, expression microarray analyses may accurately predict protein activity based on downstream effects on transcription of regulated genes. For instance, stabilized/activated p53 leads to transcription of many mediators of cell cycle arrest or apoptosis that are readily measured with mRNA-based techniques.

Utility of Gene Expression Analysis

Distinguish HNSCC Tumor Subtypes

Between and within cancers there exists a significant degree of heterogeneity of cellular makeup and genetic alteration. Fortunately, current scientific methods provide techniques to meticulously analyze the gene expression profiles of such complex tumor samples. Each tumor has a unique gene expression pattern, termed a molecular "signature" or "portrait" (Chung et al. 2002). Tumors that are morphologically similar may have significantly different molecular signatures. The ability to distinguish tumors with aberrant clinical behavior based on clinical or histological features has been a challenge in oncology. Sorlie et al. (2001) examined the gene expression profiles of 78 breast carcinomas. Hierarchical clustering of these histologically similar tumors based on microarray data revealed five unique groups. Although breast carcinomas have been previously separated into groups based on ERRB2 (HER2) expression, gene expression data identified two unique and previously undescribed subtypes of ERBB2 positive tumors. Remarkably, the data divided the two subtypes of ERBB2-positive breast carcinomas as those with good prognosis and those with poor prognosis.

Human papillomavirus has recently been etiologically linked with a subset of HNSCCs (reviewed in McKaig et al. 1998; Gillison et al. 2000; van Houten et al. 2001). The presence of HPV in HNSCC ranges from 15% to 34%. The oropharynx is the subsite within the head and neck most commonly affected by HPV-associated tumors, but squamous cell cancers of other subsites such as oral cavity and larynx may also be associated with HPV (McKaig et al. 1998; D'Souza et al. 2007). As with HPV infections of the uterine cervix, oral HPV infections are associated with sexual activity, and oral HPV infection is associated with increased risk of oropharyngeal squamous cell carcinoma (D'Souza et al. 2007). Surprisingly, HPV-associated risk is independent of the known HNSCC risk factors of tobacco and alcohol (D'Souza et al. 2007). Greater than 90% of HPV-positive oropharyngeal tumors contain HPV type 16, previously identified as high risk with respect to premalignant and malignant lesions of the cervix. HPV-positive HNSCC appears to have discrete clinical and biological characteristics when compared with HPV-negative HNSCC (Sisk et al. 2002; Ritchie et al. 2003). HPV E6 and E7 viral proteins inhibit tumor-suppressors p53 and Rb, respectively, and drive tumorigenesis. It is hypothesized that in HPV-positive HNSCC the downstream effects of loss of p53 and Rb activity on other tumor-related genes would confer a gene expression profile that is distinct from HPV-negative HNSCC (van Houten et al. 2001). Ninety-one genes that are differentially expressed between HPV-positive and -negative tumors ($p<0.01$) were identified with data from global gene expression analyses (Slebos et al. 2006). Several of the upregulated genes are involved in cell cycle regulation or transcription, and many have been previously linked with HPV-associated uterine cervical cancer (Santin et al. 2005). This set of 91 genes was able to correctly predict the HPV status in 100% of the samples tested (Slebos et al. 2006). Other studies have confirmed the biological distinction of HPV-positive HNSCC both clinically and molecularly (van Houten et al. 2001; Gillison 2004; Weinberger et al. 2006).

Predict Survival and Outcome

The AJCC staging system alone is not adequate as a prognostic indicator (Salesiotis and Cullen 2000). In fact, decreased survival and risk of recurrence portended by cervical lymphatic metastases is of such great concern that necks without clinical or radiographic signs of metastases (clinically and radiographically N0) are treated if risk of cervical metastases is deemed to be greater than 20% based on the size and site of the primary tumor. In attempts to more accurately classify HNSCC patients into high- and low-risk groups, histological evaluation of the primary tumor for growth pattern and lymphatic/vascular invasion has been examined to determine if these pathologic features correlate with risk of cervical metastases and, therefore, with overall survival. These studies have yielded mixed results, with some data indicating that vascular and lymphatic invasion may help in assessing survival and other studies suggesting that histological evidence of lymphatic invasion does not correlate with poor prognosis (Johnson et al. 1987; Fagan et al. 1998). Likewise, a microscopic invasion pattern of thin finger-like projections or single-cells has been contradictorily associated with both decreased overall survival and with improved organ preservation following induction chemotherapy (reviewed in Bradford 1999). Tumor and pathologic features have been examined in N0 oral cavity cancers to determine if they can predict metastatic potential. No parameter examined, including site (tongue vs. floor of mouth), T stage (T1 vs. T2), or tumor thickness could be correlated with the presence of cervical metastases (Kligerman et al. 1994).

Other attempts to improve prognostic accuracy in HNSCC have been driven by emerging technologies such as analyses of tumor ploidy using flow cytometry and molecular analyses for gene defects in the primary tumor. Perhaps the most common approach to augment the prognostic information provided by the TNM staging classification has been to examine individual genes within the tumor that are involved in critical pathways such as proliferation, apoptosis, immortalization, and angiogenesis. These pathways are expected to be perturbed in primary tumors, but physicians and researchers would like to know if a particular molecular defect of an individual pathway could predict metastatic potential or survival in HNSCC patients (Hahn et al. 1999). Initial excitement for this approach has been hampered by low sensitivity/specificity or by reports from follow-up studies that contradict earlier reported results. One example evaluates the apoptotic pathway in HNSCC tumors. Separate studies of Bcl-2 have suggested that overexpression is associated with improved survival, decreased survival, and increased locoregional failure and is not predictive of survival at all (Gallo et al. 1999; Klatka 2001; Wilson et al. 2001). Mutations in p53 have also been shown not to correlate with survival, to be associated with poor prognosis, and to be associated with improved survival (Sauter et al. 1992; Bradford et al. 1997; reviewed in Assimakopoulos et al. 2000; Alsner et al. 2001; Klatka 2001). Studies of proliferative oncogenes have similarly been confusing, with expression of c-erbB2 correlating with decreased survival in one study and not predictive of survival in another study (Giatromanolaki et al. 2000; Shiga et al. 2000). Taken together, these data are confusing, are not clinically useful, and suggest that individual molecular markers are inadequate to predict tumor aggressiveness, metastatic potential, or response to therapy, and that singly, molecular markers in tumors lack the power to guide therapeutic decisions (Salesiotis and Cullen 2000). Molecular analyses of HNSCC, although initially exciting, have thus far failed to be clinically useful. Ability to accurately identify primary head and neck tumors with metastatic potential will identify patients in need of aggressive therapy, as well as spare the cost and morbidity of neck therapy to patients at low risk.

After identification of a subset of HNSCC tumors related to HPV, efforts to further characterize this subtype have examined the clinical characteristics of HPV-positive HNSCC. Multiple studies have revealed prognostic implications for HPV-associated HNSCC (reviewed in Gillison 2004). Overall and disease-related survival have been found to be statistically significantly improved in patients with HPV-associated HNSCC when compared with HPV-negative tumors (Gillison et al. 2000; Sisk et al. 2002; Ritchie et al. 2003; Weinberger et al. 2006). In one large study of patients with oral cavity or oropharyngeal squamous cell carcinoma, those with HPV-positive tumors had improved overall and disease-specific survival, despite having tumors that were more advanced in stage (Schwartz et al. 2001). The ability to identify such a subset of HNSCC with improved prognosis may permit the selection of patients for less aggressive surgical and medical therapies.

Predict Tumor Behavior and Therapeutic Response of Tumors

Gene expression data from multiple tumor types may provide insight into their clinical behavior. Chung et al. (2002) compared gene expression profiles of lung and breast tumor data sets from the Stanford Microarray Database. By hierarchical clustering, a common gene expression pattern emerged from these disparate tumor types. Genes within this pattern, termed the "proliferation cluster," have been shown to be responsible for cell cycle regulation, DNA replication, and chromosomal modification. Further analysis correlated expression of this proliferation cluster with *in vitro* cellular growth in breast, lung, ovarian, prostate, liver, and gastric tumors (Perou et al. 2000; Garber et al. 2001; Welsh et al. 2001; Chen et al. 2002; Hippo et al. 2002; LaTulippe et al. 2002). Perhaps more importantly, increased expression of genes within this molecular cluster *in vivo* was linked with poor prognosis (Chung et al. 2002).

While many tumor markers have the potential to provide insight into prognosis of HNSCC, there are currently no molecular markers that predict response to conventional therapies. The identification of such markers has contributed to treatment advances in other cancer types. In breast cancer, cellular expression of the estrogen receptor correlates with a positive therapeutic response to the antiestrogen tamoxifen (Fisher et al. 1989). Activation of the Abl tyrosine kinase, as indicated by the presence of the Philadelphia chromosome, in chronic myelogenous leukemia predicts response to the Abl kinase inhibitor imatinib (Gleevac) (Druker et al. 2001). In HNSCC, recent studies suggest that the presence of HPV in the tumor is associated with improved response to therapy and survival (Mellin et al. 2000; Lindel et al. 2001; Li et al. 2003). Further exploration of the effect of HPV as a predictor of response and mechanism of action is warranted. Additional molecular markers that are predictive of treatment response or outcome in HNSCC would be of tremendous value to clinicians.

Gene Expression Analysis in HNSCC

Head and neck squamous cell carcinoma has been categorized based on histologic features, but it is clearly a group of diseases with disparate clinical behavior. Etiology related to carcinogen exposure is well documented, and the gross molecular basis of progression has been described (Sidransky et al. 2003; Hashibe et al. 2007); however, these data have not elucidated individual molecular variation that determines tumor behavior. To gain a better understanding of carcinogenesis in HNSCC, microarray technology has been applied to the analyses of normal, premalignant lesions, and HNSCC. Greater than 12,000 genes were queried using a microarray platform revealing that 334 genes had altered expression in premalignant lesions compared with histologically normal tissue (Ha et al. 2003). Remarkably, only 23 genes exhibited altered expression in the progression from premalignant to malignant, suggesting that many more gene expression changes are required for early events in tumorigenesis. Not surprisingly, the products of those genes upregulated in malignant tumors relative to normal tissue were associated with well-known tumor-related processes such as apoptosis, angiogenesis, cell cycle control, transcriptional regulation, cell adhesion, and cell-signaling pathways (Ha et al. 2003).

Cell Biology and Molecular Determinants of Metastasis

Recent advances have been made in the diagnosis and treatment of cancer, including identification of plasma or serum biomarkers, imaging techniques, local and systemic therapies, and surgical techniques. These advances have had little effect on overall cancer survival largely because disseminated disease is resistant to current therapy and is the most common cause of cancer-related death (Fidler 2003). In HNSCC, two-thirds of patients present with local or regionally advanced disease (Kim et al. 2002). Metastasis is defined as the growth of tumor cells at a site distant to the primary tumor location. Broad categorization divides metastases into either lymphatic or hematogenous. Early in the progression of OSCC, blood-borne metastases are rarely encountered; however, lymphatic metastases are very common at initial patient presentation and are frequently the only sign of cancer early in the natural history of OSCC.

Growth of metastatic tumors represents the culmination of a complex multistep process that necessitates the interaction of the tumor cells with the surrounding stroma and stromal cells, as well as with tissue components at the ultimate metastatic site (Fidler 1990). The multistep process to acquire metastatic potential can be likened to the multistep process of tumorigenesis with many necessary genetic alterations. Requirements of metastasis include: (1) invasion of a primary tumor, (2) development of new blood or lymphatic vessels, (3) detachment of the metastatic cell, (4) intravasation of tumor cells into the lymphatic or blood channels, (5) extravasation of the tumors cells from the lymphatic or blood vessel into the site of metastasis, and (6) implantation and growth of tumor cells at this distant site (Fig. 4.2). The regulation of each step is complex and can involve alteration of multiple cellular pathways (Table 4.1). For instance, blood-borne circulating tumor cells have to avoid anoikis, attach to a vessel wall within the organ capable of supporting metastatic tumor growth, extravasate, and survive and grow in a foreign environment without the benefit of conditioned tumor-associated stromal cells. As discussed by Gershenwald and Fidler (2002), one step in the metastatic pathway can occur independently and via other pathways than another. Many studies suggest that gene alterations accompany these steps necessary for metastases, and microarray gene expression analysis is particularly well suited to identify genes involved in these processes (Kitadai et al. 1996; Herbst et al. 2000; Hynes 2003).

Models of Metastasis from Primary Tumors

Clonal Selection

Despite the devastating clinical effect of metastases, it is a rare cellular event for almost all tumor types. Quite large cancers with millions of cells may lead to no metastases or only a single metastasis, indicating that only a single cell derived from the primary tumor was able to successfully metastasize. To explain the rarity

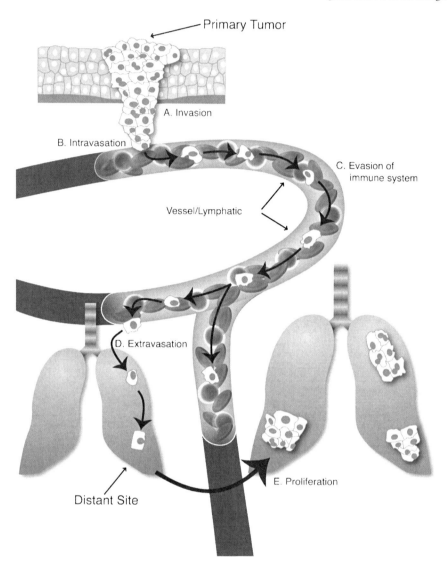

Fig. 4.2 Cellular requirements for metastasis. (**a**) Invasion of the local host tissues, (**b**) intravasation into vessels or lymphatic channels, (**c**) evasion of the host's immune system, (**d**) extravasation into and establishment within distant tissues, and (**e**) proliferation at distant sites

of metastases as well as to account for the multiple genetic alterations needed for metastases, traditional models have posited that very rare cells within the primary tumor develop metastatic potential. This model is best described as the clonal selection model (Fig. 4.3a) and accounts for the paucity of metastases even in large tumors containing 10^9–10^{12} cells (Talmadge 2007). Additionally, the clonal selection model

Table 4.1 Biologic processes involved in tumor metastasis and some respective key gene products

Biologic process	Gene products
Growth/proliferation	EGFR family members, met, IGFR and ligands, myc, ras, fos, jun, MAPK, Akt, PI3K
Cell cycle regulation	Cyclins, CDKs, p53, p16, p21, p27, E2F family, p63
Angiogenesis/lymphangiogenesis	VEGF, bFGF, IL-8, PDGF, bFGF, ET-1, COX2, ephrin, Eph receptors, NFκB
Detachment/invasion	MMPs, E-cadherin, catenins, serine proteases, HGF, TGF-β
Adherence to vessel wall	E-cadherin, selectin, integrins
Survival/apoptosis	p53, EGFR, TGF-β, Akt, met, PI3K, p14ARF, Fas, p63, p73, Bcl and family members, caspases, stress-activated protein kinase p38

Studies of multiple tumor types, including gastric carcinoma, nonsmall cell lung cancer, melanoma, and breast cancer, indicate the potential role of the above gene products in the development of tumor metastases (Webb and Vande Woude 2000; Debies and Welch 2001; Takahashi et al. 2002; Kang et al. 2003; Nyormoi and Bar-Eli 2003; Wulfing et al. 2005; Zhu et al. 2006; Nissen et al. 2007)

EGFR epidermal growth factor receptor, *IGFR* insulin-like growth factor receptor, *MAPK* mitogen-activated protein kinase, *PI3K* phosphoinositide kinase 3, *CDK* cyclin dependent kinase, *VEGF* vascular endothelial growth factor, *bFGF* basic fibroblast growth factor, *IL-8* interleukin 8, *PDGF* platelet derived growth factor, *ET-1* endothelin 1, *COX2* cytochrome c oxidase subunit II, *NFκB* nuclear factor-kappa B, *MMP* matrix metalloproteinase, *HGF* hepatocyte growth factor, *TGF-β* transforming growth factor β

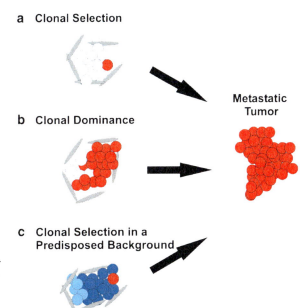

a Clonal Selection

b Clonal Dominance

Metastatic Tumor

c Clonal Selection in a Predisposed Background

Fig. 4.3 Models of metastasis. (**a**) Clonal selection, (**b**) clonal dominance, and (**c**) clonal selection in a predisposed background

assumes that alteration of genes important for metastases does not provide a selective growth or survival advantage within the primary tumor. The clonal selection model was validated when clonally derived murine melanoma cells were shown to have distinct metastatic potential when injected into the circulation of mice (Fidler and Kripke 1977). Further support for the clonal selection model derives from comparative genomic hybridization revealing that close to one-third of examined breast tumor/metastatic pairs had patterns of chromosomal alterations that did not resemble each other (Kuukasjarvi et al. 1997). Supplementary support for the clonal selection model includes additional studies confirming that characteristics of metastatic lesions differ from the parent primary tumors (Gancberg et al. 2002). Cell line subpopulations with increased metastatic potential have gene expression patterns that differ from the nonmetastatic subpopulations (Kang et al. 2003). Studies of a breast cancer cell line found that altered expression of a set of genes is associated with bony metastases and proved that forced expression of these genes increases metastatic potential (Kang et al. 2003). Many of the genes that were associated with increased metastatic potential are secreted or are cell surface proteins (interleukin [IL]-11, connective tissue growth factor [CTGF], matrix metalloproteinase [MMP]-1) that encourage angiogenesis or osteolysis.

In opposition to the clonal selection model are data from HNSCC and other tumor types suggesting that metastatic potential of a tumor can be predicted by examination of the bulk of the primary tumor (van't Veer et al. 2002; Ramaswamy et al. 2003; Chung et al. 2004a; Roepman et al. 2005). Consistent with the clonal selection model, cells with metastatic potential would be rare within the primary tumor and genetic defects that impart metastatic potential would not be represented in the bulk of the primary tumor. Accordingly, the clonal selection model predicts that gene expression profiling of the primary tumor would be incapable of predicting the ability of the tumor to form metastases.

Clonal Dominance

The clonal dominance model can be envisioned as an extension of the clonal selection model. As with the clonal selection model, rare cells with metastatic potential would arise within the primary tumor; however, unlike with the clonal selection model, the rare cell with metastatic capabilities would overgrow and eventually replace the majority of the cells within the primary tumor (Fig. 4.3b). This model would be consistent with the ability to detect metastatic potential from analyses of the primary tumor, but ignores data suggesting that metastatic tumor cells and primary tumor cells have distinct molecular differences (LaTulippe et al. 2002). The clonal dominance model does not suggest why a cell that obtains metastatic capacity would supplant nonmetastatic cells at the primary tumor site, nor would it support experimental data suggesting that only rare tumor cells within the primary tumor should be capable of metastasizing.

Furthermore, if millions of cells within a primary tumor all possessed the ability to metastasize, what would restrict widespread multiple metastases? Of course, it could be argued that even with a surfeit of fully capable metastatic cells, the process of metastasis has so many hurdles and is so arduous that, by probability alone, millions of cells must attempt metastases before one succeeds partly by chance.

Clonal Selection in a Predisposed Background

One appealing model of metastasis accounts for many clinical and research observations regarding metastases. The clonal selection in a predisposed background model (Fig. 4.3c) can justify seemingly disparate data indicating that gene expression profiles within the primary tumor can predict metastases as well as data showing that metastatic lesions have alterations seen only in rare clonal derivatives of the primary tumor. Prevailing thought suggests that tumorigenesis progresses through multiple rounds of mutagenesis and Darwinian selection. Cells obtain mutations that promote proliferation or survival, and then the "more fit" cells eventually dominate the tumor mass. This selection process is repeated as many as ten times during the development of a tumor to impart the characteristics necessary for tumor formation, such as unregulated proliferation, avoidance of apoptosis, angiogenesis, and avoidance of immune surveillance (Hanahan and Weinberg 2000). The clonal selection in a predisposed background model of metastasis hypothesizes that early genetic events during tumorigenesis not only provide a survival advantage but also impart upon the tumor characteristics necessary, but not sufficient, for metastases (Bernards and Weinberg 2002; Hynes 2003). Therefore, the majority of the tumor cells within the tumor have most, but not all, genetic alterations necessary for metastases. Tumor cells within such metastatically predisposed tumors would require only a few additional genetic alterations, or perhaps an encounter with conditioned stromal cells, to realize full metastatic potential, thus explaining the molecular differences found between metastatic deposits and the primary tumor. Gene expression data comparing primary tumors and metastases derived from the tumor detect statistically significant differences, but these differences are limited (Suzuki and Tarin 2007). Additionally, gene expression profiles and hierarchical clustering reveal that primary tumors are more closely related to their derived metastases than to other primary tumors (Weigelt et al. 2003; Roepman et al. 2006a). The clonal selection model would predict that metastatic lesions would not necessarily be more closely related to their parent primary tumors than to other metastatic tumors. The clonal selection in a predisposed background model, like the clonal dominance model, portends that gene expression profiles of the primary tumor should be capable of predicting metastases.

Cancer Stem Cell Model

Controversy remains, regarding the role or even existence of cancer stem cells in HNSCC. Cancer stem cells are described as rare cells within the cancer that are relatively undifferentiated and are capable of recreating all aspects of the tumor from very small numbers. In HNSCC, a cell surface marker, CD44, is expressed on a minority of cancer cells; when cells expressing CD44 are implanted into immune deficient diabetic SCID mice, tumors are obtained from very small numbers of cells (Prince et al. 2007).

A model of metastasis incorporating cancer stems cells could be envisioned to approximate the clonal selection model (Fig. 4.3a). In such a stem cell model, cancer stem cells would be capable of metastasizing due to their undifferentiated phenotype and genetic plasticity. However, once again, such a model would suggest that biopsy of the more differentiated cells within the tumor would not be capable of predicting metastases. Alternatively, a metastatic model incorporating cancer stem cells could be conceived that resembles the clonal selection in a predisposed background model (Fig. 4.3c). In this model, the cells with metastatic potential may be the cancer stem cells themselves or a small group of metastatically enabled cells derived from the cancer stem cells. As with the clonal selection in a predisposed background model, the majority of the cancer cells within the primary tumor would have genetic characteristics derived from the stem cells. Early gene alterations in the cancer stem cell population would impart both growth and survival advantages as well as set a foundation for metastatic potential. Of course, cancer stem cells within different tumors could either possess or lack metastatic potential explaining the variation in metastases observed between individual tumors.

Metastatic Profiles Within a Tumor

Metastatic heterogeneity within the primary tumor was described by Fidler and Kripke (1977) through their study of mouse B16 melanoma. As primary tumors demonstrate biologic heterogeneity with respect to metastatic potential, it can be extrapolated that heterogeneity of molecular metastatic profiles exists within a primary tumor. This heterogeneity may be due to variable genetic alterations within the tumor. Conversely, the heterogeneity within primary tumors may be due in part to different ratios of primary tumor cells and the tissue microenvironment. Solid tumor sections often contain components of the extracellular matrix and stromal constituents, such as fibroblasts, vascular elements, and inflammatory cells. Roepman et al. (2006b) used seven primary HNSCC samples to study the importance of sample cellular composition. Variations in the percentage of tumor vs. stromal cells within samples revealed biases that altered predictive accuracy. Those samples with less than 50% tumor cells demonstrated a clear reduction in the power to predict metastases compared to samples with 60–70% tumor cells. The samples with a lower tumor cell percentage, and conversely a higher percentage of stromal elements, exhibited a bias toward positive prediction of nodal metastases. Interestingly, the predictive power of samples with 80–100% tumor cell composition was also reduced, thereby emphasizing the contribution of stromal elements to the metastatic process.

Seed and Soil Hypothesis

As first proposed by Paget (1889) in the nineteenth century, there is a complex interaction between the cancer cell and the tissue to which it metastasizes. Each cancer cell is capable of developing into a tumor, yet different tumor types show discreet preference for metastasis to certain organs. Paget performed 735 necropsies of patients who succumbed to breast cancer. Of this group, 241 were found to have breast cancer deposits in the liver, while only 17 had cancer deposits in the spleen. This inequality is interesting as both the liver and the spleen were thought to have the same theoretical chance of metastasis based on organ size and blood flow. In other diseases, such as pyemia, the incidence of abscesses of the liver and spleen are less disproportionate, suggesting that the propensity of breast cancer metastases for the liver cannot be explained by vascular embolism alone. Consequently, the cancer cells (metaphorical seeds) are reliant on particular factors of the host environment (the soil). This observation by Paget is commonly referred to as the seed and soil hypothesis.

Data from cancer patients and mouse studies supports Paget's interrelated seed and soil hypothesis (Fidler 2003). As an example, after introduction of B16 melanoma cells into rodent circulation, tumors developed in pulmonary and ovarian tissue but not in renal tissue (Hart and Fidler 1980). Similarly, the expression of vascular endothelial growth factor-C in cutaneous melanomas and fibrosarcomas has been found to be directly correlated with the incidence of lymph node metastases but unrelated to pulmonary metastases (Padera et al. 2002). Finally, injection of syngeneic melanoma tumor cells into murine internal carotid arteries revealed that B16 melanoma cells produced meningeal tumors, whereas K-1735 melanoma cells developed brain parenchymal metastases, suggesting that even very similar tumors may have distinct organ or site preferences for metastases (Schackert and Fidler 1988). Paget's theory is also verified by the pattern of human ovarian cancer metastases. Metastatic ovarian cancer has a propensity for the peritoneal cavity but is rarely seen in other visceral organs. Autopsies performed on ovarian cancer patients with peritoneovenous shunts revealed that the introduction of metastatic cancer cells into the jugular venous circulation did not significantly alter the risk of metastasis to extraperitoneal sites (Tarin et al. 1984). Consequently, the propensity of tumors to metastasize is not solely dependent on their ability to enter the circulation. The cumulative data suggest that both tumor specific and host properties are responsible for the development of distant metastases.

Metastatic Profiles of Tumor Stroma

A complex interaction between tumor cells and the surrounding stroma within the tumor has recently been recognized as an important factor in tumor behavior. Within a cancer, epithelia and mesenchymal cells signal to one another and, through this signaling, alter or condition cellular behavior. In a molecular signature of metastasis identified by Ramaswamy et al. (2003), several expressed genes, such as collagen, actin, and myosin, appeared to be derived from the stromal tumor elements, as opposed to the epithelial components. These data contradict earlier concepts that the epithelial component of a cancer was sufficient to describe tumor behavior but are consistent with data suggesting that stromal cells within a cancer dramatically influence epithelial cell behavior even to the point of producing malignant behavior from otherwise premalignant cells (reviewed in Cunha et al. 2003). Analyses of many gene expression profiles derived from cancers suggest that both malignant epithelial and conditioned stromal elements of a primary tumor contribute to metastatic potential. Predictive metastatic profiles from primary HNSCC include contributions from genes presumptively derived from stromal elements such as vascular, immune, and mesodermal cells (Chung et al. 2004a; Roepman et al. 2005). Modulation of noncellular stromal elements in HNSCC metastases is also suggested by gene expression analyses. Genes encoding proteins responsible for binding to the extracellular matrix as well as those involved in degradation of the extracellular matrix were both overexpressed in metastatic tumors (Roepman et al. 2006c). Although these data appear incongruous, they in fact validate the complex nature of the tumor microenvironment and substantiate opinion that tumor cells likely utilize both degradation and attachment-based mechanisms of motility and invasion.

The interaction of the cancer cells and their environment is a key determinant in the site of organ metastasis. Statistical analysis of microarray profiles of metastatic lesions collected from murine lung, liver, kidney, and bone after intravenous injection of human small cell lung cancer cells clustered the lesions into organ-specific groups (Kakiuchi et al. 2003). Genes related to biological functions including growth-factor receptors, cytokines, chemokines, adhesion molecules, protein synthesis, cell motility, and metabolism distinguished the four groups. The pulmonary metastases were differentiated from those to kidney by the type of lectin, a protein that modulates cell–cell and cell–matrix interactions; the metastatic pulmonary lesions expressed LGALS1, whereas renal metastases expressed LGALS9. Several genes whose expression was increased in these experimental pulmonary deposits (e.g., RHOC, ITBG4, SDC1, C3, MT2A, and CALM) were previously associated with pulmonary metastases.

Profiles in Primary Tumors vs. Metastases

The gene expression patterns of primary tumors have been compared with those of metastatic tumors to determine if the metastatic potential of primary tumors develops from rare cells within the primary or derives from characteristics of the bulk of the primary tumor. Roepman et al. (2006a) examined the gene expression profiles of oral cavity/oropharyngeal HNSCC and their matched lymph node metastases. In 57%, the metastatic sample was most similar to its respective primary. In five of six primary tumor samples that did not cluster with their metastases, the matched metastatic nodal samples analyzed, contained less than 50% tumor cells within the lymph node. A within-pair, between-pair scatter ratio (WPBPSR) was calculated to determine the significance of similarity between matched primary tumors and lymph node metastases (Weigelt et al. 2003). Eighty-six percent of the matched pairs had a WPBPSR less than 1, indicating that the matched samples were more similar to each other than to the other primary or metastatic samples. Expression profiles between primary breast cancer tumors and distant metastases are also maintained (Weigelt et al. 2003). A single gene was differentially expressed between the primary tumors and the metastases, metastasis-associated gene 1 (MTA1). MTA1 is a regulator of epithelial-to-mesenchymal transition, a process that changes epithelial cell morphology and activities, such as motility and the decreased need for cell-to-cell contact, to more resemble mesenchymal cells.

Epithelial-to-mesenchymal transition has been shown to be predictive of poor prognosis in HNSCC and has been associated with metastatic potential (Chung et al. 2004b, 2006c; Kang and Massague 2004). Profiles from metastatic deposits of oral and oropharyngeal HNSCC were compared with two previously identified metastatic molecular signatures derived from primary tumors (Roepman et al. 2005, 2006c). Compared with their matched primary tumors, the metastatic samples had a similar expression of both sets of metastatic signature genes. Hence, the primary oral cavity and oropharyngeal HNSCC exhibit general and metastatic gene expression patterns similar to those of derived metastases. These findings indicate that gene expression profiles indicative of metastatic potential are possessed by the majority of the cells within the tumor, thereby supporting the theories of clonal dominance or clonal selection within a predisposed background.

Prediction of Metastasis

Multiple Profiles are Predictive of Metastasis

One criticism of gene expression profiling as a mechanism of predicting tumor metastases highlights the fact that different labs examining the same tumor type will arrive at predictive profiles that have minimal overlap. If gene expression of the primary tumor is responsible for tumor behaviors necessary for metastases, then why would different genes be identified that can predict metastases with similar accuracy? Explanations have varied, but detractors of expression analyses for prediction of clinical behavior suggest that microarray techniques are unreliable or that specimen processing before analyses introduces experimental variation that overwhelms biologically relevant differences. Others suggest that complex biostatistical and bioinformatic techniques used for analyses of extremely large data sets tend to "overfit" the data creating seemingly accurate prediction profiles that are not based on biologically relevant genes. In HNSCC, Roepman et al. (2006c) addressed this important question by performing multiple comparisons of an identical data set. Three thousand predictive profiles were generated. Interestingly, these distinct profiles distinguished node-negative and node-positive HNSCC with similar accuracy. Similar predictive accuracy was not solely due to a small core set of genes that was present in each profile since only 20–25% of the genes were included in all predictive profiles (Roepman et al. 2006c). Instead, it was proposed that interchanging different genes with similar expression profiles within groups, but with difference between metastatic and nonmetastatic groups, accounted for similar predictive ability despite the fact that the molecular profiles contained different genes. This explanation accounts for the observed variability of predictive genes from disparate labs. Slight differences in gene expression among distinct tumor samples or alteration of the microarray platform or the exact statistical tools used for selection of genes would be expected to result in variation in the identity of genes selected; however, if selected genes had similar expression patterns between metastatic and nonmetastatic tumors, predictive power would be similar. Thus, multiple molecular signatures may be identified with equivalent predictive outcomes.

Both the quality and the number of genes in a molecular profile affect the predictive ability of the set. After exclusion of the most frequently selected genes identified by Roepman et al. (2006c) from molecular signatures, the predictive accuracy decreased but nonetheless remained near the predictive clinical accuracy of 75%. By increasing the number of predictive genes in a molecular signature, the accuracy rose to 80–90%. Consequently, the quantity of the predictive genes in a set can counterweigh a decline in quality.

Common Genes for Metastasis Across Multiple Tumor Types

Metastatic potential of cancer cells is thought to have a common molecular basis driven by selective pressure or hurdles that the successful metastatic cell must overcome (Fig. 4.2, Table 4.1). It is clear that there are differences that affect the metastatic site or the frequency of metastases, but a core of common behaviors must be shared by metastatic cells. If a limited number of genes regulate these processes required for metastases, then a core set of genes may be found that are altered in all metastatic tumors. Ramaswamy et al. (2003) examined 64 primary adenocarcinomas from lung, breast, prostate, colorectal, uterus, and ovary and identified a shared 17 gene molecular signature for metastasis. Eight genes within this group were overexpressed, while nine were downregulated. Four of the genes that were upregulated are components of the protein translational apparatus, and one is involved in sister chromatid separation during cell division. This same 17 gene signature was applied to 279 solid tumors derived from different organ sites (lung, breast, prostate and medulloblastoma) and found to correlate with metastasis and worse clinical outcome ($p < 0.03$) (Ramaswamy et al. 2003).

Prediction of Metastasis in HNSCC

Distant metastases in HNSCC are extremely rare at initial presentation. On the other hand, metastases to regional lymph nodes are very common, and even if there are no clinical or radiographic signs of metastases, many subsites within the head and neck have occult metastatic rates approaching 25%. Sixty primary HNSCC samples were analyzed by Chung et al. (2004a) to predict prognosis and lymph node metastases. Key details of this and other microarray analyses of HNSCC metastases are shown in Table 4.2. Fifty-five of these samples were primary tumors, and five were local recurrences at the primary site. Expression of over 12,000 genes was analyzed, comparing primary HNSCC tumors, normal tonsillar epithelium, and HNSCC cell lines. Despite the fact that these tumors were indistinguishable based on all clinical, histological, and radiographic features, four distinct subtypes of HNSCC were identified. Remarkably, these four subtypes had differences in disease-free and overall survival (Chung et al. 2004a). Tumors from the group with the worst clinical outcome exhibited high expression of transforming growth factor alpha (TGFα), which has previously been linked with poor outcome in HNSCC, as well as increased expression of four genes previously identified in aggressive subtypes of breast cancer (Quon et al. 2001; Sorlie et al. 2001). Pathway analyses of the microarray data correlated activation of the EGFR pathway in the tumors with poor outcome. As previously observed in lung carcinoma, the group with the best prognosis clustered with the normal epithelial samples (Garber et al. 2001). The expression signature associated with cervical metastasis included many genes previously identified in prediction of breast cancer metastases (Huang et al. 2003; van't Veer et al. 2002). For pathologic lymph node status, the prediction accuracy was 57–60%. Interestingly, approximately half of the classification mistakes were made in prediction of tumors of oral cavity origin, suggesting that tumors of the oral cavity may be genetically distinct from or more heterogeneous than other subsites of HNSCC (Chung et al. 2004a).

Schmalbach et al. examined primary oral cavity and oropharyngeal HNSCC from 20 patients and compared gene expression of approximately 9,600 genes, to expression in HNSCC cell lines and normal oral cavity mucosa. The expression of 57 genes was recognized as distinct between tumors with and without lymph node metastases ($p < 0.01$). The tissue inhibitor of matrix metalloproteinase 1 (TIMP-1) demonstrated the greatest degree of differential expression between tumor and normal samples, and this finding was confirmed by immunohistochemistry (Schmalbach et al. 2004). As previously seen in colorectal and breast cancer, high TIMP-1 expression correlated with tumors that were metastatic to lymph nodes (Zeng et al. 1995; Ree et al. 1997). This correlation did not reach statistical significance

Table 4.2 Microarray studies of metastasis in HNSCC

Author	Tumor site	Array type	Main findings	Statistics
Nagata et al. (2003)	Oral cavity	Takara intelligene human cancer CHIP v2.1	– Altered expression of 19 genes between tumors with vs. without lymph node metastases – Increased expression of MMP-1 with lymph node metastases vs. nonmetastatic	– $U=0.0$–18.5 – $U=0.0$
Chung et al. (2004a)	All head and neck subsites	Agilent human 1 cDNA microarray	– Pathological nodal metastases prediction of 57–60% for all subsites – Pathological nodal metastasis prediction of 83% with oral cavity excluded	–
Cromer et al. (2004)	Hypopharynx	Affymetrix Hg-U95A	– 164 genes with up to 80% accuracy of predicting distant metastases vs. no distant metastases	–
Schmalbach et al. (2004)	Oral cavity, oropharynx	Affymetrix HG_U95Av2 GeneChip	– Altered expression of 57 genes between tumors with vs. without lymph node metastases – Increased nuclear TIMP-1 expression with lymph node metastases vs. nonmetastatic	– $p<0.01$ – $p=0.06$
Roepman et al. (2005)	Oral cavity, Oropharynx	Qiagen human array-ready oligo set	– 102 gene set with 86% accuracy of predicting lymph node metastases vs. nonmetastatic	– $p=0.0004$
Braakhuis et al. (2006)	All head and neck subsites	Compugen human release V.1.0 oligonucleotide library	– 150 genes with differential expression between tumors with vs. without distant metastases	$-p<0.01$

Details of microarray analyses of cervical lymph node and distant metastases in HNSCC
MMP-1 matrix metalloproteinase 1, *TIMP-1* tissue inhibitor of metalloproteinase 1

($p=0.06$), and disease-free survival did not correlate with increased TIMP-1 levels (Schmalbach et al. 2004).

A larger study of primary oral cavity and oropharyngeal cancers was performed by Roepman et al. (2005). The expression of over 21,000 genes was examined for 82 tumors (45 metastatic and 37 nonmetastatic). A set of 102 genes was identified with an overall nodal metastasis predictive accuracy of 86% ($p=0.0004$) compared with a 68% accuracy of clinical diagnosis. Functional grouping of the predictive gene products identified epithelial markers, extracellular matrix components, cell adhesion molecules, and genes involved in cell death, cell growth, and maintenance. Interestingly, the majority of the genes in this set were downregulated in the regionally metastatic tumors (Roepman et al. 2005).

Microarray studies have also been performed to determine if prediction of distant metastases was possible in HNSCC. Cromer et al. (2004) identified a set of 164 genes that was able to correctly predict up to 80% of distant metastases in hypopharyngeal HNSCC. In examining HNSCC from all subsites, Braakhuis et al. (2006) detected 150 genes with differential expression in tumors that developed distant metastases ($p<0.01$).

Future of Oral Cancer Treatment

Identify Molecular Signatures of Patient Tumors

Despite the relative consistency in treatment strategies for similar stages of HNSCC, individual clinical outcomes and prognoses vary significantly. Because clinical behavior of HNSCC has been poorly predicted based on clinical staging, histology, or single molecular markers, efforts to improve prediction and patient outcomes have been directed toward global genome analyses (Chung et al. 2006b). A molecular classification based on gene expression profiles may more accurately predict treatment response and overall prognosis (Chung et al. 2002). The behavioral heterogeneity of HNSCC correlates with distinct subtypes based on microarray analyses. Chung et al. (2004a) identified four distinct groups whose molecular signatures correlated with disease-free and overall survival. While the majority of HNSCC express epidermal growth factor receptor (EGFR), the subgroup associated with the worst clinical outcome exhibited a gene expression pattern consistent with activation of the EGFR pathway. Consequently, this group may benefit most from therapeutic strategies that incorporate EGFR inhibition. Tumors clustering in the normal epithelial group had the best clinical outcome, delineating a HNSCC group in which suspension of multimodality therapy may be considered. Belbin et al. (2002) identified 375 genes which separated HNSCC into two distinct groups with differences in cause-specific survival that approached statistical significance ($p=0.057$). Interestingly, the group with the higher TNM stage had the better cause-specific and overall survival, indicating that classification by gene expression profiling was more accurate in predicting outcome than clinicopathologic variables.

Gene expression profiles may also be used to guide clinical decision making by predicting the response of HNSCC to therapy. Akervall et al. (2004) examined the in vitro sensitivity of HNSCC cell lines to treatment with cisplatin. Gene expression analysis of five sensitive and five resistant cell lines detected approximately 60 genes with differential expression patterns between the two groups. Several genes known to be involved in drug resistance, metastasis and tumor proliferation (timp-2, caveolin-2, and the met oncogene) were found within this group. Immunohistochemical analysis of tumors from patients with complete responses to induction chemotherapy with cisplatin showed decreased expression of met validating decreased met gene expression found in cisplatin sensitive cell lines (Akervall et al. 2004). Consequently, patients with decreased expression of the met oncogene may be expected to benefit from cisplatin therapy. Similar studies have correlated gene expression analysis with the prediction of response to chemotherapy in esophageal cancer and breast cancer (Kihara et al. 2001; Chang et al. 2005). Identification of such biomarkers by global gene expression analysis will continue to facilitate individualization of treatment regimens.

Targeted Therapy

Oncology drug development should ideally target genes or pathways responsible for aggressive tumor behavior and poor prognosis (Liotta and Kohn 2003). One obvious molecular target in HNSCC is the EGFR pathway. The majority of HNSCC express EGFR and activation of EGFR as well as expression and amplification of the EGFR gene have been associated with poor prognosis (Grandis et al. 1998; Etienne et al. 1999; Ang et al. 2002; Chung et al. 2006a). Unfortunately, studies of EGFR inhibitors used as monotherapy have indicated low response rates in advanced HNSCC. Providentially, combinatorial therapy with EGFR inhibitors has shown more promise and addition of cetuximab as a radiation sensitizer improves survival (Robert et al. 2001; reviewed in Pomerantz and Grandis 2004; Bonner et al. 2006; Curran et al. 2007). Through identification of tumors that are most dependent on EGFR signaling, microarray analyses may be used to predict which tumors may respond best to EGFR inhibition.

Other targets of potential value in HNSCC include EGFR family members, src, nuclear factor kappa B (NF-κB), met, cyclooxygenase (COX)-2, phosphoinositide 3-kinase (PI3K), insulin-like growth factor (IGF)-1 receptor, vascular endothelial growth factor receptor (VEGFR), mammalian target of rapamycin (mTOR), Akt, cyclin-dependent kinases (CDKs), mutant p53, E2Fs, ephrin, myc, ras, and many more. A great challenge impeding clinical implementation of targeted therapies is our current inability to determine which targeted agents, or combinations of targeted agents, may be most active in a particular tumor. Clinical trials to test combinations of targeted therapies with one another or with more traditional therapies are impractical due to expense and the requirement for large numbers of patients. Additionally, the percentage of selected patients that may benefit from a targeted agent may be low. Traditional clinical trial design would discard an agent, active in only a small percentage of patients, when in fact it may be very active, but for only a particular group of tumors. Hypothetically, short-term therapy followed by biopsy to assess response, *in vitro* studies of primary HNSCC, or human-in-mouse models of primary HNSCC could be used to determine effectiveness of combinations of targeted agents. Response could then be correlated with gene expression profiles derived from the pretreatment primary tumors. Gene expression profiles found to predict response could then be used to guide clinical trials enrolling only patients with profiles predictive of response.

Reduction of Treatment Morbidity

Use of a metastatic gene profile to predict those HNSCC patients with a higher likelihood of metastasis would spare those patients at low risk the morbidity associated with unnecessary treatment. Currently in oncologic practice, many low-stage tumors are treated based on the worst clinical scenario. However, only approximately 10–20% of cancer patients succumb to disseminated disease (Liotta and Kohn 2003). For example, current chemotherapeutic guidelines for breast cancer treatment are based on histological and clinical characteristics. With these criteria, van't Veer et al. (2002) calculated that up to 90% of patients younger than 35 years of age at diagnosis would be candidates for chemotherapy. However, 70–80% of these patients would not have developed metastasis within 5 years without adjuvant chemotherapy. In this group of patients, treatment may not have provided any clinical benefit but was associated with patient morbidity as well as expense. For HNSCC of the oral cavity and oropharynx, cervical nodal therapy is performed in patients without clinical or radiographic indication of metastases if the risk of nodal metastases is greater than 20% based on historical data. This condemns up to 80% of patients to neck therapy with associated morbidity despite the fact that their tumors may have never metastasized. Molecular expression profiling of HNSCC has a predictive accuracy of 86%, suggesting that the number of patients unnecessarily treated may be dramatically reduced (Roepman et al. 2005). The use of metastatic molecular profiles to predict cervical lymph node metastasis would reduce the number of patients exposed to adverse side effects of surgery, radiation or combined chemotherapy and radiation.

References

Akervall J, Guo X, Qian CN, Schoumans J, Leeser B, Kort E, Cole A, Resau J, Bradford C, Carey T et al (2004) Genetic and expression profiles of squamous cell carcinoma of the head and neck correlate with cisplatin sensitivity and resistance in cell lines and patients. Clin Cancer Res 10:8204–8213

Alsner J, Sorensen SB, Overgaard J (2001) TP53 mutation is related to poor prognosis after radiotherapy, but not surgery, in squamous cell carcinoma of the head and neck. Radiother Oncol 59:179–185

Anderson PE, Shah JP, Cambronero E, Spiro RH (1994) The role of comprehensive neck dissection with preservation of the spinal accessory nerve in the clinically positive neck. Am J Surg 168:499–502

Ang KK, Berkey BA, Tu X, Zhang HZ, Katz R, Hammond EH, Fu KK, Milas L (2002) Impact of epidermal growth factor receptor expression on survival and pattern of relapse in patients with advanced head and neck carcinoma. Cancer Res 62:7350–7356

Assimakopoulos D, Kolettas E, Zagorianakou N, Evangelou A, Skevas A, Agnatis NJ (2000) Prognostic significance of p53 in the cancer of the larynx. Anticancer Res 20:3555–3564

Becker MT, Shores CG, Yu KK, Yarbrough WG (2004) Molecular assay to detect metastatic head and neck squamous cell carcinoma. Arch Otolaryngol Head Neck Surg 130:21–27

Belbin TJ, Singh B, Barber I, Socci N, Wenig B, Smith R, Prystowsky MB, Childs G (2002) Molecular classification of head and neck squamous cell carcinoma using cDNA microarrays. Cancer Res 62:1184–1190

Bernards R, Weinberg RA (2002) A progression puzzle. Nature 418:823

Bonner JA, Harari PM, Giralt J, Azarnia N, Shin DM, Cohen RB, Jones CU, Sur R, Raben D, Jassem J et al (2006) Radiotherapy plus cetuximab for squamous-cell carcinoma of the head and neck. N Engl J Med 354:567–578

Braakhuis BJ, Senft A, de Bree R, de Vries J, Ylstra B, Cloos J, Kuik DJ, Leemans CR, Brakenhoff RH (2006) Expression profiling and prediction of distant metastases in head and neck squamous cell carcinoma. J Clin Pathol 59:1254–1260

Bradford CR (1999) Predictive factors in head and neck cancer. Hematol Oncol Clin North Am 13:777–785

Bradford CR, Zhu S, Poore J, Fisher SG, Beals TF, Thoraval D, Hanash SM, Carey TE, Wolf GT (1997) p53 mutation as a prognostic marker in advanced laryngeal carcinoma Department of Veterans Affairs Laryngeal Cancer Cooperative Study Group. Arch Otolaryngol Head Neck Surg 123:605–609

Butte A (2002) The use and analysis of microarray data. Nat Rev Drug Discov 1:951–960

Chang JC, Wooten EC, Tsimelzon A, Hilsenbeck SG, Gutierrez MC, Tham YL, Kalidas M, Elledge R, Mohsin S, Osborne CK et al (2005) Patterns of resistance and incomplete response to docetaxel by gene expression profiling in breast cancer patients. J Clin Oncol 23:1169–1177

Chen X, Cheung ST, So S, Fan ST, Barry C, Higgins J, Lai KM, Ji J, Dudoit S, Ng IO et al (2002) Gene expression patterns in human liver cancers. Mol Biol Cell 13:1929–1939

Chung CH, Bernard PS, Perou CM (2002) Molecular portraits and the family tree of cancer. Nat Genet 32(Suppl):533–540

Chung CH, Parker JS, Karaca G, Wu J, Funkhouser WK, Moore D, Butterfoss D, Xiang D, Zanation A, Yin X et al (2004) Molecular classification of head and neck squamous cell carcinomas using patterns of gene expression. Cancer Cell 5:489–500

Chung CH, Ely K, McGavran L, Varella-Garcia M, Parker J, Parker N, Jarrett C, Carter J, Murphy BA, Netterville J et al (2006a) Increased epidermal growth factor receptor gene copy number is associated with poor prognosis in head and neck squamous cell carcinomas. J Clin Oncol 24:4170–4176

Chung CH, Levy S, Yarbrough WG (2006b) Clinical applications of genomics in head and neck cancer. Head Neck 28:360–368

Chung CH, Parker JS, Ely K, Carter J, Yi Y, Murphy BA, Ang KK, El-Naggar AK, Zanation AM, Cmelak AJ et al (2006c) Gene expression profiles identify epithelial-to-mesenchymal transition and activation of nuclear factor-kappaB signaling as characteristics of a high-risk head and neck squamous cell carcinoma. Cancer Res 66:8210–8218

Cromer A, Carles A, Millon R, Ganguli G, Chalmel F, Lemaire F, Young J, Dembele D, Thibault C, Muller D et al (2004) Identification of genes associated with tumorigenesis and metastatic potential of hypopharyngeal cancer by microarray analysis. Oncogene 23:2484–2498

Cunha GR, Hayward SW, Wang YZ, Ricke WA (2003) Role of the stromal microenvironment in carcinogenesis of the prostate. Int J Cancer 107:1–10

Curran D, Giralt J, Harari PM, Ang KK, Cohen RB, Kies MS, Jassem J, Baselga J, Rowinsky EK, Amellal N et al (2007) Quality of life in head and neck cancer patients after treatment with high-dose radiotherapy alone or in combination with cetuximab. J Clin Oncol 25:2191–2197

Debies MT, Welch DR (2001) Genetic basis of human breast cancer metastasis. J Mammary Gland Biol Neoplasia 6:441–451

Druker BJ, Sawyers CL, Kantarjian H, Resta DJ, Reese SF, Ford JM, Capdeville R, Talpaz M (2001) Activity of a specific inhibitor of the BCR-ABL tyrosine kinase in the blast crisis of chronic myeloid leukemia and acute lymphoblastic leukemia with the Philadelphia chromosome. N Engl J Med 344:1038–1042

D'Souza G, Kreimer AR, Viscidi R, Pawlita M, Fakhry C, Koch WM, Westra WH, Gillison ML (2007) Case-control study of human papillomavirus and oropharyngeal cancer. N Engl J Med 356:1944–1956

Etienne MC, Pivot X, Formento JL, Bensadoun RJ, Formento P, Dassonville O, Francoual M, Poissonnet G, Fontana X, Schneider M et al (1999) A multifactorial approach including tumoural epidermal growth factor receptor, p53, thymidylate synthase and dihydropyrimidine dehydrogenase to predict treatment outcome in head and neck cancer patients receiving 5-fluorouracil. Br J Cancer 79:1864–1869

Fagan JJ, Collins B, Barnes L, D'Amico F, Myers EN, Johnson JT (1998) Perineural invasion in squamous cell carcinoma of the head and neck. Arch Otolaryngol Head Neck Surg 124:637–640

Ferris RL, Xi L, Raja S, Hunt JL, Wang J, Gooding WE, Kelly L, Ching J, Luketich JD, Godfrey TE (2005) Molecular staging of cervical lymph nodes in squamous cell carcinoma of the head and neck. Cancer Res 65:2147–2156

Fidler IJ (1990) Critical factors in the biology of human cancer metastasis: twenty-eighth G.H.A. Clowes memorial award lecture. Cancer Res 50:6130–6138

Fidler IJ (2003) The pathogenesis of cancer metastasis: the 'seed and soil' hypothesis revisited. Nat Rev Cancer 3:453–458

Fidler I, Kripke M (1977) Metastasis results from preexisting variant cells within a malignant tumor. Science 197:893–895

Fisher B, Costantino J, Redmond C, Poisson R, Bowman D, Couture J, Dimitrov NV, Wolmark N, Wickerham DL, Fisher ER et al (1989) A randomized clinical trial evaluating tamoxifen in the treatment of patients with node-negative breast cancer who have estrogen-receptor-positive tumors. N Engl J Med 320:479–484

Gallo O, Chiarelli I, Boddi V, Bocciolini C, Bruschini L, Porfirio B (1999) Cumulative prognostic value of p53 mutations and bcl-2 protein expression in head and neck cancer treated by radiotherapy. Int J Cancer 84:573–579

Gancberg D, Di Leo A, Cardoso F, Rouas G, Pedrocchi M, Paesmans M, Verhest A, Bernard-Marty C, Piccart MJ, Larsimont D (2002) Comparison of HER-2 status between primary breast cancer and corresponding distant metastatic sites. Ann Oncol 13:1036–1043

Garber ME, Troyanskaya OG, Schluens K, Petersen S, Thaesler Z, Pacyna-Gengelbach M, van de Rijn M, Rosen GD, Perou CM, Whyte RI et al (2001) Diversity of gene expression in adenocarcinoma of the lung. Proc Natl Acad Sci USA 98:13784–13789

Gershenwald JE, Fidler IJ (2002) Cancer. Targeting lymphatic metastasis. Science 296:1811–1812

Giatromanolaki A, Koukourakis MI, Sivridis E, Fountzilas G (2000) c-erbB-2 oncoprotein is overexpressed in poorly vascularised squamous cell carcinomas of the head and neck, but is not associated with response to cytotoxic therapy or survival. Anticancer Res 20:997–1004

Gillison ML (2004) Human papillomavirus-associated head and neck cancer is a distinct epidemiologic, clinical, and molecular entity. Semin Oncol 31:744–754

Gillison ML, Koch WM, Capone RB, Spafford M, Westra WH, Wu L, Zahurak ML, Daniel RW, Viglione M, Symer DE et al (2000) Evidence for a causal association between human papillomavirus and a subset of head and neck cancers. J Natl Cancer Inst 92:709–720

Grandis J, Melhem M, Gooding W, Day R, Holst V, Wagener M, Drenning S, Tweardy D (1998) Levels of TGF-alpha and EGFR protein in head and neck squamous cell carcinoma and patient survival. J Natl Cancer Inst 90:824–832

Ha PK, Benoit NE, Yochem R, Sciubba J, Zahurak M, Sidransky D, Pevsner J, Westra WH, Califano J (2003) A transcriptional progression model for head and neck cancer. Clin Cancer Res 9:3058–3064

Hahn WC, Counter CM, Lundberg AS, Beijersbergen RL, Brooks MW, Weinberg RA (1999) Creation of human tumor cells with defined genetic elements. Nature 400:464–468

Hanahan D, Weinberg RA (2000) The hallmarks of cancer. Cell 100:57–70

Hart IR, Fidler IJ (1980) Role of organ selectivity in the determination of metastatic patterns of B16 melanoma. Cancer Res 40:2281–2287

Hashibe M, Brennan P, Benhamou S, Castellsague X, Chen C, Curado MP, Dal Maso L, Daudt AW, Fabianova E, Wunsch-Filho V et al (2007) Alcohol drinking in never users of tobacco, cigarette smoking in never drinkers, and the risk of head and neck cancer: pooled analysis in the International Head and Neck Cancer Epidemiology Consortium. J Natl Cancer Inst 99:777–789

He YD, Friend SH (2001) Microarrays-the 21st century divining rod? Nat Med 7:658–659

Herbst RS, Yano S, Kuniyasu H, Khuri FR, Bucana CD, Guo F, Liu D, Kemp B, Lee JJ, Hong WK, Fidler IJ (2000) Differential expression of E-cadherin and type IV collagenase genes predicts outcome in patients with stage I non-small cell lung carcinoma. Clin Cancer Res 6:790–797

Hippo Y, Taniguchi H, Tsutsumi S, Machida N, Chong JM, Fukayama M, Kodama T, Aburatani H (2002) Global gene expression analysis of gastric cancer by oligonucleotide microarrays. Cancer Res 62:233–240

Huang E, Cheng SH, Dressman H, Pittman J, Tsou MH, Horng CF, Bild A, Iversen ES, Liao M, Chen CM et al (2003) Gene expression predictors of breast cancer outcomes. Lancet 361:1590–1596

Hynes RO (2003) Metastatic potential: generic predisposition of the primary tumor or rare, metastatic variants-or both? Cell 113:821–823

Jemal A, Siegel R, Ward E, Murray T, Xu J, Thun MJ (2007) Cancer Statistics, 2007. CA Cancer J Clin 57:43–66

Johnson JT, Myers EN, Schramm VL, NMayernik DG, Nolan TA, Sigler BA, Wagner RL (1987) Adjuvant chemotherapy for high-risk squamous-cell carcinoma of the head and neck. J Clin Oncol 5:456–458

Kakiuchi S, Daigo Y, Tsunoda T, Yano S, Sone S, Nakamura Y (2003) Genome-wide analysis of organ-preferential metastasis of human small cell lung cancer in mice. Mol Cancer Res 1:485–499

Kang Y, Massague J (2004) Epithelial-mesenchymal transitions: twist in development and metastasis. Cell 118:277–279

Kang Y, Siegel PM, Shu W, Drobnjak M, Kakonen SM, Cordon-Cardo C, Guise TA, Massague J (2003) A multigenic program mediating breast cancer metastasis to bone. Cancer Cell 3:537–549

Kihara C, Tsunoda T, Tanaka T, Yamana H, Furukawa Y, Ono K, Kitahara O, Zembutsu H, Yanagawa R, Hirata K et al (2001) Prediction of sensitivity of esophageal tumors to adjuvant chemotherapy by cDNA microarray analysis of gene-expression profiles. Cancer Res 61:6474–6479

Kim ES, Kies M, Herbst RS (2002) Novel therapeutics for head and neck cancer. Curr Opin Oncol 14:334–342

Kitadai Y, Ellis LM, Tucker SL, Greene GF, Bucana CD, Cleary KR, Takahashi Y, Tahara E, Fidler IJ (1996) Multiparametric in situ mRNA hybridization analysis to predict disease recurrence in patients with colon carcinoma. Am J Pathol 149:1541–1551

Klatka J (2001) Prognostic value of the expression of p53 and bcl-2 in patients with laryngeal carcinoma. Eur Arch Otorhinolaryngol 258:537–541

Kligerman J, Lima RA, Soares JR, Prado L, Dias FL, Freitas EQ, Olivatto LO (1994) Supraomohyoid neck dissection in the treatment of T1/T2 squamous cell carcinoma of oral cavity. Am J Surg 168:391–394

Kovacs AF (2007) Head and neck squamous cell carcinoma: sentinel node or selective neck dissection. Surg Oncol Clin N Am 16:81–100

Kuukasjarvi T, Karhu R, Tanner M, Kahkonen M, Schaffer A, Nupponen N, Pennanen S, Kallioniemi A, Kallioniemi O-P, Isola J (1997) Genetic heterogeneity and clonal evolution underlying development of asynchronous metastasis in human breast cancer. Cancer Res 57:1597–1604

LaTulippe E, Satagopan J, Smith A, Scher H, Scardino P, Reuter V, Gerald WL (2002) Comprehensive gene expression analysis of prostate cancer reveals distinct transcriptional programs associated with metastatic disease. Cancer Res 62:4499–4506

Li W, Thompson CH, O'Brien CJ, McNeil EB, Scolyer RA, Cossart YE, Veness MJ, Walker DM, Morgan GJ, Rose BR (2003) Human papillomavirus positivity predicts favourable outcome for squamous carcinoma of the tonsil. Int J Cancer 106:553–558

Lindel K, Beer KT, Laissue J, Greiner RH, Aebersold DM (2001) Human papillomavirus positive squamous cell carcinoma of the oropharynx: a radiosensitive subgroup of head and neck carcinoma. Cancer 92:805–813

Liotta LA, Kohn EC (2003) Cancer's deadly signature. Nat Genet 33:10–11

McKaig RG, Baric RS, Olshan AF (1998) Human papillomavirus and head and neck cancer: epidemiology and molecular biology. Head Neck 20:250–265

Mellin H, Friesland S, Lewensohn R, Dalianis T, Munck-Wikland E (2000) Human papillomavirus (HPV) DNA in tonsillar cancer: clinical correlates, risk of relapse, and survival. Int J Cancer 89:300–304

Mohr S, Leikauf GD, Keith G, Rihn BH (2002) Microarrays as cancer keys: an array of possibilities. J Clin Oncol 20:3165–3175

Nagata M, Fujita H, Ida H, Hoshina H, Inoue T, Seki Y, Ohnishi M, Ohyama T, Shingaki S, Kaji M et al (2003) Identification of potential biomarkers of lymph node metastasis in oral squamous cell carcinoma by cDNA microarray analysis. Int J Cancer 106:683–689

Nissen LJ, Cao R, Hedlund EM, Wang Z, Zhao X, Wetterskog D, Funa K, Brakenhielm E, Cao Y (2007) Angiogenic factors FGF2 and PDGF-BB synergistically promote murine tumor neovascularization and metastasis. J Clin Invest 117:2766–2777

Nyormoi O, Bar-Eli M (2003) Transcriptional regulation of metastasis-related genes in human melanoma. Clin Exp Metastasis 20:251–263

Padera TP, Kadambi A, di Tomaso E, Carreira CM, Brown EB, Boucher Y, Choi NC, Mathisen D, Wain J, Mark EJ et al (2002) Lymphatic metastasis in the absence of functional intratumor lymphatics. Science 296:1883–1886

Paget S (1889) Distribution of secondary growths in cancer of the breast. Lancet 133:571–573

Perou CM, Sorlie T, Eisen MB, van de Rijn M, Jeffrey SS, Rees CA, Pollack JR, Ross DT, Johnsen H, Akslen LA et al (2000) Molecular portraits of human breast tumors. Nature 406:747–752

Pomerantz RG, Grandis JR (2004) The epidermal growth factor receptor signaling network in head and neck carcinogenesis and implications for targeted therapy. Semin Oncol 31:734–743

Prince ME, Sivanandan R, Kaczorowski A, Wolf GT, Kaplan MJ, Dalerba P, Weissman IL, Clarke MF, Ailles LE (2007) Identification of a subpopulation of cells with cancer stem cell properties in head and neck squamous cell carcinoma. Proc Natl Acad Sci USA 104:973–978

Quon H, Liu FF, Cummings BJ (2001) Potential molecular prognostic markers in head and neck squamous cell carcinomas. Head Neck 23:147–159

Ramaswamy S, Ross KN, Lander ES, Golub TR (2003) A molecular signature of metastasis in primary solid tumors. Nat Genet 33:49–54

Ree AH, Florenes VA, Berg JP, Maelandsmo GM, Nesland JM, Fodstad O (1997) High levels of messenger RNAs for tissue inhibitors of metalloproteinases (TIMP-1 and TIMP-2) in primary breast carcinomas are associated with development of distant metastases. Clin Cancer Res 3:1623–1628

Ritchie J, EM S, Summersgill K, HT H, Wang D, Klussmann J, Turek L, Haugen T (2003) Human papillomavirus infection as a prognostic factor in carcinomas of the oral cavity and oropharynx. Int J Cancer 104:336–344

Robert F, Ezekiel MP, Spencer SA, Meredith RF, Bonner JA, Khazaeli MB, Saleh MN, Carey D, LoBuglio AF, Wheeler RH et al (2001) Phase I study of anti-epidermal growth factor receptor antibody cetuximab in combination with radiation therapy in patients with advanced head and neck cancer. J Clin Oncol 19:3234–3243

Roepman P, Wessels LF, Kettelarij N, Kemmeren P, Miles AJ, Lijnzaad P, Tilanus MG, Koole R, Hordijk GJ, van der Vliet PC et al (2005) An expression profile for diagnosis of lymph node metastases from primary head and neck squamous cell carcinomas. Nat Genet 37:182–186

Roepman P, de Jager A, Groot Koerkamp MJ, Kummer JA, Slootweg PJ, Holstege FC (2006a) Maintenance of head and neck tumor gene expression profiles upon lymph node metastasis. Cancer Res 66:11110–11114

Roepman P, de Koning E, van Leenen D, de Weger RA, Kummer JA, Slootweg PJ, Holstege FC (2006b) Dissection of a metastatic gene expression signature into distinct components. Genome Biol 7:R117

Roepman P, Kemmeren P, Wessels LF, Slootweg PJ, Holstege FC (2006c) Multiple robust signatures for detecting lymph node metastasis in head and neck cancer. Cancer Res 66:2361–2366

Ross G, Shoaib T, Soutar DS, Camilleri IG, Gray HW, Bessent RG, Robertson AG, MacDonald DG (2002) The use of sentinel node biopsy to upstage the clinically N0 neck in head and neck cancer. Arch Otolaryngol Head Neck Surg 128:1287–1291

Ross GL, Soutar DS, Gordon MacDonald D, Shoaib T, Camilleri I, Roberton AG, Sorensen JA, Thomsen J, Grupe P, Alvarez J et al (2004) Sentinel node biopsy in head and neck cancer: preliminary results of a multicenter trial. Ann Surg Oncol 11:690–696

Salesiotis AN, Cullen KJ (2000) Molecular markers predictive of response and prognosis in the patients with advanced squamous cell carcinoma of the head and neck: evolution of a model beyond TNM staging. Curr Opin Oncol 12:229–239

Santin AD, Zhan F, Bignotti E, Siegel ER, Cane S, Bellone S, Palmieri M, Anfossi S, Thomas M, Burnett A et al (2005) Gene expression profiles of primary HPV16- and HPV18-infected early stage cervical cancers and normal cervical epithelium: identification of novel candidate molecular markers for cervical cancer diagnosis and therapy. Virology 331:269–291

Sauter ER, Ridge JA, Gordon J, Eisenberg BL (1992) p53 overexpression correlates with increased survival in patients with squamous carcinoma of the tongue base. Am J Surg 164:651–653

Schackert G, Fidler IJ (1988) Site-specific metastasis of mouse melanomas and a fibrosarcoma in the brain or meninges of syngeneic animals. Cancer Res 48:3478–3484

Schmalbach CE, Chepeha DB, Giordano TJ, Rubin MA, Teknos TN, Bradford CR, Wolf GT, Kuick R, Misek DE, Trask DK, Hanash S (2004) Molecular profiling and the identification of genes associated with metastatic oral cavity/pharynx squamous cell carcinoma. Arch Otolaryngol Head Neck Surg 130:295–302

Schuller DE, McGuirt WF, McCabe BF, Young D (1980) The prognostic significance of metastatic cervical lymph nodes. Laryngoscope 40:557–570

Schwartz SR, Yueh B, McDougall JK, Daling JR, Schwartz SM (2001) Human papillomavirus infection and survival in oral squamous cell cancer: a population-based study. Otolaryngol Head Neck Surg 125:1–9

Sessions DG, Spector GJ, Lenox J, Parriott S, Haughey B, Chao C, Marks J, Perez C (2000) Analysis of treatment results for floor-of-mouth cancer. Laryngoscope 110:1764–1772

Sessions DG, Spector GJ, Lenox J, Haughey B, Chao C, Marks J (2002) Analysis of treatment results for oral tongue cancer. Laryngoscope 112:616–625

Sessions DG, Lenox J, Spector GJ, Chao C, Chaudry OA (2003) Analysis of treatment results for base of tongue cancer. Laryngoscope 113:1252–1261

Shiga H, Rasmussen AA, Johnston PG, Langmacher M, Baylor A, Lee M, Cullen KJ (2000) Prognostic value of c-erbB2 and other markers in patients treated with chemotherapy for recurrent head and neck cancer. Head Neck 22:599–608

Sidransky D, Irizarry R, Califano JA, Li X, Ren H, Benoit N, Mao L (2003) Serum protein MALDI profiling to distinguish upper aerodigestive tract cancer patients from control subjects. J Natl Cancer Inst 95:1711–1717

Sisk EA, Soltys SG, Zhu S, Fisher SG, Carey TE, Bradford CR (2002) Human papillomavirus and p53 mutational status as prognostic factors in head and neck carcinoma. Head Neck 24:841–849

Slebos RJ, Yi Y, Ely K, Carter J, Evjen A, Zhang X, Shyr Y, Murphy BM, Cmelak AJ, Burkey BB et al (2006) Gene expression differences associated with human papillomavirus status in head and neck squamous cell carcinoma. Clin Cancer Res 12:701–709

Sorlie T, Perou CM, Tibshirani R, Asas T, Geisler SA, Johnsen H, Hastie T, Eisen MB, van de Rijn M, Jeffrey SS et al (2001) Gene expression patterns of breast carcinomas distinguish tumor subclasses with clinical implications. Proc Natl Acad Sci USA 98:10869–10874

Spiro RH, Alfonso AE, Farr HW, Strong EW (1974) Cervical node metastasis from epidermoid carcinoma of the oral cavity and oropharynx. Am J Surg 128:562–567

Stoeckli SJ (2007) Sentinel node biopsy for oral and oropharyngeal squamous cell carcinoma of the head and neck. Laryngoscope 117:1539–1551

Suzuki M, Tarin D (2007) Gene expression profiling of human lymph node metastases and matched primary breast carcinomas: clinical implications. Mol Oncol 1:172–180

Takahashi Y, Kitadai Y, Ellis LM, Bucana CD, Fidler IJ, Mai M (2002) Multiparametric in situ mRNA hybridization analysis of gastric biopsies predicts lymph node metastasis in patients with gastric carcinoma. Jpn J Cancer Res 93:1258–1265

Talmadge JE (2007) Clonal selection of metastasis within the life history of a tumor. Cancer Res 67:11471–11475

Tarin D, Price JE, Kettlewell MG, Souter RG, Vass AC, Crossley B (1984) Clinicopathological observations on metastasis in man studied in patients treated with peritoneovenous shunts. Br Med J (Clin Res Ed) 288:749–751

Taylor RJ, Wahl RL, Sharma PK, Bradford CR, Terrell JE, Teknos TN, Heard EM, Wolf GT, Chepeha DB (2001) Sentinel node localization in oral cavity and oropharynx squamous cell cancer. Arch Otolaryngol Head Neck Surg 127:970–974

van Houten VM, Snijders PJ, van den Brekel MW, Kummer JA, Meijer CJ, van Leeuwen B, Denkers F, Smeele LE, Snow GB, Brakenhoff RH (2001) Biological evidence that human papillomaviruses are etiologically involved in a subgroup of head and neck squamous cell carcinomas. Int J Cancer 93:232–235

van't Veer LJ, Dai H, van de Vijver MJ, He YD, Hart AAM, Mao M, Peterse HL, van der Kooy K, Marton MJ, Witteveen AT et al (2002) Gene expression profiling predicts clinical outcome of breast cancer. Nature 415:530–536

Warner GC, Reis PP, Makitie AA, Sukhai MA, Arora S, Jurisica I, Wells RA, Gullane P, Irish J, Kamel-Reid S (2004) Current applications of microarrays in head and neck cancer research. Laryngoscope 114:241–248

Webb CP, Vande Woude GF (2000) Genes that regulate metastasis and angiogenesis. J Neurooncol 50:71–87

Weigelt B, Glas AM, Wessels LF, Witteveen AT, Peterse JL, van't Veer LJ (2003) Gene expression profiles of primary breast tumors maintained in distant metastases. Proc Natl Acad Sci USA 100:15901–15905

Weinberger PM, Yu Z, Haffty BG, Kowalski D, Harigopal M, Brandsma J, Sasaki C, Joe J, Camp RL, Rimm DL, Psyrri A (2006) Molecular classification identifies a subset of human papillo-mavirus-associated oropharyngeal cancers with favorable prognosis. J Clin Oncol 24:736–747

Welsh JB, Zarrinkar PP, Sapinoso LM, Kern SG, Behling CA, Monk BJ, Lockhart DJ, Burger RA, Hampton GM (2001) Analysis of gene expression profiles in normal and neoplastic ovarian tissue samples identifies candidate molecular markers of epithelial ovarian cancer. Proc Natl Acad Sci USA 98:1176–1181

Werner JA, Dunne AA, Ramaswamy A, Dalchow C, Behr T, Moll R, Folz BJ, Davis RK (2004) The sentinel node concept in head and neck cancer: solution for the controversies in the N0 neck? Head Neck 26:603–611

Wilson GD, Saunders MI, Dische S, Richman PI, Daley FM, Bentzen SM (2001) bcl-2 Expression in head and neck cancer: an enigmatic prognostic marker. Int J Radiat Oncol Biol Phys 49:435–441

Wulfing P, Kersting C, Buerger H, Mattsson B, Mesters R, Gustmann C, Hinrichs B, Tio J, Bocker W, Kiesel L (2005) Expression patterns of angiogenic and lymphangiogenic factors in ductal breast carcinoma in situ. Br J Cancer 92:1720–1728

Zeng ZS, Cohen AM, Zhang ZF, Stetler-Stevenson W, Guillem JG (1995) Elevated tissue inhibitor of metalloproteinase 1 RNA in colorectal cancer stroma correlates with lymph node and distant metastases. Clin Cancer Res 1:899–906

Zhu CQ, Shih W, Ling CH, Tsao MS (2006) Immunohistochemical markers of prognosis in non-small cell lung cancer: a review and proposal for a multiphase approach to marker evaluation. J Clin Pathol 59:790–800

Chapter 5
The Role of High Throughput Molecular Analysis of Biofluids and Tumors in Patients with Oral Cancer

Shen Hu, Zhanzhi Hu, Xiaofeng Zhou, and David T. Wong

Abstract Oral cancer, predominantly oral squamous cell carcinoma, is considered as the 6th most common human cancer in the world. The American Cancer Society estimated that 35,310 new cases of oral cancer were diagnosed in 2008 and 7,590 patients died from the disease in the US. Worldwide, oral cancer is a major cancer problem, with an estimated 300,000 new cases diagnosed annually. Patients with OSCC are often diagnosed at a late stage, and there is a high recurrence rate after treatment, especially in those with neck lymph node metastasis. The overall 5-year survival rates for oral cancer have remained low and stagnant during the past few decades. The high mortality rate can be attributed to factors including nonresponsiveness to chemotherapy and radiation therapy, late presentation of the lesions, and the lack of biological markers for the early detection of these lesions. In this chapter, we have provided a brief introduction on current genomic and proteomic technologies and review their applications in molecular analysis of oral cancer. A precise molecular portrait of oral carcinogenesis will improve diagnosis, treatment, and monitoring of the disease.

Overview of High Throughput Molecular Approaches

DNA Copy Number Analysis

Comparative genomic hybridization (CGH) was developed to survey DNA copy-number abnormalities (amplifications and deletions) across a whole genome (Kallioniemi et al. 1992). In a typical CGH analysis, differentially labeled test/

D.T. Wong (✉)
School of Dentistry, Dental Research Institute, Jonsson Comprehensive Cancer Center, and Molecular Biology Institute, University of California at Los Angeles, Los Angeles, CA, USA
e-mail: dwong@dentistry.ucla.edu

J. Myers (ed.), *Oral Cancer Metastasis,*
DOI 10.1007/978-1-4419-0775-2_5, © Springer Science+Business Media, LLC 2010

disease and reference genomic DNAs are cohybridized to normal metaphase chromosomes to generate fluorescence ratios along the length of chromosomes that provide DNA copy-number measurement (Pinkel and Albertson 2005a, b). However, chromosome-based CGH has a limited mapping resolution (~10–20 Mb). Array-based CGH has been introduced to improve the mapping resolution. Several array platforms have been utilized for array-based CGH analysis, including arrays that contain large genomic clones (for example bacterial artificial chromosomes [BACs]) (Pinkel et al. 1998; Ishkanian et al. 2004), cDNA arrays (Pollack et al. 1999; Zhou et al. 2004c), oligonucleotide arrays (Lucito et al. 2003; Brennan et al. 2004), tiling arrays (Ishkanian et al. 2004), and high-density single nucleotide polymorphism (SNP) microarrays (Bignell et al. 2004; Zhao et al. 2004, 2005; Zhou et al. 2004e). Tiling and SNP array-based approaches have drawn the most attention due to their high resolution. Tiling arrays have the potential to resolve small (gene level) gains and losses (resolution ~40 kb) that may be missed by marker-based genomic arrays that contain large number of gaps due to the distance between the targeted probes (Ishkanian et al. 2004; Davies et al. 2005). It is conceivable that even higher resolution tiling arrays will become available in the future, providing an opportunity to map genomic alterations at close to base pair resolution. The SNP array-based approach provides the unique advantage of concurrent CGH and loss of heterozygosity (LOH) analysis, which is discussed in further details below (Zhao et al. 2004; Zhou et al. 2004e).

Loss of Heterozygosity Analysis

Allelic losses, which are caused by mitotic recombination, gene conversion, or non-disjunction, cannot be detected by CGH and thus require additional methods (such as LOH) for their identification. The LOH approach is "favored" by the Knudson two-hit hypothesis (Knudson 1971, 1996) for hunting tumor suppressor genes. The discovery of the first tumor suppressor gene, RB1 (Friend et al. 1986), followed the Knudson two-hit hypothesis that tumor suppressor genes are inactivated by a recessive mutation in one allele followed by the loss of the other wild-type allele, which can be detected by LOH. Polymorphic markers, such as restriction fragment length polymorphisms (RFLPs), microsatellite markers, and SNPs, have been used to detect LOH through allelotypic comparisons of DNA from a cancer sample and a matched normal sample.

Because of their abundance, even spacing, and stability across the genome, SNPs have significant advantages over RFLPs and microsatellite markers, as a basis for high-resolution whole genome allelotyping with accurate copy number measurements. It is now possible to genotype approximately one million SNP markers using the Affymetrix Mapping SNP oligonucleotide array platform (Affymetrix). LOH patterns generated by SNP array analysis have a high degree of concordance with previous microsatellite analyses of the same cancer samples (Lindblad-Toh et al. 2000). Additionally, shared regions of LOH from SNP arrays can be used to cluster lung cancer samples into subtypes (Janne et al. 2004), and distinct patterns of LOH are found to associate with clinical features in primary breast, bladder, head and neck, and prostate tumors (Hoque et al. 2003; Lieberfarb et al. 2003; Wang et al. 2004; Zhou et al. 2004d, e). One unique advantage of this SNP array-based approach is that the intensity of sample hybridization to the array probes can also be used to infer copy number changes (similar to CGH) (Bignell et al. 2004; Zhao et al. 2004;Zhou et al. 2004e). This unique feature has been explored by algorithms implemented in several independent bioinformatics/statistical software packages, including dChipSNP (Zhao et al. 2004), Copy Number Analysis Tool (Affymetrix) (Huang et al. 2004) and FASeg (fragment assembling segmentation) (Yu et al. 2007). Application of these novel bioinformatics tools to high-density SNP array data now allows the analysis of DNA copy number to be combined with LOH analysis to distinguish copy number gains, copy number neutral allelic losses, and copy number losses and to comprehensively map out the configuration of tumor genomes (Zhao et al. 2004).

Cytogenetic Analysis

The cytogenetic techniques represent a collection of chromosome staining methods that were initially introduced in the 1960s (Caspersson et al. 1969a, b). One common drawback of these methods is the requirement for in vitro culture and metaphase preparation of the cells of interest, which limits its application to many studies of solid cancers. Nevertheless, cytogenetic approaches continue to play an important role in genomic profiling because they facilitate direct visualization of chromosomal abnormalities. They complement CGH and LOH analyses by providing information on chromosomal structural rearrangements that are not resolved by DNA copy number analyses. For example, translocations are one of the most common genomic abnormalities in cancer (Futreal et al. 2004), but they cannot be detected by CGH or LOH. An experienced cytogeneticist, however, can readily detect many forms of chromosomal translocations using classical cytogenetic techniques, such as karyotyping (chromosome banding). A karyotype analysis usually involves blocking cells in mitosis and microscopically visualizing condensed chromosomes stained with Giemsa dye, which stains regions of chromosomes that are rich in the base pairs adenine (A) and thymine (T) to produce a dark band. However, many cancer cells have complex karyotypes that are difficult to interpret. Recently, several new labeling techniques have been introduced in the field of molecular cytogenetics, including spectral karyotyping (SKY), multiple fluorescence in situ hybridization (M-FISH), cross-species color banding (Rx-FISH), color-changing karyotyping (CCK) (Henegariu et al. 1999), and multicolor chromosome banding. These techniques permit the simultaneous visualization of all chromosomes in different colors and thus considerably improve the detection of subtle rearrangements.

Microarray and Serial Analysis of Gene Expression

A mere 15–20 years ago, the prevalent mode of biological and medical research was centered on the "one gene at a time" model: cloning and characterizing a single gene or a few closely related genes. This had been the gold standard for biomedical research until the mid 1990s, when the "genomics era" began with the establishment of several epoch-making genomic techniques: DNA microarray and serial analysis of gene expression (SAGE). Together with the completion of the Human Genome Project in 2003, the resulting exponential boom of new knowledge brought us into the "post-genomics" era.

Both DNA microarray and SAGE are powerful tools targeted at global gene expression. While the microarray technology requires prior knowledge of the gene sequence for analysis, SAGE technology can analyze gene expression in organisms with uncharacterized genomes. The obvious advantage of the microarray is the ability to measure gene expression in cell and tissue samples, and commercial platforms (e.g., GeneChip from Affymetrix, Inc.) are available for flexible research design. With the Human Genome Project completed, the microarray takes center stage in investigating global gene expression in all aspects of human cancer.

A DNA microarray is typically a small solid support, usually a glass microscope slide, on which known sequences of tens of thousands of genes are immobilized. Commonly used methods of immobilization of gene sequences include "ink-jet" printing, pin-spotting, and various methods of direct synthesis. The parallel presence of so many genes (often covering the whole genome of an organism) on a single microarray has allowed genomic studies to be performed in a high-throughput fashion. For example, gene expression changes on the whole genome scale can be monitored simultaneously. Doing this "one gene at a time" would be unworkable.

The continuously evolving microarray technology has the potential to revolutionize both clinical research and the healthcare practice. Physicians in the future may be empowered with a handheld device to monitor health status in real time during a routine physical examination, to detect any abnormalities at an early stage and even to suggest the best treatment options based on the particular individual's genome. With the powerful microarray technology for molecular profiling, we are witnessing the dawn of the personalized medicine era.

Exon-Level Resolution Expression Profiling

A major focus in the emerging field of personalized medicine is the search for biomarkers that can help classify and subgroup patients, preferably in the early stages of disease. Ideally, such markers should exist in clinical specimens (e.g., blood and saliva) that are easy to collect and involve minimally invasive procedures. Such clinical testing should also be inexpensive to enable population-scale screening. In this sense, saliva has gained increased recognition as an appealing body fluid for human disease diagnosis and normal health surveying (Li et al. 2004a, b).

Microarray profiling is a useful strategy to identify disease-associated mRNA biomarkers during the initial discovery phase. In model systems such as cell lines, 3′-based arrays employing poly-dT priming and in vitro transcription (IVT) amplification have been successful. However, most body fluids including saliva contain nonintegral RNAs, where a large amount of information is missing due to the fragmentation and degradation of RNAs (Park et al. 2007). The degradation also deprives many RNAs of their poly-A tails, making poly-dT priming impossible. On the other hand, random priming approaches result in additional shortening of the fragments and thus further loss of information.

Using nanogram-scale salivary RNA as a proof-of-principle example, our group has optimized the protocol for the linear amplification of RNA fragments that can be applied to the expression profiling using the new Human Exon arrays (Affymetrix). This novel mRNA amplification strategy is independent of the poly-A tail, yet capable of amplifying any mRNA fragments close to full length. The exon arrays contain potentially all the exons that may be expressed, leaving no bias against any particular transcribed sequence. The technical advantage of this approach is clearly demonstrated with the discovery of a salivary exon core transcriptome (SECT) that contains seven times as much information as in a previous study that was based on the old 3′-base approach (Hu et al. 2008). Importantly, the diagnostic potential of this approach is highlighted with salivary exon biomarkers that accurately discriminated sex in healthy individuals. This study, as part of the ongoing effort to fully reveal the clinical diagnostic value of body fluids such as saliva, has demonstrated the feasibility of high-resolution genome-wide expression profiling with whole transcript coverage from samples containing fragmented RNAs. As we get one step closer to the goal of accurate and affordable health surveillance using body fluids, there is every reason to believe that the full realization of personalized medicine is not far away.

Mass Spectrometry-Based Proteomics

Proteomics refers to global analysis and characterization of the proteome – the protein complement to the genome. Proteomic analysis of disease specimens and model cell lines and organisms is used to identify new protein targets, to explore mechanisms of action or toxicology of pharmaceuticals, and to discover new disease biomarkers for clinical and diagnostic applications. Due to its exquisite sensitivity and highly accurate mass measurements, mass spectrometry (MS) has become one of the core technologies for proteomics. A very common proteomics approach is to map out proteins using two-dimensional (2-D) gel electrophoresis (2-DE) followed by in-gel digestion and MS measurement of resulting peptide fragments, either by peptide mass fingerprinting (PMF) or tandem MS, to identify proteins from each gel spot. Such global analysis can also be performed by using a "shotgun" proteomics approach, in which 2-D liquid chromatography (LC) with tandem MS are typically used to analyze a fully digested proteomic sample (Washburn et al. 2001). These approaches are conceptually known as "bottom-up" proteomics, and they typically require the use of database search engines to investigate an existing proteomic or genomic database to identify proteins. In contrast, "top-down" proteomics involves direct analysis of intact proteins, without previous proteolytic digestion. It mainly relies on high-resolution measurement of intact molecular weight and direct fragmentation of protein ions in the gas phase for protein identification (Kelleher 2004). Although bottom-up proteomics is very frequently used, top-down proteomics has been found as promising for interpreting protein isoforms and post-translational modifications.

Global analysis of disease-associated protein changes requires quantitative proteomics tools. Differentially expressed proteins can be revealed by 2-DE or 2-D differential gel electrophoresis and subsequently identified using tandem MS or PMF. Tandem MS with stable isotope labeling represents an emerging technology for quantitative proteome analysis (Gygi et al. 1999a; Zhou et al. 2004a). In this approach, two protein samples of interest are labeled with "heavy" or "light" isotopes, respectively. The relative levels of a protein in the two samples can then be quantified based on the MS measurement of the isotope-labeled versions of the protein or the labeled peptides that originated from the protein. Prior to the development of quantitative proteomics tools, the study of cellular protein changes was limited to the investigation of either a limited numbers of proteins or gross morphological changes. Quantitative studies were largely dependent on western blotting or immunohistology by the use of antibodies, and this was semiquantitative due to the variation in antibody binding affinities. With the newly developed quantitative proteomics tools, biologists now have the ability to monitor global protein expression and obtain much-needed quantitative molecular data about cellular changes.

Integrating Data Streams from Multiple Biological Levels

A critical biological difficulty confronting the identification and eventual translation of genomic markers/targets for cancer prediction, diagnostics, treatment, and prognostics is how to distinguish the genomic aberrations driving malignant cell growth from those that are byproducts of abnormal proliferation. Among these key processes are germline variations that lead to hereditary cancer predispositions, the acquisition of transforming DNA or RNA sequences from cancer viruses, somatic mutations in the cancer genome, and epigenetic mechanisms (such as DNA methylation or histone modification) that promote oncogenesis by modifying cancer-related genes and altered expression of these genes at RNA and protein levels. While a variety of high-throughput technologies have been developed enabling the identification of a broad range of molecular abnormalities, none of the existing techniques can capture all of these changes in a single analysis. This represents a major obstacle to the comprehensive analysis of tumor genomes and their relationship to clinical phenotypes. A central goal in cancer research is to comprehensively delineate the complex genomic aberrations that shape tumor cell behavior and clinical outcomes. One potential approach to this problem would be to combine molecular genetic technologies (such as CGH and LOH) for comprehensive screening of genomic alterations. Each of these techniques has its own unique advantages, but each also has individual limitations that motivate efforts to combine multiple approaches (see Zhou et al. 2006b for a review on this topic).

Microarray expression profiling has proven to be a powerful approach for characterizing the changes associated with biological processes such as disease states. However, expression arrays measure only the alterations at the mRNA level. Most biological functions are executed by proteins rather than mRNAs. While the expression of many genes is controlled at the transcriptional level, some genes also employ post-transcriptional regulation involving mRNA stability, translation initiation, and protein stability. Thus, an important question is how these two expression data correlate with each other, and this analysis provides deeper insight into a biological process. Integrated analysis, by combining microarray profiling with quantitative proteomics, allows us to not only identify genes that are regulated at the transcription level but also unveil important post-transcriptional regulatory mechanisms that would not be evident by examining either mRNA or protein expression alone. Moderate to poor correlation of mRNA and protein expression data was reported for yeast and Halobacterium (Gygi et al. 1999b; Baliga et al. 2002). However, these prior studies only examined steady-state levels of mRNA and proteins. Discordant expression of protein and mRNA in lung adenocarcinomas was also observed, although the heterogeneity of tumor tissue was not considered (Chen et al. 2002). With the improvement of coverage, sensitivity, and throughput for proteomics and genomics technologies, we may expect a higher degree of concordance for correlation analysis of mRNA and protein expression (Hu et al. 2006b).

Due to the multifactorial nature of oncogenesis, it is of particular interest to identify the biological pathways that contribute to these oncogenetic events, rather than a single gene. Bioinformatics tools have been developed to investigate the involvements of biological pathways by combining our observational results (e.g., microarray expression dataset) with the vast existing knowledge of biological pathways at molecular levels. These tools essentially consist of a library containing all known events that make up biological processes, regulation, interaction and modifications among thousands of proteins, as well as statistical algorithms to identify associated pathways based on the integration of the library with the observational results. This approach has been successfully applied to identify relevant pathways for cancer cell migration, spread, and invasion (Donninger et al. 2004).

The continuing development of microarray-based expression analysis and large public depositories of microarray data have motivated new efforts to extract additional biological information from these data in addition to the static RNA transcript levels. One such attempt involves inferring chromosomal structural changes from spatially linked alterations in microarray expression data. Several array CGH studies have shown a genome-wide correlation of gene expression with copy number alterations and have proved useful in individual amplicon refinement (Pollack et al. 2002; Wolf et al. 2004). For example, through tissue microarray FISH and reverse transcriptase–polymerase chain reaction (RT-PCR), a minimally amplified region around ERBB2 (Her2) was identified in a large number of breast tumors; in addition, gene amplification was found to be correlated with increased gene expression in a subset of those samples (Kauraniemi et al. 2003). Recently, several groups have observed that chromosomal alterations can lead to regional gene expression biases in human tumors and tumor-derived cell lines. A fraction of gene expression values (15–25%) were found regulated in concordance with chromosomal DNA content (Phillips et al. 2001; Virtaneva et al. 2001; Crawley and Furge 2002; Zhou et al. 2004b, 2005). The developed statistical methods also appeared to be useful for detecting DNA copy number abnormalities based on differential gene expression (Crawley and Furge 2002; Myers et al. 2004; Zhou et al. 2004b, 2005).

Additional functional genomic information can be derived from microarray gene expression data using bioinformatics analysis of upstream transcription factor dynamics. Tools have recently been developed to identify aberrant transcription factor activity based on sequence similarities in the promoters of large groups of genes showing altered expression (Frith et al. 2004; Cole et al. 2005). Aberrant transcription factor activity plays a central role in many solid tumors, and reverse-inference of such alterations from microarray gene expression data provides an approach to cross-validating the results of structural genomic surveys, suggesting that a particular transcription control pathway might be altered in a tumor.

Molecular Analysis of Biofluids and Tumor Tissues

Discovery of Salivary mRNA Biomarkers for OSCC

We recently discovered that human saliva contains cell-free mRNAs (salivary transcriptome) that may be highly informative and discriminatory for disease detection. By using Affymetrix U133 microarrays for genome-wide profiling of saliva from ten healthy subjects, we found all subjects' saliva had approximately 3,000 different mRNA molecules, including 185 that were common among all the subjects (Li et al. 2004b). We further investigated the source and integrity of RNA in saliva. Most of the salivary RNA is generally fragmented and originates from both nucleus and mitochondria (Park et al. 2007). The notion of using salivary genomic targets for potential applications in human diseases has been demonstrated in our recent studies on discovery of salivary mRNA markers for detection of OSCC. Initial microarray profiling followed by real-time quantitative PCR revealed that four salivary mRNAs (OAZ, SAT, IL8, and IL1b) collectively have a discriminatory power of 91% sensitivity and specificity for oral cancer detection, and the area under the receiver operating characteristic (ROC) curve measuring 95% (Li et al. 2004a). These markers are currently being validated according to the guidelines of early disease detection network (EDRN). The clinical potential of these salivary mRNA markers has also been compared with the serum-based prediction model established with the same methodology and patient cohorts (Li et al. 2006). The panel of four mRNA biomarkers collectively exhibited an ROC value of 0.95 versus an ROC value of 0.88 from the serum-derived marker panel. These results show that saliva testing may not only be less invasive but also provide a slightly better diagnostic value than blood for oral cancer.

Systematic Identification of Salivary Proteins

Human whole saliva typically contains about 1 mg/ml of total proteins, which are expressed and secreted from the parotid, submandibular, sublingual, and some minor glands. These polypeptides not only play important roles in maintaining oral and general health but may also serve as biomarkers to survey human disease status. Supported by the National Institute of Dental and Craniofacial Research (NIDCR), a consortium of the Human Saliva Proteome Project was established to conduct in-depth analysis of the human saliva proteome (the total proteins/peptides present in saliva). To date, there have been approximately 1900 saliva that have been identified by using the combination of a variety of prefractionation techniques with tandem MS (Hu et al. 2004, 2005, 2007a; Xie et al. 2005; Guo et al. 2006). However, the post-translational modifications of salivary proteins, such as glycosylation and phosphorylation (Ramachandran et al. 2006; Helmerhorst and Oppenheim 2007), remain to be elucidated. A 3-year collaborative effort from the consortium has also led to the identification of over 1,100 nonredundant proteins from parotid sand submandibular/sublingual saliva (Hardt et al. 2007). The data have been consolidated in a central repository (www.hspp.ucla.edu) and linked to public annotated protein databases, providing a valuable resource for researchers within the fields of oral biology and saliva diagnostics.

Serum/Saliva Protein Biomarkers for OSCC

Biomarkers are measurable biological and physiological parameters that can serve as indices for health-related assessments. Saliva/serum protein biomarkers are particularly valuable because they are amenable to simple clinical tools for disease applications. For patients, noninvasive saliva collection dramatically reduces anxiety and discomfort and simplifies procurement of repeated samples for monitoring over time. Compared with tissue biopsies, saliva is an easily accessible fluid, and, therefore, a large number of saliva samples can be enrolled for clinical studies. This allows enough statistical power for a robust study design, and true signatures can be revealed as disease biomarkers (Hu et al. 2006a, 2007b; Streckfus and Dubinsky 2007).

Currently, there are no reliable blood or saliva biomarkers in the clinic for OSCC, but recent studies have suggested the potential of using serum/saliva protein biomarkers for possible detection of OSCC/HNSCC. For instance, multiplexed serum profiles of cytokines, growth factors, and tumor antigens have been found promising for early detection or screening of HNSCC/OSCC patients at high risk (Hathaway et al. 2005; Linkov et al. 2007). Identification of markers in saliva is intrinsically challenging because the saliva constituents are constantly changing due to the variance in salivary flow and a differential contribution from the different salivary glands within the oral cavity. Saliva proteins including CD44, fibronectin, tumor necrosis factor (TNF)-alpha, interleukin (IL)-1, IL-6, IL-8, thioredoxin, cytokeratin 19 fragment (CYFRA 21-1), tissue polypeptide antigen, and cancer antigen CA125, have been shown to have diagnostic potential to distinguish OSCC patients from healthy subjects (Lyons and Cui 2000; St. John et al. 2004; Franzmann et al. 2005; Rhodus et al. 2005; Nagler et al. 2006). Nevertheless, these candidates need to be further validated through long-term longitudinal studies with large populations of individuals with oral cancer and those who are at high risk for developing oral cancer. Our group is pursuing this currently in conjunction with the National Cancer Institute (NCI) Early Disease Research Network (EDRN) for a panel of proteomic and transcriptomic salivary biomarkers for oral cancer.

The presence of lymph node metastasis in OSCC is an important prognostic factor and crucial in making clinical treatment decisions. Currently, the detection of nodal metastasis is based on routine histopathological evaluation of the lymph nodes in the neck, and there is an immediate need for developing preoperative molecular biomarkers for prediction of lymph node metastases in OSCC. These biomarkers will certainly help identify patients who clinically have no detectable disease but are potential candidates for lymph nodes metastasis and should have prophylactic neck dissection and/or adjuvant radiotherapy. Conversely, such a set of reliable biomarkers would also help avoid unnecessary surgery for those who are metastasis free.

The notion of using such markers in serum for possible detection of cancer metastasis has been demonstrated in several recent studies. For instance, cysteine proteinases cathepsins B and L and their endogenous inhibitors stefins A and B were implicated in HNSCC invasion and metastasis and could be potential markers (Strojan et al. 2000). Overexpression of cathepsin-D, matrix metalloproteinases (MMPs) and tissue inhibitors of matrix metalloproteinases (TIMPs) had significant correlation with local or distant metastasis in patients with oral tongue cancer (Gandour-Edwards et al. 1999; Kurahara et al. 1999). These preliminary studies have suggested exciting possibilities of using serum protein biomarker for metastasis detection.

Analysis of Oral Cancer Tumor Tissue

The high recurrence and low survival rates of OSCC reflect the need to understand molecular mechanisms contributing to this malignancy so that molecular diagnostics and targeted therapeutics can be improved for successful treatment. By using proteomics to monitor the global protein alterations in OSCC tissues, a number of tumor-associated proteins have been identified (Chen et al. 2004; He et al. 2004; Lo et al. 2007). In terms of biological processes, the majority of the proteins are related to cell adhesion, interaction, growth, and apoptosis or are related to stress and anti-oxidation. These studies also indicate that multiple cellular and etiological pathways are involved in the process of oral oncogenesis and suggest that multiple protein molecules should be simultaneously targeted as an effective strategy to counter the disease (Chen et al. 2004).

Gene expression signatures may also exist in primary tumors that can be used for predicting increased risk of metastasis (van 't Veer et al. 2002; Ramaswamy et al. 2003). The metastasis of the HNSCCs is unique in that they metastasize mainly to regional lymph nodes through the draining lymphatics, where metastasis to distant sites is relatively uncommon. Several recent gene expression studies have suggested the existence of such "fingerprints" in the primary tumor for metastasis of HNSCC (Schmalbach et al. 2004; O'Donnell et al. 2005; Roepman et al. 2005). In a recent study, we identified CTTN and MMP9 as consistently overexpressed genes in the primary tumor tissue samples of the tongue with lymph node metastasis (Zhou et al. 2006a). These genes also provide predictive values for extracapsular spread (ECS) of lymph node metastasis, one of the most important negative prognostic factors of OSCC (Myers et al. 2001; Greenberg et al. 2003).

Future Directions

In summary, molecular profiling tools such as microarrays and proteomics will significantly accelerate the translational research in oral cancer. With the maturation of these novel technologies, future applications may focus on the following aspects of the disease.

First, similarly as with other major cancers, early detection is key for successful treatment of OSCC. Considering that approximately 10% of the general population have oral mucosal abnormalities and precancerous and early cancerous lesions that are not readily detectable by visual inspection (Lingen 2007), it is critical to develop molecular biomarkers for early cancer screening. This, in turn, can identify targeted high-risk populations for more definitive tests.

Second, the low survival rate of patients with OSCC is largely due to the high metastatic potential of the tumor. Molecular analysis of metastatic and nonmetastatic OSCCs should be explored in order to understand the molecular mechanism of OSCC metastasis and to develop molecular biomarkers for prediction of lymph node metastases.

Third, there is an enormous need to develop more effective and less toxic therapeutic approaches to treat patients with OSCC. The opportunities for molecular profiling tools to impact the study of differential gene expression applied to drug discovery and optimization can be remarkable. These advances will likely include the discovery of new molecular targets, the confirmation of suspected mechanism of drug action, the assessment of drug efficacy and toxicity, the identification of disease subgroups, and prediction of treatment responses of individual patients. These applications may eventually lead to simple tools for clinical decision making and facilitate the development of molecular-targeted chemotherapies for this devastating disease.

References

American Cancer Society (2006) Cancer facts and figures 2006. Atlanta, GA

Baliga NS, Pan M, Goo YA, Yi EC, Goodlett DR, Dimitrov K, Shannon P, Aebersold R, Ng WV, Hood L (2002) Coordinate regulation of energy transduction modules in Halobacterium sp. analyzed by a global systems approach. Proc Natl Acad Sci U S A 99:14913–14918

Bignell GR, Huang J, Greshock J, Watt S, Butler A, West S, Grigorova M, Jones KW, Wei W, Stratton MR et al (2004) High-resolution analysis of DNA copy number using oligonucleotide microarrays. Genome Res 14:287–295

Brennan C, Zhang Y, Leo C, Feng B, Cauwels C, Aguirre AJ, Kim M, Protopopov A, Chin L (2004) High-resolution global profiling of genomic alterations with long oligonucleotide microarray. Cancer Res 64:4744–4748

Caspersson T, Zech L, Modest EJ, Foley GE, Wagh U, Simonsson E (1969a) Chemical differentiation with fluorescent alkylating agents in Vicia faba metaphase chromosomes. Exp Cell Res 58:128–140

Caspersson T, Zech L, Modest EJ, Foley GE, Wagh U, Simonsson E (1969b) DNA-binding fluorochromes for the study of the organization of the metaphase nucleus. Exp Cell Res 58:141–152

Chen G, Gharib TG, Huang CC, Taylor JM, Misek DE, Kardia SL, Giordano TJ, Iannettoni MD, Orringer MB, Hanash SM, Beer DG (2002) Discordant protein and mRNA expression in lung adenocarcinomas. Mol Cell Proteomics 1:304–313

Chen J, He QY, Yuen AP, Chiu JF (2004) Proteomics of buccal squamous cell carcinoma: the involvement of multiple pathways in tumorigenesis. Proteomics 4:2465–2475

Cole SW, Yan W, Galic Z, Arevalo J, Zack JA (2005) Expression-based monitoring of transcription factor activity: the TELiS database. Bioinformatics 21:803–810

Crawley JJ, Furge KA (2002) Identification of frequent cytogenetic aberrations in hepatocellular carcinoma using gene-expression microarray data. Genome Biol 3:RESEARCH0075

Davies JJ, Wilson IM, Lam WL (2005) Array CGH technologies and their applications to cancer genomes. Chromosome Res 13:237–248

Donninger H, Bonome T, Radonovich M, Pise-Masison CA, Brady J, Shih JH, Barrett JC, Birrer MJ (2004) Whole genome expression profiling of advance stage papillary serous ovarian cancer reveals activated pathways. Oncogene 23:8065–8077

Franzmann EJ, Reategui EP, Carraway KL, Hamilton KL, Weed DT, Goodwin WJ (2005) Salivary soluble CD44: a potential molecular marker for head and neck cancer. Cancer Epidemiol Biomarkers Prev 14:735–739

Friend SH, Bernards R, Rogelj S, Weinberg RA, Rapaport JM, Albert DM, Dryja TP (1986) A human DNA segment with properties of the gene that predisposes to retinoblastoma and osteosarcoma. Nature 323:643

Frith MC, Fu Y, Yu L, Chen JF, Hansen U, Weng Z (2004) Detection of functional DNA motifs via statistical over-representation. Nucleic Acids Res 32:1372–1381

Futreal PA, Coin L, Marshall M, Down T, Hubbard T, Wooster R, Rahman N, Stratton MR (2004) A census of human cancer genes. Nat Rev Cancer 4:177–183

Gandour-Edwards R, Trock B, Donald PJ (1999) Predictive value of cathepsin-D for cervical lymph node metastasis in head and neck squamous cell carcinoma. Head Neck 21:718–722

Greenberg JS, Fowler R, Gomez J, Mo V, Roberts D, El Naggar AK, Myers JN (2003) Extent of extracapsular spread: a critical prognosticator in oral tongue cancer. Cancer 97:1464–1470

Greenlee RT, Murray T, Bolden S, Wingo PA (2000) Cancer statistics, 2000. CA Cancer J Clin 50:7–33

Guo T, Rudnick PA, Wang W, Lee CS, Devoe DL, Balgley BM (2006) Characterization of the human salivary proteome by capillary isoelectric focusing/nanoreversed-phase liquid chromatography coupled with ESI-tandem MS. J Proteome Res 5(6):1469–1478

Gygi SP, Rochon B, Gerber SA, Turecek F, Gelb MH, Aebersold R (1999a) Quantitative analysis of complex protein mixtures using isotope-coded affinity tags. Nat Biotechnol 17:994–999

Gygi SP, Rochon Y, Franza BR, Aebersold R (1999b) Correlation between protein and mRNA abundance in yeast. Mol Cell Biol 19:1720–1730

Hathaway B, Landsittel DP, Gooding W, Whiteside TL, Grandis JR, Siegfried JM, Bigbee WL, Ferris RL (2005) Multiplexed analysis of serum cytokines as biomarkers in squamous cell carcinoma of the head and neck patients. Laryngoscope 115:522–527

He QY, Chen J, Kung HF, Yuen AP, Chiu JF (2004) Identification of tumor-associated proteins in oral tongue squamous cell carcinoma by proteomics. Proteomics 4(1):271–278

Helmerhorst EJ, Oppenheim F (2007) Saliva: a dynamic proteome. J Dent Res 86:680–693

Henegariu O, Heerema NA, Bray-Ward P, Ward DC (1999) Colour-changing karyotyping: an alternative to M-FISH/SKY. Nat Genet 23:263–264

Hoque MO, Lee CC, Cairns P, Schoenberg M, Sidransky D (2003) Genome-wide genetic characterization of bladder cancer: a comparison of high-density single-nucleotide polymorphism arrays and PCR-based microsatellite analysis. Cancer Res 63:2216–2222

Hu S, Denny P, Denny P, Xie Y, Loo JA, Wolinsky LE, Li Y, McBride J, Loo RR, Navazesh M, Wong DT (2004) Differentially expressed protein markers in human submandibular and sublingual secretions. Int J Oncol 25:1423–1430

Hu S, Loo J, Wong DT (2006a) Human body fluid proteome analysis. Proteomics 6:6326–6353

Hu S, Loo J, Wong DT (2007a) Human saliva proteome analysis. Ann N Y Acad Sci 1098:323–329

Hu S, Loo Y, Wang J, Xie Y, Tjon K, Wolinsky L, Loo RR, Loo JA, Wong DT (2006b) Human saliva proteome and transcriptome. J Dent Res 85:1129–1133

Hu S, Xie Y, Ramachandran P, Loo RR, Li Y, Loo JA, Wong DT (2005) Large-scale identification of proteins in human salivary proteome by liquid chromatography/mass spectrometry and two-dimensional gel electrophoresis-mass spectrometry. Proteomics 5:1714–1728

Hu S, Yu T, Xie Y, Yang Y, Li Y, Zhou X, Tsung S, Loo RR, Loo JR, Wong DT (2007b) Discovery of oral fluid biomarkers for human oral cancer by mass spectrometry. Cancer Genomics Proteomics 4:55–64

Hu Z, Zimmermann BG, Zhou H, Wang J, Henson BS, Yu Y, Elashoff D, Krupp G, Wong DT (2008) Exon level expression profiling: a comprehensive transcriptome analysis for body fluids. Clin Chem 54:824–832

Huang J, Wei W, Zhang J, Liu G, Bignell GR, Stratton MR, Futreal PA, Wooster R, Jones KW, Shapero MH (2004) Whole genome DNA copy number changes identified by high density oligonucleotide arrays. Hum Genomics 1:287–299

Ishkanian AS, Malloff CA, Watson SK, DeLeeuw RJ, Chi B, Coe BP, Snijders A, Albertson DG, Pinkel D, Marra MA et al (2004) A tiling resolution DNA microarray with complete coverage of the human genome. Nat Genet 36:299–303

Janne PA, Li C, Zhao X, Girard L, Chen TH, Minna J, Christiani DC, Johnson BE, Meyerson M (2004) High-resolution single-nucleotide polymorphism array and clustering analysis of loss of heterozygosity in human lung cancer cell lines. Oncogene 23:2716–2726

Kallioniemi A, Kallioniemi OP, Sudar D, Rutovitz D, Gray JW, Waldman F, Pinkel D (1992) Comparative genomic hybridization for molecular cytogenetic analysis of solid tumors. Science 258:818–821

Kauraniemi P, Kuukasjarvi T, Sauter G, Kallioniemi A (2003) Amplification of a 280-kilobase core region at the ERBB2 locus leads to activation of two hypothetical proteins in breast cancer. Am J Pathol 163:1979–1984

Kelleher NL (2004) Top-down proteomics. Anal Chem 76:197A–203A

Knudson AG (1996) Hereditary cancer: two hits revisited. J Cancer Res Clin Oncol 122:135–140

Knudson AG Jr (1971) Mutation and cancer: statistical study of retinoblastoma. Proc Natl Acad Sci U S A 68:820–823

Kurahara S, Shinohara M, Ikebe T, Nakamura S, Beppu M, Hiraki A, Takeuchi H, Shirasuna K (1999) Expression of MMPS, MT-MMP, and TIMPs in squamous cell carcinoma of the oral cavity: correlations with tumor invasion and metastasis. Head Neck 21(7):627–638

Li Y, Elashoff D, Oh M, Sinha U, St John MAR, Zhou X, Abemayor E, Wong DT (2006) Serum circulating human mRNA profiling and its utility for oral cancer detection. J Clin Oncol 24:1754–1760

Li Y, St John MA, Zhou X, Kim Y, Sinha U, Jordan RC, Eisele D, Abemayor E, Elashoff D, Park NH et al (2004a) Salivary transcriptome diagnostics for oral cancer detection. Clin Cancer Res 10:8442–8450

Li Y, Zhou X, St John MA, Wong DT (2004b) RNA profiling of cell-free saliva using microarray technology. J Dent Res 83:199–203

Lieberfarb ME, Lin M, Lechpammer M, Li C, Tanenbaum DM, Febbo PG, Wright RL, Shim J, Kantoff PW, Loda M et al (2003) Genome-wide loss of heterozygosity analysis from laser capture microdissected prostate cancer using single nucleotide polymorphic allele (SNP) arrays and a novel bioinformatics platform dChipSNP. Cancer Res 63:4781–4785

Lindblad-Toh K, Tanenbaum DM, Daly MJ, Winchester E, Lui WO, Villapakkam A, Stanton SE, Larsson C, Hudson TJ, Johnson BE et al (2000) Loss-of-heterozygosity analysis of small-cell lung carcinomas using single-nucleotide polymorphism arrays. Nat Biotechnol 18:1001–1005

Lingen M (2007) Oral cancer screening aids: where is the science? Oral Surg Oral Med Oral Pathol Oral Radiol Endod 103:153–154

Linkov F, Lisovich A, Yurkovetsky Z, Marrangoni A, Velikokhatnaya L, Nolen B, Winan M, Bigbee W, Siegfried J, Lokshin A, Ferris RL (2007) Early detection of head and neck cancer: development of a novel screening tool using multiplexed immunobead-based biomarker profiling. Cancer Epidemiol Biomarkers Prev 16:102–107

Lippman SM, Hong WK (2001) Molecular markers of the risk of oral cancer. N Engl J Med 344:1323–1326

Lo WY, Tsai M, Tsai Y, Hua CH, Tsai FJ, Huang SY, Tsai CH, Lai CC (2007) Identification of over-expressed proteins in oral squamous cell carcinoma (OSCC) patients by clinical proteomic analysis. Clin Chim Acta 376:101–107

Lucito R, Healy J, Alexander J, Reiner A, Esposito D, Chi M, Rodgers L, Brady A, Sebat J, Troge J et al (2003) Representational oligonucleotide microarray analysis: a high-resolution method to detect genome copy number variation. Genome Res 13:2291–2305

Lyons AJ, Cui N (2000) Salivary oncofoetal fibronectin and oral squamous cell carcinoma. J Oral Pathol Med 29:267–270

Hardt M, Yan WH, Niles R, Robinson S, Witkowska HE, Miroshnychenko O, Prakobphol A, Hall SC, Sullivan MA, Hagen FK, Bedi GS, Gonzalez-Begne M, Park SK, Delahunty CM, Xu T, Hewel J, Liao L, Han X, Cociorva D, Hu S, Boontheung P, Ramachandran P, Xie Y, Dunsmore J, Loo RR, Sondej M, Arellanno M, Wang J, Henson B, Wolinsky L, Jeffrey S, Richert M, Jiang J, Yu W, Than S, Halgand F, Bassilian S, Souda P, Faull KF, Whitelegge JP, Denny P, Denny T, Gilligan J, Malamud D, Melvin JE, Loo JA, Wong DT, Yates JR, Fisher SJ (2008) The proteomes of human parotid and submandibular/sublingual gland salivas collected as the ductal secretions. J Proteome Res 7:1994–2006

Myers CL, Dunham MJ, Kung SY, Troyanskaya OG (2004) Accurate detection of aneuploidies in array CGH and gene expression microarray data. Bioinformatics 20:3533–3543

Myers JN, Greenberg JS, Mo V, Roberts D (2001) Extracapsular spread. A significant predictor of treatment failure in patients with squamous cell carcinoma of the tongue. Cancer 92:3030–3036

Nagler R, Bahar G, Shpitzer T, Feinmesser R (2006) Concomitant analysis of salivary tumor markers – a new diagnostic tool for oral cancer. Clin Cancer Res 12:3979–3984

O'Donnell RK, Kupferman M, Wei SJ, Singhal S, Weber R, O'Malley B, Cheng Y, Putt M, Feldman M, Ziober B et al (2005) Gene expression signature predicts lymphatic metastasis in squamous cell carcinoma of the oral cavity. Oncogene 24:1244–1251

Park NJ, Zhou X, Yu T, Brinkman BM, Zimmermann BG, Palanisamy V, Wong DT (2007) Characterization of salivary RNA by cDNA library analysis. Arch Oral Biol 52:30–35

Parkin DM, Bray F, Ferlay J, Pisani P (2005) Global cancer statistics, 2002. CA Cancer J Clin 55:74–108

Phillips JL, Hayward SW, Wang Y, Vasselli J, Pavlovich C, Padilla-Nash H, Pezullo JR, Ghadimi BM, Grossfeld GD, Rivera A et al (2001) The consequences of chromosomal aneuploidy on gene expression profiles in a cell line model for prostate carcinogenesis. Cancer Res 61:8143–8149

Pinkel D, Albertson DG (2005a) Array comparative genomic hybridization and its applications in cancer. Nat Genet 37(Suppl):S11–S17

Pinkel D, Albertson DG (2005b) Comparative genomic hybridization. Annu Rev Genomics Hum Genet 6:331–354

Pinkel D, Segraves R, Sudar D, Clark S, Poole I, Kowbel D, Collins C, Kuo WL, Chen C, Zhai Y et al (1998) High resolution analysis of DNA copy number variation using comparative genomic hybridization to microarrays. Nat Genet 20:207–211

Pollack JR, Perou CM, Alizadeh AA, Eisen MB, Pergamenschikov A, Williams CF, Jeffrey SS, Botstein D, Brown PO (1999) Genome-wide analysis of DNA copy-number changes using cDNA microarrays. Nat Genet 23:41–46

Pollack JR, Sorlie T, Perou CM, Rees CA, Jeffrey SS, Lonning PE, Tibshirani R, Botstein D, Borresen-Dale AL, Brown PO (2002) Microarray analysis reveals a major direct role of DNA copy number alteration in the transcriptional program of human breast tumors. Proc Natl Acad Sci U S A 99(20):12963–12968

Ramachandran P, Boontheung P, Xie Y, Sondej M, Wong DT, Loo JA (2006) Identification of N-linked glycoproteins in human saliva by glycoprotein capture and mass spectrometry. J Proteome Res 5:1493–1503

Ramaswamy S, Ross KN, Lander ES, Golub TR (2003) A molecular signature of metastasis in primary solid tumors. Nat Genet 33:49–54

Rhodus NL, Ho V, Miller CS, Myers S, Ondrey F (2005) NF-kappaB dependent cytokine levels in saliva of patients with oral preneoplastic lesions and oral squamous cell carcinoma. Cancer Detect Prev 29:42–45

Roepman P, Wessels LF, Kettelarij N, Kemmeren P, Miles AJ, Lijnzaad P, Tilanus MG, Koole R, Hordijk GJ, van der Vliet PC et al (2005) An expression profile for diagnosis of lymph node metastases from primary head and neck squamous cell carcinomas. Nat Genet 37:182–186

Schmalbach CE, Chepeha DB, Giordano TJ, Rubin MA, Teknos TN, Bradford CR, Wolf GT, Kuick R, Misek DE, Trask DK et al (2004) Molecular profiling and the identification of genes associated with metastatic oral cavity/pharynx squamous cell carcinoma. Arch Otolaryngol Head Neck Surg 130:295–302

St. John M, Li Y, Zhou X, Denny P, Ho CM, Montemagno C, Shi W, Qi F, Wu B, Sinha U, Jordan R, Wolinsky L, Park NH, Liu H, Abemayor E, Wong DT (2004) Interleukin 6 and interleukin 8 as potential biomarkers for oral cavity and oropharyngeal squamous cell carcinoma. Arch Otolaryngol Head Neck Surg 130(8):929–935

Streckfus CF, Dubinsky WP (2007) Proteomic analysis of saliva for cancer diagnosis. Expert Rev Proteomics 4:329–332

Strojan P, Budihna M, Smid L, Svetic B, Vrhovec I, Kos J, Skrk J (2000) Prognostic significance of cysteine proteinases cathepsins B and L and their endogenous inhibitors stefins A and B in patients with squamous cell carcinoma of the head and neck. Clin Cancer Res 6:1052–1062

van 't Veer LJ, Dai H, van de Vijver MJ, He YD, Hart AA, Mao M, Peterse HL, van der Kooy K, Marton MJ, Witteveen AT et al (2002) Gene expression profiling predicts clinical outcome of breast cancer. Nature 415:530–536

120 S. Hu et al.

Virtaneva K, Wright FA, Tanner SM, Yuan B, Lemon WJ, Caligiuri MA, Bloomfield CD, de La
Chapelle A, Krahe R (2001) Expression profiling reveals fundamental biological differences
in acute myeloid leukemia with isolated trisomy 8 and normal cytogenetics. Proc Natl Acad
Sci U S A 98:1124–1129

Vokes EE, Weichselbaum RR, Lippman SM, Hong WK (1993) Head and neck cancer. N Engl J
Med 328:184–194

Wang ZC, Lin M, Wei LJ, Li C, Miron A, Lodeiro G, Harris L, Ramaswamy S, Tanenbaum DM,
Meyerson M et al (2004) Loss of heterozygosity and its correlation with expression profiles in
subclasses of invasive breast cancers. Cancer Res 64:64–71

Washburn MP, Wolter D, Yates JR (2001) Large-scale analysis of the yeast proteome by multidi-
mensional protein identification technology. Nat Biotechnol 19:242–247

Wolf M, Mousses S, Hautaniemi S, Karhu R, Huusko P, Allinen M, Elkahloun A, Monni O, Chen
Y, Kallioniemi A et al (2004) High-resolution analysis of gene copy number alterations in
human prostate cancer using CGH on cDNA microarrays: impact of copy number on gene
expression. Neoplasia 6:240–247

Xie H, Rhodus N, Griffin RJ, Carlis JV, Griffin TJ (2005) A catalogue of human saliva proteins
identified by free flow electrophoresis-based peptide separation and tandem mass spectrometry. Mol Cell Proteomics 4:1826–1830

Yu T, Ye H, Sun W, Li KC, Chen Z, Jacobs S, Bailey DK, Wong DT, Zhou X (2007) A forward-
backward fragment assembling algorithm for the identification of genomic amplification and
deletion breakpoints using high-density single nucleotide polymorphism (SNP) array. BMC
Bioinformatics 8:145

Zhao X, Li C, Paez JG, Chin K, Janne PA, Chen TH, Girard L, Minna J, Christiani D, Leo C et al
(2004) An integrated view of copy number and allelic alterations in the cancer genome using
single nucleotide polymorphism arrays. Cancer Res 64:3060–3071

Zhao X, Weir BA, LaFramboise T, Lin M, Beroukhim R, Garraway L, Beheshti J, Lee JC, Naoki
K, Richards WG et al (2005) Homozygous deletions and chromosome amplifications in
human lung carcinomas revealed by single nucleotide polymorphism array analysis. Cancer
Res 65:5561–5570

Zhou H, Boyle R, Aebersold R (2004a) Quantitative protein analysis by solid phase isotope tag-
ging and mass spectrometry. Methods Mol Biol 261:511–518

Zhou X, Cole SW, Chen Z, Li Y, Wong DT (2005) Identification of discrete chromosomal deletion by
binary recursive partitioning of microarray differential expression data. J Med Genet 42:416–419

Zhou X, Cole SW, Hu S, Wong DT (2004b) Detection of DNA copy number abnormality by
microarray expression analysis. Hum Genet 114:464–467

Zhou X, Jordan RCK, Mok S, Birrer MJ, Wong DT (2004c) DNA copy number abnormality of
oral squamous cell carcinoma detected by cDNA array-based CGH. Cancer Genet Cytogenet
151:90–92

Zhou X, Li C, Mok SC, Chen Z, Wong DTW (2004d) Whole genome loss of heterozygosity
profiling on oral squamous cell carcinoma by high-density single nucleotide polymorphic
allele (SNP) array. Cancer Genet Cytogenet 151:82–84

Zhou X, Mok SC, Chen Z, Li Y, Wong DT (2004e) Concurrent analysis of loss of heterozygosity
(LOH) and copy number abnormality (CNA) for oral premalignancy progression using the
Affymetrix 10K SNP mapping array. Hum Genet 115:327–330

Zhou X, Temam S, Oh M, Pungpravat N, Huang BL, Mao L, Wong DT (2006a) Global expression-based classification of lymph node metastasis and extracapsular spread of oral tongue
squamous cell carcinoma. Neoplasia 8:925–932

Zhou X, Yu T, Cole SW, Wong DT (2006b) Advancement in characterization of genomic alterations for improved diagnosis, treatment and prognostics in cancer. Expert Rev Mol Diagn
6:39–50

Chapter 6
Adjuvant Therapy for Patients with Oral Cavity Cancer

C. Wesley Hodge, Deepak Khuntia, Rafael Manon, and Paul M. Harari

Abstract Locoregionally advanced oral cavity cancer is commonly treated using a combined modality approach in an effort to maximize tumor control. Radiotherapy, either alone or in combination with chemotherapy, is generally administered following surgery. Radiation doses on the order of 60 Gy are typically recommended post-operatively, although higher doses may be advisable in cases of extracapsular nodal extension or gross residual disease. Advances in radiation delivery techniques including intensity modulated radiation therapy (IMRT) have the potential to reduce normal tissue toxicities without compromising the likelihood of tumor control. The role of concomitant chemotherapy in the adjuvant setting has evolved considerably in the last 10 years, and its use has recently been validated for selected high-risk patients on the basis of two large multi-institutional randomized trials. Newer approaches include the evaluation of targeted agents, with the goal of preserving a beneficial effect with radiation while further diminishing treatment related side effects.

General Management

Surgery, radiation, and chemotherapy, either singly or in combination, are classical treatment options for patients with oral cavity cancer. Treatment recommendations depend on tumor stage and specific anatomic location, as well as relevant patient factors, including performance status, comorbid illness, and motivation for organ preservation. Broadly speaking, single-modality treatment (i.e., surgery or radiation) is generally preferred for early-stage lesions The control rates are similar for T1–T2 lesions with either modality delivered as monotherapy (Hintz et al. 1979). For more advanced lesions a combined-modality treatment approach is generally preferred to maximize locoregional tumor control. Several other treatment approaches, including definitive radiotherapy with or without chemotherapy, and

P.M. Harari (✉)
Department of Human Oncology, University of Wisconsin School of Medicine and Public Health, 600 Highland Avenue, K4/336, Madison, WI, 53792, USA
e-mail: harari@humonc.wisc.edu

J. Myers (ed.), *Oral Cancer Metastasis*,
DOI 10.1007/978-1-4419-0775-2_6, © Springer Science+Business Media, LLC 2010

neoadjuvant chemotherapy followed by surgery with or without radiotherapy, are areas of active clinical investigation. These approaches remain primarily investigational and are beyond the scope of the current summary.

The timing of radiation, before or after surgery, has been the subject of some debate. Notable disadvantages of preoperative radiation therapy include limitations on the dose of radiation that can be delivered due to the risk of postoperative wound complications, and the compromise of precise pathologic data, particularly as it pertains to occult nodal disease. Postoperative radiation treatment has the advantage of less relative dose limitation, no delay in definitive surgical resection, and preservation of complete pathologic tumor staging. However, it is recognized that postoperative wound complications may delay adjuvant radiation and that, compared with normal oxygenation, regional hypoxia following surgery may diminish the effectiveness of radiation. A single randomized trial including 59 oral cavity cancers in a population of 320 evaluable patients, identified no significant survival, locoregional control, or toxicity difference between preoperative and postoperative radiation (Snow et al. 1981). However, the preponderance of data as well as global practice patterns suggest that postoperative radiation is commonly preferred. Further, emerging data for selected patients with high-risk pathologic features indicate that the addition of concurrent chemotherapy during the postoperative radiation treatment course may further augment tumor control rates (Bernier et al. 2004; Cooper et al. 2004; Day et al. 2003). High-risk features commonly include advanced T stage, multiple positive nodes, extracapsular tumor spread, positive resection margins, and perineural invasion (Bernier et al. 2004; Cooper et al. 2004).

Combined-Modality Therapy

Disease control outcomes for advanced lesions of the oral cavity (T3, T4) are less than satisfactory with surgery or radiation alone, thereby prompting the common implementation of combined-modality therapy (Fu et al. 1976; Shah and Lydiatt 1995; Vikram et al. 1980). With steadily improving reconstruction techniques, surgery has emerged as the preferred initial treatment approach for the majority of patients with tumors of the oral cavity, with adjuvant radiation (or, in selected cases, chemoradiation) employed to enhance the likelihood of locoregional tumor control.

Adjuvant Radiation Technique

Carcinoma of the oral cavity has traditionally been treated with opposed lateral fields, using either two-dimensional or three-dimensional CT-based techniques. During simulation and treatment, patients are typically immobilized with a thermoplastic mask. Patients are placed in the supine position with a bite block (for oral tongue and floor of mouth cases) to depress the tongue away from the palate. The oral cavity tumor bed with a 1.5–2.0-cm margin and upper cervical lymph nodes constitute the initial lateral fields. The inferior border of the field resides at approximately the thyroid notch (or aryepiglottic folds when using CT-based planning), just above the true vocal cords. The posterior border is set at the mid-vertebral body level if level V nodal coverage is not required. For patients with more advanced neck disease or positive level V lymph nodes, the initial fields should be set behind the C1 vertebral body spinous process to facilitate coverage of the posterior triangle. The lateral fields are reduced at 40–45 Gy, depending upon patient anatomy, to spare the spinal cord from doses in excess of tolerance. Treatment of the low neck generally consists of a single half-beam-blocked anteroposterior field matched to the inferior border of the opposed lateral fields. An anterior larynx block is used, which functions to protect the central larynx from unnecessary radiation dose and to protect against spinal cord overdose due to field overlap. Beam energies between 4 and 6 MV are most suitable for treatment of cancers involving the oral cavity. Bolus material may be necessary to bring dose to the surface as required for tumors that extend to the skin, particularly in patients with large volume nodal disease or extracapsular extension (ECE) where adequate dosing of superficial tissues is crucial to the success of the treatment. All fields should be treated daily, with at least five scheduled treatment days per week.

In recent years, intensity-modulated radiation therapy (IMRT) has increasingly been used for the treatment of head and neck tumors (Fig. 6.1), with the goal of

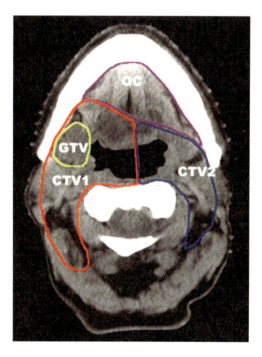

Fig. 6.1 Treatment volume delineation for a patient with stage IVA (T3 N2b M0) cancer of the right retromolar trigone receiving definitive IMRT. The gross tumor volume (GTV, *yellow*), high-risk clinical target volume (CTV1, *red*), low-risk clinical target volume (CTV2, *blue*), and oral cavity (OC, *magenta*) are shown. (From Chao KS, Ozygit G, (eds) *Intensity modulated radiation therapy for head & neck cancer*. Philadelphia: Lippincott, 2003, with permission)

preserving treatment outcome while diminishing normal tissue toxicities, including damage to major salivary glands and mandible, which result in xerostomia or osteo-radionecrosis, respectively (Yao et al. 2005; Studer et al. 2006; Daly et al. 2006). Dosimetric analysis of radiation dose to the parotid glands with evaluation of resultant salivary function suggests that limiting the mean parotid dose to <26 Gy may result in improved post-radiation salivary function (Eisbruch et al. 2003). In light of the steep dose gradients that often accompany IMRT plans, successful delivery is highly dependent on accurate and reproducible localization and immobilization. At several centers, an optically guided localization system is used to enhance daily treatment precision for IMRT delivery. Tomotherapy, which involves the helical delivery of intensity-modulated radiation, enables a high degree of target conformality coupled with the capacity for megavoltage CT scanning, thereby allowing image guidance for precise daily set-up verification (Fig. 6.2) (Sheng et al. 2006; Fiorino et al. 2006; Harari et al. 2004). Other treatment platforms have developed similar integrated CT-based imaging capabilities.

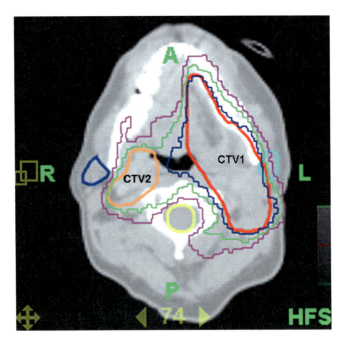

Fig. 6.2 Radiation dose distribution for an IMRT treatment plan delivered via helical tomotherapy to a patient with stage IVA (T2 N2b M0) squamous cell carcinoma of the left lateral oral tongue; status, postsurgical resection of the primary tumor. The high-risk clinical target volume (CTV1, *red*) and low-risk clinical target volume (CTV2, *orange*) are shown, with radiation dose distribution demonstrated by the 63 Gy (*blue*), 54 Gy (*green*), and 45 Gy (*magenta*) isodose lines. Critical normal structures, which have been contoured in this view, are the left parotid gland (*light blue*), right parotid gland (*dark blue*), and spinal cord (*yellow*)

Dose and Fractionation

When postoperative radiation is used for oral cavity cancer, the most common dose fractionation in the United States is 1.8–2.0 Gy per day. The postoperative tumor bed should generally receive a total dose of 60 Gy. However, for close or positive microscopic margins, or extracapsular nodal extension, a 4- to 6-Gy localized boost should be considered. Peters and colleagues conducted a prospective randomized trial of radiation dose escalation in the postoperative setting. They concluded that a minimum dose of 57.6 Gy was necessary to achieve satisfactory tumor control and that doses in excess of 63 Gy were indicated in the setting of nodal ECE (Peters et al. 1993). If there is gross residual disease, either further surgical resection or focal boosting up to 70 Gy is advisable. Regions of somewhat lesser risk (i.e., clinically or pathologically uninvolved necks) should receive 50–54 Gy. As IMRT techniques are increasingly employed, simultaneous in-field boosts (Miller et al. 2005) are used to deliver these different doses in a comprehensive treatment plan composed of differential doses per fraction to the areas of high, intermediate, and low risk.

Altered Fractionation

It is well understood that head and neck squamous cell carcinomas (HNSCCs) are rapidly proliferating. There has been significant interest in the use of intensified radiation fractionation schedules to counter rapid tumor cell repopulation and potentially improve outcome in HNSCC treated with radiation. Altered fractionation regimens such as hyperfractionation or accelerated fractionation have been demonstrated to improve the likelihood of locoregional tumor control when used as definitive therapy (Peters et al. 1988). These altered fractionation regimens were associated with a higher incidence of grade 3 or worse acute mucosal toxicity, but no significant difference in overall toxicity at 2 years after completion of treatment. However, oral cavity carcinoma constituted a minority of cases enrolled in these studies (Fu et al. 2000), and data addressing the use of hyperfractionated radiation in the postoperative setting is sparse and heterogeneous in the conclusions reached (Ang et al. 2001; Awwad et al. 1992; Niewald et al. 1996), with some reports of excess morbidity in the form of osteoradionecrosis using this approach (Niewald et al. 1996). A single randomized study comparing conventional vs. accelerated fractionation in the postoperative setting showed no advantage to accelerated fractionation except in patients whose treatment initiation was delayed by postoperative complications (Sanguineti et al. 2005).

Brachytherapy

Historically, brachytherapy has played a key role in the treatment for oral cavity carcinoma, primarily as a boost to the primary site in the oral cavity before or after external beam radiation. Traditionally, radiation has been delivered using low dose rates of 0.4–0.6 Gy/h to the target volume (Mohanti et al. 2001; Strnad 2004). Treatments can be delivered using either rigid cesium needles or with ^{192}Ir sources afterloaded into angiocatheters (Fig. 6.3). The most common technique is after loading with [192]Ir (Wang et al. 1976). Guide needles can be inserted either free-hand or with the aid of a custom template to help maintain optimal source spacing.

Gradual improvements in both radiation and reconstructive surgery techniques have diminished the use of brachytherapy in the treatment of oral cavity carcinoma. Single-institution studies have evaluated brachytherapy techniques in the context of adjuvant therapy for locally advanced disease but have typically demonstrated unsatisfactory results in node-positive patients (Lapeyre et al. 2004). Further, the evolution

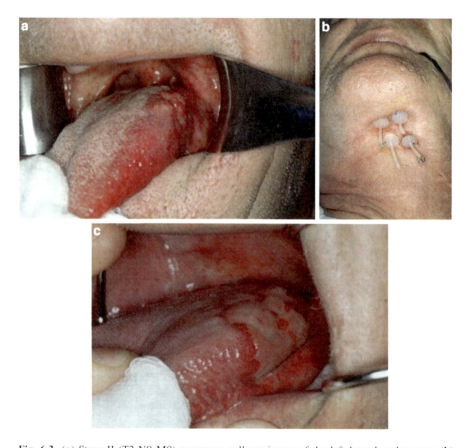

Fig. 6.3 (**a**) Stage II (T2 N0 M0) squamous cell carcinoma of the left lateral oral tongue. (**b**) Submental view of interstitial implantation catheters containing ^{192}Ir sources for delivery of a 25 Gy tumor boost after previous external beam radiation to a dose of 50 Gy. (**c**) Implantation bed mucositis conforming to the tumor distribution 7 days after 25 Gy implant boost. (From Halperin EC, Perez CA, Brady LW, eds., *Principles and practice of radiation oncology, fifth edition.* Philadelphia: Lippincott Williams & Wilkins, 2008, with permission)

of highly conformal external beam techniques such as IMRT has contributed to less frequent practice of brachytherapy in head and neck cancer overall.

Outcomes with Adjuvant Radiotherapy

Several randomized trials have evaluated surgery alone or in combination with radiotherapy. Robertson and colleagues conducted a phase III study in the United Kingdom of 350 patients with T2-4 N0-2 oral cavity or oropharyngeal cancers comparing surgery and postoperative radiation vs. radiation alone. Because a difference in survival was identified, the study was closed early. The authors found that after 23 months, overall survival, cause-specific survival, and local control were all improved on the surgery plus radiation arm (Robertson et al. 1998). Mishra et al. conducted a prospective randomized trial of surgery with or without adjuvant radiation 6 weeks after surgery in patients with carcinoma of the buccal mucosa (Mishra et al. 1996). They reported a 30% absolute improvement in disease-free survival, although there was no difference in overall survival with the use of adjuvant radiation therapy. Indications for postoperative radiation therapy include multiple cervical lymph node metastases, positive or close surgical margins, extracapsular nodal extension, perineural invasion, advanced T stage, and suspicion of mandibular cortical involvement.

Much of the outcome data for postoperative radiotherapy in regionally metastatic oral cavity cancer is gleaned from single-institution retrospective reports, which generally assess a specific subsite of the oral cavity (e.g., oral tongue, floor of mouth, buccal mucosa), and frequently include postoperative patients as only a small subset of the total cohort (Byers et al. 1981; Shibuya et al. 1984; Zelefsky et al. 1990; Rodgers et al. 1993; Hicks et al. 1997). These studies are all concordant with the limited randomized data in showing a locoregional control advantage to postoperative radiotherapy, providing additional clinical support for the use of combined-modality treatment.

Chemotherapy and Radiation

The role of chemotherapy in head and neck cancer has evolved considerably in recent years and is currently an important component of treatment in the definitive setting. Several studies demonstrate the benefit of radiation with concurrent chemotherapy administration in this setting (Adelstein et al. 2003; Brizel et al. 1998; Calais et al. 1999; Denis et al. 2004; Merlano et al. 1996; Staar et al. 2001; Wendt et al. 1998). Although these trials vary with respect to radiation dose, fractionation schedule, and chemotherapy regimen employed, they are all randomized comparisons between radiotherapy alone and radiotherapy plus chemotherapy. The advantage of concurrent chemotherapy with radiation has been further evaluated in several meta-analyses (Browman et al. 2001; El-Sayed and Nelson 1996; Munro 1995; Pignon et al. 2000). These meta-analyses generally identify a small overall survival benefit (1–8%) for the use of chemotherapy (Harari et al. 2003). Summary analyses suggest no significant survival benefit for the use of neoadjuvant and adjuvant chemotherapy but do suggest a clear benefit for the use of concurrent chemoradiation (Pignon et al. 2007). However, in many of the randomized studies comparing radiation alone to chemoradiation, oral cavity cancer patients are once again either excluded or make up only a small fraction of the study population.

The use of concurrent chemoradiation in the postoperative setting initially demonstrated encouraging locoregional control outcomes but failed to demonstrate an improvement in overall survival (Marcial et al. 1990; Al-Sarraf et al. 1997). These findings prompted several institutions to analyze both retrospective and prospective patient databases in an attempt to identify a population at high risk of local recurrence, with the hypothesis that treatment of appropriately selected high-risk patients with chemoradiation may confer an overall survival benefit. The findings of several of these studies are relatively homogeneous in nature, identifying positive surgical margins, ECE, and presence of two or more involved lymph nodes as being most strongly predictive of local recurrence (Ang et al. 2001; Cooper et al. 1998; Rosenthal et al. 2002; Langendijk et al. 2003). These findings provided impetus for two randomized multicenter trials to study the outcome in high-risk patients treated with postoperative chemoradiation.

Cooper et al. reported the results of a randomized study in North America comparing radiation alone (60–66 Gy) with chemoradiation (same radiation dose plus three cycles of 100 mg/m² cisplatin) in patients with head and neck carcinoma demonstrating high-risk features after gross total resection (Cooper et al. 2004). High-risk disease was defined as any or all of the following: two or more involved lymph nodes, ECE of nodal disease, and microscopically involved resection margins. This study demonstrated a benefit in locoregional control and disease-free survival at 2 years, favoring the chemoradiation arm, but no overall survival benefit was appreciated (Fig. 6.4a). A recent update of this trial with extended follow-up failed to show a difference between treatment arms in 5-year locoregional control and disease-free survival, although an unplanned subgroup analysis suggested a benefit in patients with positive margins or ECE (Cooper et al. 2006).

Fig. 6.4 Kaplan-Meier estimates for overall survival from EORTC 22931 (**a**), and RTOG 95-01 (**b**). (**c**) Comparative analysis of hazard ratio values for overall survival using pooled data from the European Organization for Research and Treatment of Cancer (EORTC) and RTOG trials in patients eligible for both trials or one trial only. Patients eligible for both trials included those with positive surgical margins and extracapsular nodal extension (ECE). (From Bernier J, Domenge C, Ozsahin M et al., Postoperative irradiation with or without concomitant chemotherapy for locally advanced head and neck cancer, *N Engl J Med.* 2004 May 6; 350(19):1945–1952, Cooper JS, Pajak TF, Forastiere AA et al., Postoperative concurrent radiotherapy and chemotherapy for high-risk squamous-cell carcinoma of the head and neck, *N Engl J Med.* 2004 May 6; 350(19):1937–1944, with permission; and Bernier J, Cooper JS, Pajak TF et al., Defining risk levels in locally advanced head and neck cancers: a comparative analysis of concurrent postoperative radiation plus chemotherapy trials of the EORTC (#22931) and RTOG (# 9501) *Head Neck,* 2005 Oct; 27(10):843–850, © 2005, J. Bernier, reprinted with permission of John Wiley & Sons, Inc.)

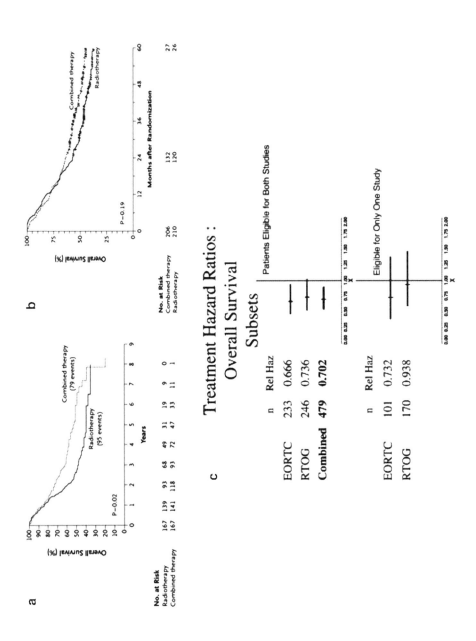

A parallel study in Europe by Bernier et al. randomized patients to essentially equivalent treatment arms following head and neck cancer surgery (Bernier et al. 2004). Eligibility criteria included patients with pathologic T3 or T4 disease (except T3 N0), or patients with any T stage disease with two or more involved lymph nodes, or patients with T1/T2 and N0/N1 disease with unfavorable pathologic findings (extranodal spread, positive margins, perineural involvement, or vascular embolism). Local control, progression-free survival, and overall survival were superior for patients on the chemoradiation arm (Fig. 6.4b). Both of these randomized trials demonstrate a significant increase in treatment-related toxicity in the chemoradiation arms, reinforcing the concept that the outcome benefit observed is a consequence of more aggressive treatment, with no appreciable change to the existing therapeutic ratio. A pooled data analysis of these two trials demonstrates a small but statistically significant improvement in locoregional control, disease-free survival, and overall survival in the chemoradiation arm for all enrolled patients but confirms that patients with positive surgical margins and/or ECE derived the majority of the outcome benefit (Fig. 6.4c) (Bernier et al. 2005). It should be noted that the pooled analysis does not incorporate updated outcome data from either trial, thereby limiting the evidence-based recommendation for postoperative chemoradiation to patients with positive margins and/or ECE.

Targeted Agents Combined with Radiation

In recent years, there has been a substantial increase in the exploration of targeted agents in an effort to improve the therapeutic ratio by alleviating some of the treatment-related toxicities commonly associated with cytotoxic chemotherapy. One such agent, cetuximab, was shown in initial laboratory studies to be an effective radiosensitizing agent in head and neck cancer cell lines (Huang et al. 1999; Milas et al. 2000). A randomized clinical trial comparing radiation alone or in combination with cetuximab as definitive treatment for head and neck cancer demonstrated an absolute survival benefit of 10% at 3 years with the use of cetuximab, with little substantial additive toxicity over radiation alone (Bonner et al. 2006). This led to the subsequent US Food and Drug Administration (FDA)-approval for this agent in the treatment of head and neck cancer.

A phase II randomized clinical trial recently conducted by the Radiation Therapy Oncology Group (RTOG) evaluated two cetuximab-based postoperative chemoradiation regimens in the patient population defined as high-risk by the Cooper study discussed previously (positive margins, two or more involved lymph nodes or ECE). Initial feasibility and toxicity reports show that the cetuximab-containing regimens are tolerable, with an incidence of grade 4–5 toxicity (9.2–10.1%) that compares favorably to the 15% estimate for radiation plus cisplatin from RTOG 95-01 (Harari et al. 2007).

Although the efficacy data from this trial are still maturing, it is hoped that this and other trials of targeted agents in combination with radiation will continue to suggest a widening of the therapeutic ratio, with preservation or improvement of outcomes and minimal additive toxicity for patients with high-risk disease.

References

Adelstein DJ, Li Y, Adams GL et al (2003) An intergroup phase III comparison of standard radiation therapy and two schedules of concurrent chemoradiotherapy in patients with unresectable squamous cell head and neck cancer. J Clin Oncol 21(1):92–98

Al-Sarraf M, Pajak TF, Byhardt RW et al (1997) Postoperative radiotherapy with concurrent cisplatin appears to improve locoregional control of advanced, resectable head and neck cancers: RTOG 88-24. Int J Radiat Oncol Biol Phys 37(4):777–782

Ang KK, Trotti A, Brown BW et al (2001) Randomized trial addressing risk features and time factors of surgery plus radiotherapy in advanced head-and-neck cancer. Int J Radiat Oncol Biol Phys 51(3):571–578

Awwad HK, Khafagy Y, Barsoum M et al (1992) Accelerated versus conventional fractionation in the postoperative irradiation of locally advanced head and neck cancer: Influence of tumour proliferation. Radiother Oncol 25(4):261–266

Bernier J, Domenge C, Ozsahin M et al (2004) Postoperative irradiation with or without concomitant chemotherapy for locally advanced head and neck cancer. N Engl J Med 350:1945–1952

Bernier J, Cooper JS, Pajak TF et al (2005) Defining risk levels in locally advanced head and neck cancers: A comparative analysis of concurrent postoperative radiation plus chemotherapy trials of the EORTC (#22931) and RTOG (# 9501). Head Neck 27(10):843–850

Bonner JA, Harari PM, Giralt J et al (2006) Radiotherapy plus cetuximab for squamous-cell carcinoma of the head and neck. N Engl J Med 354(6):567–78

Brizel DM, Albers ME, Fisher SR et al (1998) Hyperfractionated irradiation with or without concurrent chemotherapy for locally advanced head and neck cancer. N Engl J Med 338(25):1798–1804

Browman GP, Hodson DI, Mackenzie RJ et al (2001) Choosing a concomitant chemotherapy and radiotherapy regimen for squamous cell head and neck cancer: A systematic review of the published literature with subgroup analysis. Head Neck 23(7):579–589

Byers RM, Newman R, Russell N et al (1981) Results of treatment for squamous carcinoma of the lower gum. Cancer 47(9):2236–2238

Calais G, Alfonsi M, Bardet E et al (1999) Randomized trial of radiation therapy versus concomitant chemotherapy and radiation therapy for advanced-stage oropharynx carcinoma. J Natl Cancer Inst 91(24):2081–2086

Cooper JS, Pajak TF, Forastiere A et al (1998) Precisely defining high-risk operable head and neck tumors based on RTOG #85-03 and #88-24: Targets for postoperative radiochemotherapy? Head Neck 20(7):588–594

Cooper JS, Pajak TF, Forastiere AA et al (2004) Postoperative concurrent radiotherapy and chemotherapy for high-risk squamous-cell carcinoma of the head and neck. N Engl J Med 350:1937–1944

Cooper JS, Pajak TF, Forastiere AA et al (2006) Long-term survival results of a phase III Intergroup trial (RTOG 95-01) of surgery followed by radiotherapy vs. radiochemotherapy for resectable high risk squamous cell carcinoma of the head and neck. Int J Radiat Oncol Biol Phys 66(3):S14

Daly ME, Lieskovsky Y, Pawlicki T et al (2006) Evaluation of patterns of failure and subjective salivary function in patients treated with intensity modulated radiotherapy for head and neck squamous cell carcinoma. Head Neck

Day TA, Davis BK, Gillespie MB et al (2003) Oral cancer treatment. Curr Treat Options Oncol 4:27–41

Denis F, Garaud P, Bardet E et al (2004) Final results of the 94–01 French Head and Neck Oncology and Radiotherapy Group randomized trial comparing radiotherapy alone with concomitant radiochemotherapy in advanced-stage oropharynx carcinoma. J Clin Oncol 22(1):69–76

Eisbruch A, Ship JA, Dawson LA et al (2003) Salivary gland sparing and improved target irradiation by conformal and intensity modulated irradiation of head and neck cancer. World J Surg 27(7):832–837

El-Sayed S, Nelson N (1996) Adjuvant and adjunctive chemotherapy in the management of squamous cell carcinoma of the head and neck region. A meta-analysis of prospective and randomized trials. J Clin Oncol 14(3):838–847

Fiorino C, Dell'Oca I, Pierelli A et al (2006) Significant improvement in normal tissue sparing and target coverage for head and neck cancer by means of helical tomotherapy. Radiother Oncol 78(3):276–282

Fu KK, Ray JW, Chan EK et al (1976) External and interstitial radiation therapy of carcinoma of the oral tongue. A review of 32 years' experience. AJR Am J Roentgenol 126(1):107–115

Fu KK, Pajak TF, Trotti A et al (2000) A Radiation Therapy Oncology Group (RTOG) phase III randomized study to compare hyperfractionation and two variants of accelerated fractionation to standard fractionation radiotherapy for head and neck squamous cell carcinomas: First report of RTOG 9003. Int J Radiat Oncol Biol Phys 48(1):7–16

Harari PM, Mehta MP, Ritter MA et al (2003) Clinical promise tempered by reality in the delivery of combined chemoradiation for common solid tumors. Semin Radiat Oncol 13(1):3–12

Harari PM, Jaradat HA, Connor NP et al (2004) Refining target coverage and normal tissue avoidance with helical tomotherapy vs linac-based IMRT for oropharyngeal cancer. Int J Radiat Oncol Biol Phys 60(1):S160

Harari PM, Harris J, Kies MS et al (2007) Phase II randomized trial of surgery followed by chemoradiation plus cetuximab for high-risk squamous cell carcinoma of the head and neck (RTOG 0234). Int J Radiat Oncol Biol Phys 69(3):S13

Hicks WL Jr, Loree TR, Garcia RI et al (1997) Squamous cell carcinoma of the floor of mouth: A 20-year review. Head Neck 19(5):400–405

Hintz B, Charyulu K, Chandler JR et al (1979) Randomized study of local control and survival following radical surgery or radiation therapy in oral and laryngeal carcinomas. J Surg Oncol 12:61–74

Huang SM, Bock JM, Harari PM (1999) Epidermal growth factor receptor blockade with C225 modulates proliferation, apoptosis, and radiosensitivity in squamous cell carcinomas of the head and neck. Cancer Res 59(8):1935–1940

Langendijk JA, de Jong MA, Leemans CR et al (2003) Postoperative radiotherapy in squamous cell carcinoma of the oral cavity: The importance of the overall treatment time. Int J Radiat Oncol Biol Phys 57(3):693–700

Lapeyre M, Bollet MA, Racadot S et al (2004) Postoperative brachytherapy alone and combined postoperative radiotherapy and brachytherapy boost for squamous cell carcinoma of the oral cavity, with positive or close margins. Head Neck 26(3):216–223

Marcial VA, Pajak TF, Mohiuddin M et al (1990) Concomitant cisplatin chemotherapy and radiotherapy in advanced mucosal squamous cell carcinoma of the head and neck Long-term results of the Radiation Therapy Oncology Group study 81–17. Cancer 66(9):1861–1868

Merlano M, Benasso M, Corvo R et al (1996) Five-year update of a randomized trial of alternating radiotherapy and chemotherapy compared with radiotherapy alone in treatment of unresectable squamous cell carcinoma of the head and neck. J Natl Cancer Inst 88(9):583–589

Milas L, Mason K, Hunter N et al (2000) In vivo enhancement of tumor radioresponse by C225 antiepidermal growth factor receptor antibody. Clin Cancer Res 6(2):701–708

Miller KL, Shafman TD, Anscher MS et al (2005) Bronchial stenosis: An underreported complication of high-dose external beam radiotherapy for lung cancer? Int J Radiat Oncol Biol Phys 61(1):64–69

Mishra RC, Singh DN, Mishra TK (1996) Post-operative radiotherapy in carcinoma of buccal mucosa, a prospective randomized trial. Eur J Surg Oncol 22(5):502–504

Mohanti BK, Bansal M, Bahadur S et al (2001) Interstitial brachytherapy with or without external beam irradiation in head and neck cancer: Institute Rotary Cancer Hospital experience. Clin Oncol (R Coll Radiol) 13(5):345–352

Munro AJ (1995) An overview of randomised controlled trials of adjuvant chemotherapy in head and neck cancer. Br J Cancer 71(1):83–91

Niewald M, Barbie O, Schnabel K et al (1996) Risk factors and dose-effect relationship for osteoradionecrosis after hyperfractionated and conventionally fractionated radiotherapy for oral cancer. Br J Radiol 69(825):847–851

Peters LJ, Ang KK, Thames HD Jr (1988) Accelerated fractionation in the radiation treatment of head and neck cancer. A critical comparison of different strategies. Acta Oncol 27(2):185–194

Peters LJ, Goepfert H, Ang KK et al (1993) Evaluation of the dose for postoperative radiation therapy of head and neck cancer: First report of a prospective randomized trial. Int J Radiat Oncol Biol Phys 26(1):3–11

Pignon JP, Bourhis J, Domenge C et al (2000) Chemotherapy added to locoregional treatment for head and neck squamous-cell carcinoma: Three meta-analyses of updated individual data. MACH-NC Collaborative Group. Meta-analysis of chemotherapy on head and neck cancer. Lancet 355(9208):949–955

Pignon JP, le Maitre A, Bourhis J (2007) Meta-analyses of chemotherapy in head and neck cancer (MACH-NC): An update. Int J Radiat Oncol Biol Phys 69(Suppl 2):S112–S114

Robertson AG, Soutar DS, Paul J et al (1998) Early closure of a randomized trial: Surgery and postoperative radiotherapy versus radiotherapy in the management of intra-oral tumours. Clin Oncol (R Coll Radiol) 10(3):155–160

Rodgers LW Jr, Stringer SP, Mendenhall WM et al (1993) Management of squamous cell carcinoma of the floor of mouth. Head Neck 15(1):16–19

Rosenthal DI, Liu L, Lee JH et al (2002) Importance of the treatment package time in surgery and postoperative radiation therapy for squamous carcinoma of the head and neck. Head Neck 24(2):115–126

Sanguineti G, Richetti A, Bignardi M et al (2005) Accelerated versus conventional fractionated postoperative radiotherapy for advanced head and neck cancer: results of a multicenter Phase III study. Int J Radiat Oncol Biol Phys 61(3):762–771

Shah JP, Lydiatt W (1995) Treatment of cancer of the head and neck. CA Cancer J Clin 45(6):352–368

Sheng K, Molloy JA, Read PW (2006) Intensity-modulated radiation therapy (IMRT) dosimetry of the head and neck: A comparison of treatment plans using linear accelerator-based IMRT and helical tomotherapy. Int J Radiat Oncol Biol Phys 65(3):917–923

Shibuya H, Horiuchi J, Suzuki S et al (1984) Oral carcinoma of the upper jaw. Results of radiation treatment. Acta Radiol Oncol 23(5):331–335

Snow JB, Gelber RD, Kramer S et al (1981) Comparison of preoperative and postoperative radiation therapy for patients with carcinoma of the head and neck. Interim report. Acta Otolaryngol 91:611–626

Staar S, Rudat V, Stuetzer H et al (2001) Intensified hyperfractionated accelerated radiotherapy limits the additional benefit of simultaneous chemotherapy-results of a multicentric randomized German trial in advanced head-and-neck cancer. Int J Radiat Oncol Biol Phys 50(5):1161–1171

Strnad V (2004) Treatment of oral cavity and oropharyngeal cancer. Indications, technical aspects, and results of interstitial brachytherapy. Strahlenther Onkol 180(11):710–717

Studer G, Studer SP, Zwahlen RA et al (2006) Osteoradionecrosis of the mandible: Minimized risk profile following intensity-modulated radiation therapy (IMRT). Strahlenther Onkol 182(5):283–288

Vikram B, Strong EW, Shah J et al (1980) Elective postoperative radiation therapy in stages III and IV epidermoid carcinoma of the head and neck. Am J Surg 140(4):580–584

Wang CC, Boyer A, Mendiondo O (1976) Afterloading interstitial radiation therapy. Int J Radiat Oncol Biol Phys 1(3–4):365–368

Wendt TG, Grabenbauer GG, Rodel CM et al (1998) Simultaneous radiochemotherapy versus radiotherapy alone in advanced head and neck cancer: A randomized multicenter study. J Clin Oncol 16(4):1318–1324

Yao M, Dornfeld KJ, Buatti JM et al (2005) Intensity-modulated radiation treatment for head-and-neck squamous cell carcinoma – the University of Iowa experience. Int J Radiat Oncol Biol Phys 63(2):410–421

Zelefsky MJ, Harrison LB, Fass DE et al (1990) Postoperative radiotherapy for oral cavity cancers: Impact of anatomic subsite on treatment outcome. Head Neck 12(6):470–475

Chapter 7
Animal Models of Oral Cancer Metastasis

Zvonimir Milas, Jeffrey Myers, and Carlos Caulin

Abstract Metastasis is a complex, highly coordinated series of events in which cells from a primary tumor invade lymphatic and/or blood vessels and spread to regional lymph nodes and/or distant organs, establishing proliferating tumor deposits. Because this process requires the interaction of tumor cells with many types of normal cells, tissues, and systems of an intact organism, in vitro model systems provide very limited information regarding the biology of metastasis. Therefore, in vivo model systems are needed to further our understanding of the metastatic process. Several major types of murine model systems have been most informative and include those in which tumor cells are implanted into tissues or injected into the blood system. Also useful are autochthonous models, in which tumors with metastatic potential are induced at the primary site, in this case, the oral cavity, through treatment of the oral mucosa with chemical carcinogens or by genetically engineering changes in the expression of oncogenes and tumor suppressor genes in the oral epithelia. This chapter summarizes the progress that has been made in the development of mouse models of metastasis in oral cancer and the contributions of these models to our understanding of the biology of oral cancer metastasis.

Introduction

Metastasis, the establishment of secondary growths at sites distant from the primary tumor, results from a cascade of sequential steps, including the entry of tumor cells into the blood or lymphatic circulation, their transit within the circulation, and the lodging and growth of these cells at remote tissues and organs. The metastatic process includes a complex, highly coordinated series of events involving tumor cells and their interactions with host tissues and systems including the basement membrane; the surrounding stroma; the lymphatic and systemic vasculature; the immune

J. Myers (✉)
Department of Head and Neck Surgery-Unit 441, University of Texas M D Anderson Cancer, 1515 Holcombe Blvd, Houston, TX, 77030, USA
e-mail: jmyers@mdanderson.org

J. Myers (ed.), *Oral Cancer Metastasis*,
DOI 10.1007/978-1-4419-0775-2_7, © Springer Science+Business Media, LLC 2010

system; the lymph nodes; and distant organs such as the lungs, liver, brain, and bones. In vitro analyses of the molecular and cellular processes constituting the hallmarks of cancer cells, including unchecked cell proliferation, loss of growth inhibitory signals, loss of apoptotic mechanisms, and elaboration of proteolytic enzymes, are not sufficient to fully demonstrate the complex interplay between tumor cells and the organism in which tumors develop and spread. Rather, in vivo metastatic models are needed to better identify the multiple molecular and cellular interactions between tumor cells and host tissues that are required for the development of metastases. Mouse models have been particularly helpful in this regard and comprise a wide array of model systems, including human tumor or cell line implantation in orthotopic or heterotopic sites in immunosuppressed animals, tumor implantation studies in syngeneic animals, chemical carcinogenesis models, and genetically engineered mouse models. Each of these systems has been used in the study of oral cancer metastases and has provided insights into the metastatic process. In this chapter, we will summarize the relative merits and deficiencies of the different types of metastatic models and the progress that has been with each of these in the study of oral cancer metastases.

Historical Background

Toward the end of the nineteenth century, Dr. Stephen Paget, a British surgeon, proposed the "seed and soil" hypothesis of cancer metastasis, wherein he postulated that cancer cells are the "seeds" that have the variant capacity to escape from the primary tumor, spread to, and implant in a distant tissue and that specific qualities of the recipient tissues determine the condition of "the soil," which enables a metastasis to proliferate, survive, and progress in that tissue (Paget 1889). Paget described the preference of tumor metastasis and the locations as a result of specific organs providing a more suitable growth environment for that specific tumor cell type. This was supported by his observations of breast cancer cases in which metastases from breast cancers were more often observed to occur in the liver as opposed to other organs examined, indicating that the site of metastasis development did not occur by chance.

Experimental evidence for Dr. Paget's astute clinical observations and clearly stated hypothesis came from the investigations of Dr. Isaiah Fidler and his colleagues, who used an elegant animal model of melanoma, in which subcutaneously implanted tumors metastasized preferentially to the lungs and ovaries (Hart and Fidler 1980). In this work, they went on to show that even though tumor cells initially became trapped in multiple organs, they ultimately took root and grew only in selected sites.

This work demonstrated that the process of metastasis is relatively inefficient, as only a small subset of cells can overcome each of the multiple successive limiting steps and actually form viable metastases (Weiss 1996). The initial steps of metastasis include the loss of cell–cell contacts, adhesion to the extracellular matrix

(ECM), and the capacity to survive detachment from the ECM (Swan et al. 2003). Once this is achieved, tumor cells must be motile enough to migrate through the surrounding stroma and express proteases in order to invade through the basement membrane (Zucker et al. 2000). Next, cells must be able to bind to and transverse the lymphatic and systemic vasculature (Ji 2006). Once within the circulation, the tumor cells must survive the kinetic and shear forces in order to progress to the next step of metastasis formation. Also within the circulatory or lymphatic system, the tumor cells are exposed to increased immune system surveillance. The tumor cells must avoid detection or identification by natural killer cells and cytotoxic T lymphocytes, which have been implicated in the reduction of tumor metastases (Habu et al. 1981; Kasai et al. 1981). Once the tumor cells have spread through the circulatory system, they can become embedded through embolization within a capillary bed or extravasate through a process of adhesion and migration into distant sites. Within this new locale, the tumor cells must receive adequate growth factors via autocrine or paracrine signaling that ensure their survival and proliferation (Hill 2002). Finally, establishment of angiogenesis is important for sustaining the continued growth of metastatic foci.

To study the complicated, multifactorial process of metastasis, examination of the characteristics of the local tissue and the host factors is as important as the study of the tumor cell characteristics. Therefore, despite many technological advances, in vitro experiments cannot entirely recreate the local tissue conditions necessary to study the later stages of the metastatic process. Consequently, research into the mechanisms of tumor metastasis has required in vivo models to reproduce clinical conditions and host factors as closely as possible.

Several major types of murine model systems have been used to study the complex interplay of tumor cell and host factors in vivo, and these include implantation models in which tumor cells are implanted into tissues or injected into the circulation. The other major class of murine models that have been useful for studies of metastasis are autochthonous tumors models. In these models, tumors with metastatic potential are induced at the primary site, in this case, the oral cavity, through treatment of the oral mucosa with chemical carcinogens or by genetically engineering changes in the expression of oncogenes and tumor suppressor genes in the oral epithelia.

Implantation Metastasis Models

There are two major classes of in vivo tumor implantation models of metastasis, specifically, spontaneous metastasis models and experimental metastasis models, both of which have been used with syngeneic murine tumor cells in immunocompetent mice as well as xenogenic human tumor cell lines in immunosupressed mice. In the experimental metastasis model, tumor cells are prepared in single cell suspension from excised tumors or in vitro cultured cell lines and are then injected into the circulation via an intravenous (commonly tail vein), intra-arterial or intraportal route.

An illustrative example of this model is the generation of metastases of the murine B16 melanoma in syngeneic C57BL mice (Fidler 1973; Fidler and Kripke 1977). B16 melanoma cells were injected intravenously into syngeneic mice with resultant lung tumor nodules observable at about 2 weeks after tumor cell inoculation. The cells from these nodules were cultured and re-injected into mice. With each successive injection from cultured metastases, the average number of resultant pulmonary tumors increased. Subsequent research used multiple cultured sub-clones of the B16 melanoma cell line to look for phenotypic changes in the subclones' ability to produce lung metastases after intravenous injection (Fidler and Kripke 1977). Through these seminal studies, Fidler and Kripke demonstrated that the original B16 melanoma tumor was heterogeneous and contained clonal cell populations of variant metastatic potential, and this has become one of the key principles of metastatic tumor biology.

Momose et al. confirmed this principle of clonal heterogeneity in oral squamous cell carcinoma (HSC-3) using both experimental metastasis and spontaneous metastasis models (Momose et al. 1989). More recently, the experimental metastasis model of syngeneic B16 melanoma has been combined with cDNA microarrays to identify a metastasis related gene, RhoC, in the B16 melanoma clonal population (Clark et al. 2000). Clark's study demonstrates that the experimental metastasis model continues to yield important information as newer methods of molecular characterization are used to distinguish differences in the expression of molecules critical to the metastatic process between highly metastatic cells derived from a minimally metastatic heterogeneous cell line.

Experimental metastasis models, however, have not been used commonly in the study of oral squamous cell carcinomas for several reasons (Momose et al. 1989). The experimental metastasis model bypasses the early determinants of tumor metastasis, notably tumor cell adhesion and invasion. It evaluates the metastatic process only after tumor cells have gained vascular access, and it does not evaluate loss of tumor cell adhesion, ECM proteolysis, and the subsequent tumor cell vascular or lymphatic invasion (Hill 2002). The metastases that form from direct intravascular injection of tumor cells can be a result of tumor embolization or from tumor cell adhesion and diapedesis, and the experimental metastasis model cannot accurately distinguish between these two mechanisms. Nonetheless, the experimental metastasis model does appropriately re-approximate tumors and condition that result in hematogenous metastasis.

Experimental metastatic models have several significant advantages. For example, the number of tumor cells injected can be controlled allowing for easier comparison and study of tumor metastasis efficiency in a specific tumor cell line. In addition, in the experimental model, tumor metastasis formation is generally synchronous in animals injected simultaneously allowing for larger-scale experiments, and the metastases formed tend to preserve the phenotypic characteristics of the injected cells.

Although the experimental metastasis model remains a very powerful tool with significant advantages and certain limitations, research in oral squamous cell carcinoma and its metastases has predominantly relied on spontaneous tumor models. A major reason for this is that the major clinical problem in the metastasis of oral cancer is regional lymphatic metastasis more than systemic metastatic spread through the hematogenous route. However, clinical trials of the nonsurgical treatment of squamous cell cancers of nonoral upper aerodigestive tract (UADT) sites indicate that as local-regional control improves, the rate of death as a result of development of metastasis also increases. Thus, the issue of distant metastasis in UADT cancer is becoming clinically more relevant and will require additional preclinical studies in appropriate complementary model systems.

In spontaneous tumor models, cell suspensions or explanted tumor fragments are implanted within a particular tissue, and this allows for local tumor establishment and the possibility for the development of regional and/or systemic metastases. In spontaneous tumor models, either syngeneic murine tumor cells or human explants or cell lines can be implanted in orthotopic or heterotopic locations, and then the spontaneous development of tumor metastases can be studied. A major advantage then of spontaneous tumor models in contrast to experimental metastasis models, is that the spontaneous tumor model does not abrogate the initial steps needed for a tumor to form metastases. However, there are relative disadvantages to spontaneous tumor models, which are dependent on the particular tumor model. Creating a large cohort of metastasized tumors for investigation can be difficult because metastasis development is not assured, nor is it temporally identical between test animals. Local injection may create a breakdown in the basement membrane, thereby bypassing the initial invasion steps through the basement membrane and facilitating the escape of tumor cells. Metastases tend to be late events, in animal models and humans. A risk of the spontaneous tumor model is that the mouse may succumb to local effects from the primary tumor implant, particularly if the tumor is implanted orthotopically (Bibby 2004). This is highly relevant to the study of oral squamous cell carcinoma in which orthotopic implantation often creates difficulties in an animal's ability to eat, which may threaten the animal's survival prior to the development of metastasis.

Orthotopic Models and Metastasis

In one of the first investigations demonstrating the feasibility of orthotopic implantation, Tan et al. (1977) successfully performed orthotopic transplantation of murine colon adenocarcinomas into the colon of syngeneic mice (Tan et al. 1977). At the time, they also noted an increase in liver metastases in this model, thus setting the stage for the use of orthotopic modeling in metastasis research.

In the late 1980s and early 1990s, several reports emerged describing the development of orthotopic models of oral squamous cell carcinoma with varying degrees of success (Fitch et al. 1988; Dinesman et al. 1990; Kawashiri et al. 1995). Fitch et al. aspirated cells from fresh human tumors growing subcutaneously in nude mice and then injected these cells into the tongues of nude mice (Fitch et al. 1988).

This model demonstrated comparable tumorigenicity between the subcutaneous and orthotopic site probably because of the method of harvesting cells from already growing and implanted subcutaneous tumors. Dinesman et al. developed a slightly different model implanting cells into the floor of the mouth in nude mice to imitate the physiologic environment of the oral cavity (Dinesman et al. 1990). Tumor cells were injected via a submandibular route into the tissue, deep in to the mylohyoid muscle beneath the floor of the mouth. They observed that only 5% of the mice had lymph node metastases, whereas 40% had pulmonary metastases. This finding contrasted both clinical human patterns of oral squamous cell carcinoma and prior murine subcutaneous oral squamous cell carcinoma models. The discrepancy in tumor metastases between lung and lymph nodes in Dinesman's model is not fully understood. That notwithstanding, the floor of the mouth model captured significant attention for its tremendous potential in oral cancer research.

Dinesman's floor of the mouth model was slightly modified by Simon et al. who implanted SCC cells into the floor of the mouth, at a depth superficial to the mylohyoid muscle (Simon et al. 1998). Kawashiri et al. and Myers et al. were the first to describe orthotopic lingual models of oral squamous cell carcinoma (Kawashiri et al. 1999; Kawashiri et al. 1995; Myers et al. 2002). Both groups injected nude mice with variable numbers of tumor cells in the submucosa of the tongue through a transoral approach. These mice reliably developed local tumors with lymph node metastases. Qui et al. modified this lingual model by transplanting 1 mm^3 fresh human specimen, instead of tumor cell suspensions, into nude mice (Qiu et al. 2003). The rationale of this model was to maintain the cell-to-cell interactions whose disruption is the prerequisite to metastasis.

The use of orthotopic transplantation models can also expose factors of clinical significance to the disease process not seen in subcutaneous models. In nonoral squamous cell tumors, Kuo and Fidler independently established the stark differences between subcutaneous tumors and orthotopic tumors in response to chemotherapy (Fidler et al. 1994; Kuo et al. 1993). Kawashiri et al. observed another difference between the subcutaneous and orthotopic implantation site. They injected nude mice with well-established oral squamous cell carcinoma cell lines, OSC19 and OSC20, and then compared the histological difference of the tumors between the implantation sites. The heterotopic subcutaneous tumor had a more expansive but poorly invasive growth pattern. In contrast, the orthotopic implanted tumors expressed a more locally invasive pattern, similar to the original tumors (Kawashiri et al. 1995). This observation of variable growth between subcutaneous and orthotopic tumors in oral squamous cell tumors has been validated by other authors (Myers et al. 2002). These experiments substantiated the principle in oral squamous cell carcinoma that the orthotopic transplantation of tumor cells produce tumors that better mimic the phenotypic properties of the original tumor, compared to heterotopic injection.

With the clear establishment of the value of orthotopic models in the study of oral squamous cell carcinoma metastasis, a body of literature has developed specifically investigating diverse aspects of the biology of metastasis and their response to therapeutics. In addition, metastatic oral squamous cell carcinoma explanted from cervical lymph nodes generated more aggressive clones with a higher metastatic potential after sequential re-culturing and orthotopic re-implantation, as previously observed with the melanoma B16 model (Myers et al. 2002; Qiu et al. 2003; Matsui et al. 1998). This process can lead to the outgrowth of tumor subclones with different metastatic potential, which can be used to identify gene expression patterns and epigenetic changes predisposing tumors to metastasize. Others have used the orthotopic model to develop preclinical models to test targeted therapy for oral squamous cell carcinoma metastasis. Thus, molecular targeting of epidermal growth factor receptor (EGFR) and vascular endothelial growth factor receptor (VEGFR) has been found to reduce metastasis formation (Yazici et al. 2005; Shintani et al. 2003). In addition, Lee et al. observed that lupeol, a nuclear factor kappa B (NF-κB) inhibitor, used with the combination of chemotherapy resulted in tumor size reduction and decreased metastasis formation (Lee et al. 2007). In another example, Marimastat, a broad matrix metalloproteinase (MMP) inhibitor, decreased the rate of cervical lymph node metastasis even though it did not reduce the original tumor volume (Maekawa et al. 2002). These studies and many others highlight the depth and breadth of investigations being carried out in oral cancer tumor models.

Xenograft and Syngeneic Models

Most of the models discussed so far have used human cancer cell lines that have been transplanted into immunosuppressed mice. Nude, athymic mice (nu/nu) and severe combined immunodeficient (SCID) mice that are T and B lymphocyte cell deficient tolerate engraftment of human xenografted tissue including malignant tumors. Indeed, xenografts of oral squamous cell carcinoma were first reported in the mid 1980s with very good success (Braakhuis et al. 1984; Baker 1985), and they have since been the most commonly used models in the study of oral squamous cell carcinoma. However, the relevance of using immunosuppressed mice in xenograft models for human cancer has been a topic of much discussion.

There are certainly disadvantages with using immunosuppressed mice and xenografted tumors. Although nude mice retain innate immunity, natural killer (NK) lymphocytes and macrophages, they are T-lymphocyte cell deficient. In early studies, NK cells were found to limit tumor growth and potentially prevent metastasis (Habu et al. 1981; Kasai et al. 1981). Later, Xie et al. compared SCID mice and nude mice with three different tumor cell lines and found no significant difference between the two immunosuppressed mouse strains in tumor growth rates or cytotoxicity induced by NK cells. They did, however, observe a higher metastasis rate in all the three cell lines in the SCID mice (Xie et al. 1992). Immunosuppressed mice also lack the human stroma and immune cells, which are important to the metastatic process (Varney et al. 2002). Considering the advantages and limitations of the xenograft models, it is not surprising to find that their use as preclinical models for testing drug efficacy has produced contrasting results. While there are studies that suggest a good correlation between xenograft data and clinical activity of drugs (Fiebig and Berger 1995), other studies are not as supportive (Johnson et al. 2001).

Regardless of the positive findings, legitimate concerns regarding the interpretation of studies using immune deficient mice still remain.

Studies in immunocompetent models would, theoretically, more accurately replicate the human clinical condition. Therefore, several investigators have developed syngeneic tumor models for oral squamous cell carcinoma. However, the widespread development of these models has been limited by the relatively rare occurrence of spontaneous oral cancers in immunocompetent mice. O'Malley et al. devised an attractive immunocompetent murine model for oral cancer by injecting cells from the murine cutaneous squamous cell carcinoma cell line, SCC VII, into the floor of the mouth of syngeneic C3H/HeJ mice (O'Malley et al. 1997). They observed cervical lymph node and pulmonary metastases usually by the third week from injection. Interestingly, a subsequent study further characterized this tumor cell line and did not find any systemic metastases following intradermal (subcutaneous) injection in the flank (Khurana et al. 2001). The SCC VII syngeneic squamous cell carcinoma arose spontaneously in the abdominal wall of a C3H mouse and is, therefore, technically not a squamous cell carcinoma of oral mucosa origin (Hirst et al. 1982). Regardless, this was an important development that has allowed research into a syngeneic model with an intact immune system using a squamous cell carcinoma.

Another spontaneous squamous cell carcinoma, AT-84, in the C3H mouse was identified (Hier et al. 1995). This cell line was initially used in a subcutaneous model. Later, Lou et al. implanted AT-84 in an orthotopic tongue model and compared it to the subcutaneous model used previously (Lou et al. 2003; Lou et al. 2002). Their findings were very similar to those seen with SCC VII tumor cell line; the tumor was not regionally metastatic with subcutaneous implantation. They saw only lung metastases and did not observe lymph node metastases, leading them to believe the mechanism of metastasis for AT-84 was primarily hematogenous (Lou et al. 2003). Both AT-84 and SCC VII represent tremendous potential for investigation of squamous cell carcinomas in an immunocompetent system. However, their metastases seem to be predominantly hematogenous, unlike human oral squamous cell carcinoma tumors and xenografts.

Detection of Metastasis

Detection of metastatic foci, whether in lymph nodes or distant organs, can present a significant challenge. Classically, the presence of metastasis has been evaluated at necropsy in euthanized mice after completion of the experimental protocol. In oral squamous cell carcinoma, most investigators resect both the draining lymph node basins and the lungs for pathological evaluation. The histology slides are then stained and examined in detail to identify foci of metastasis. At the molecular level, metastatic cells can be detected by using molecular markers present in the metastasis but not in the host tissue. For instance, Komori et al. developed a polymerase chain reaction (PCR) technique using specific primers for human β-globin and mutant p53 genes to identify the presence of metastases in lymph node and lung samples from xenografted oral squamous carcinomas (Komatsubara et al. 2002; Shigeta et al. 2007). Although very valuable for metastasis detection, these techniques require tissue processing and are not feasible for the detection of tumor cells in viable tissues. Another classical approach to metastasis identification is the use of pigmented cells, such as B16 melanoma, to macroscopically identify metastases. Unfortunately, oral squamous cell carcinomas do not innately have such an advantage.

Several techniques have been adapted for visualization of metastasis in mice, including the generation of xenografts using cell lines modified to express molecular markers that can be readily detected in host tissues, such as the Escherichia coli beta-galactosidase (lacZ) gene (Lin et al. 1990). This technique allows the visualization of tumor and metastatic cells at the single cell level. However, the detection of lacZ activity requires histological preparation of tissues and cannot be used for cellular imaging in live animals. Subsequently, newer technologies have been developed to detect tumor cells in live cells, allowed to visualize in vivo oral squamous cell carcinoma formation and the metastases derived from them.

The green fluorescent protein (GFP) was cloned from the bioluminescent jellyfish *Aequorea Victoria* in the early 1970s (Morin and Hastings 1971), and was more recently applied as a marker for gene expression in animal models in the mid 1990s (Chalfie et al. 1994; Cheng et al. 1996). This technology was quickly applied to the tumor cell imaging of GFP-transfected cells xenografted in animal models, which can be visualized with intravital microscopy using a multiphoton confocal microscope, facilitated by the long-term half-life of the GFP protein (Hoffman 2002). This provided an opportunity for the real-time observation of tumors, angiogenesis, and metastasis. Initially, this technique was limited to the investigation of ectopic primary tumors or exteriorized organs using multiphoton confocal microscopy.

Several studies have used GFP for imaging primary oral squamous cell carcinoma and metastasis. Myers et al. demonstrated the feasibility of imaging exteriorized lymph nodes to determine the presence of lymph node metastases in an orthotopic tongue model (Fig. 7.1) (Myers et al. 2002). This was later reproduced and verified by other authors (Shintani et al. 2002). Advances in technology of whole body imaging and higher resolution imaging increased the versatility of GFP-based visualization approaches (Hoffman 2002; Yang et al. 2001). Although GFP imaging is not widely used in oral squamous cell carcinoma models, it remains a powerful tool for metastasis monitoring and animal imaging.

In essentially synchronous development with GFP, bioluminescence with the enzyme firefly luciferase (luc) has been applied to noninvasive in vivo tumor measurement. The gene encoding luciferase, a photoprotein from the *photinus pyralis* firefly is transfected into human tumor cells and its expression can be used to monitor tumor growth and response to antineoplastic agents (Zhang et al. 1994). Unlike GFP, detection of luciferase activity requires that the substrate, luciferin, be administered to mice prior to detection; but due to its relatively short half-life it is a real-time indicator of transcription and a better reporter to monitor changes in gene expression, compared to the longer lived and expressed GFP (Contag et al. 2000). These properties make tumor cells transfected with luciferase, a valuable tool for monitoring tumor kinetics, growth, and response to treatment in real-time.

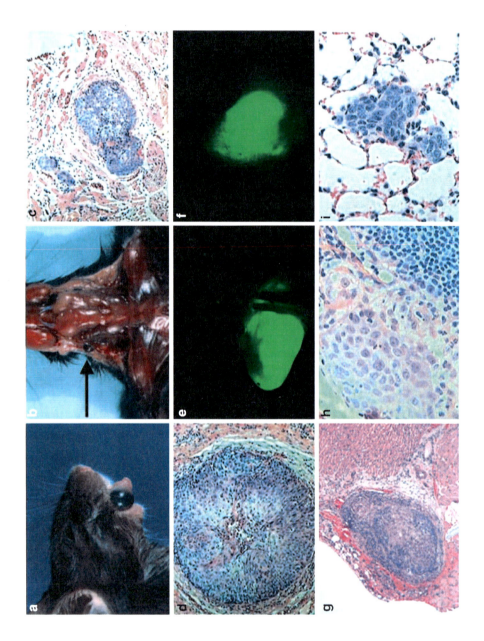

A major advantage of using luciferase for tumor studies in animal models is provided by current optical systems that allow specific and sensitive detection of luciferase activity in internal tissues, critical to identifying tumor metastasis. Application of this technology to oral squamous cell carcinomas has been carried out by Sano and Myers, who have found that an orthotopic tongue tumor and subsequent regional metastases can be monitored via luciferase imaging both before and after partial glossectomy (Fig. 7.2) (Sano and Myers 2007). The use of the luciferase gene in in vivo models for oral cancer is gaining in popularity (Patel et al. 2004; Henson et al. 2007).

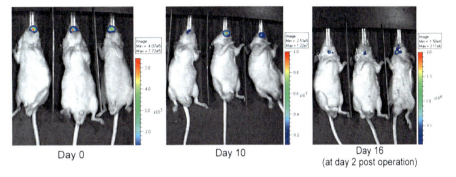

Day 0   Day 10   Day 16
(at day 2 post operation)

Fig. 7.2 Bioluminescence imaging of mice orthotopically transplanted with luciferase-transduced cells. The tips of the mice tongues were injected with OSC19Luc + cells. The mice were imaged using the IVIS 200 imaging system (Xenogen Corporation, Berkeley, CA). Initial imaging (day 0) demonstrates engraftment of the orthotopic transplanted xenografted OSC19Luc + cells. Repeat bioluminescent imaging (day 10) shows continued localized photon emission at the site of tongue tumor growth. Glossectomy was performed on day 14, and 2 days after glossectomy. Cervical lymph node metastases are identified in vivo without animal sacrifice through the bioluminescence of the tumors (day 16)

◀

Fig. 7.1 Orthotopic Tongue Model: Histology and Imaging Techniques with GFP. Panels (**a**) and (**b**) demonstrate regional metastasis from orthotopic sublingual implantation of B16-BL6 melanoma. The tongues of C57BL/6 black mice were inoculated with syngeneic B16-BL6 melanoma cells; the mice were killed after 14 days and necropsy performed. An obvious tumor is seen in the tongue. Bilateral metastases are easily identified by melanotic pigmentation within the cervical lymph nodes. Comparative histopathology illustrates the resemblance between orthotopically transplanted, xenografted Tu167 human SCC implanted into the oral tongue of a nude mouse, panel (**c**), with a pathology specimen of human squamous cell carcinoma of the tongue, panel (**d**). Panels (**e**)–(**g**) demonstrate green fluorescent protein's (GFP's) role in visualization of orthotopic tongue tumors and regional metastasis. Tu159GFP was inoculated submucosally in the tongue of each mouse; the mouse was sacrificed, and the tumor was visualized under a dissecting fluorescence microscope. The primary tumor in the tongue (**e**) is readily apparent. An area of fluorescence, noted in the submandibular region (**f**), was resected, revealing metastatic tumor on microscopic examination (**g**). The final two panels are hematoxylin-eosin-stained slides of metastasis found with GFP imaging. Panel (**h**) shows a cervical lymph node with subcapsular metastatic tumor in a nude mouse in which the Tu167G-LN1 line was grown orthotopically. Panel (**i**) is an image of distant metastatic tumor in the lungs from the same experiment

Other techniques have been developed to assist in identification and evaluation of metastases including computed tomography (CT) and three-dimensional image reconstruction which have been miniaturized to image mice and other rodents. Several authors have used microCT to characterize the locally invasive and destructive nature of oral cancers in the xenograft orthotopic model (Cui et al. 2005; Henson et al. 2007; Nomura et al. 2007). Other novel and miniaturized imaging modalities have been applied to in vivo animal research of oral squamous cell carcinoma. For example, Melancon et al. developed and tested novel imaging compounds designed for dual magnetic resonance (MR)-optical imaging in mice bearing orthotopic tongue tumors. They then applied this compound with the dual MR-optical imaging to more sensitively detect, localize, and characterize sentinel lymph nodes in an orthotopic tumor mouse model (Melancon et al. 2007). Erdem et al. has used micropositron emission tomography (PET)/CT imaging to identify and compare the locally invasive characteristics and metastatic capacities of several oral squamous cell carcinoma cell lines after injecting into the masseter muscle in SCID mice (Erdem et al. 2008).

Autochthonous Mouse Models

Mouse models generated by transplantation of tumors or cell lines into immunosuppressed or immunocompetent mice have provided significant progress in understanding biological mechanisms and molecular pathways involved in oral cancer metastasis, as detailed in previous sections of this chapter. However, metastasis is a complex process that starts in the primary tumor and involves the interaction of tumor cells with surrounding normal epithelial cells and a variety of cells of different lineages that make up the tumor microenvironment. During tumor progression, cancer cells accumulate genetic alterations that contribute to invasion and metastasis in processes that involve the interaction of the tumor cells with the stroma. The significance of these interactions in metastasis development can only be fully evaluated in tumors that develop endogenously in the context of a functional immune system.

Initially, autochthonous oral tumors were generated in animal models by using chemical carcinogenesis protocols on rodents, including hamsters, rats and mice. These models have been extensively used to study the biology of oral tumor formation, molecular alterations that contribute to oral tumor formation and malignant progression and as preclinical models for testing the efficiency of potential antitumor agents. Chemical carcinogenesis models have contributed to the concept that oral cancers result from the accumulation of multiple genetic alterations. When the technology to manipulate the mouse genome became available, the first transgenic mouse models for oral cancer were developed. In these models, potential oncogenes are targeted for expression in the oral epithelium to determine their role during oral carcinogenesis. More recently, technological advances have allowed replacement of normal mouse genes for mutant forms similar to those found in human oral cancers. In addition, the ability to activate endogenous mutations exclusively in the oral epithelium allows the generation of models that closely recapitulate in the mouse, the genetic events identified in human oral cancers. In the next sections, we will discuss some of the advances in understanding oral tumor progression and metastasis provided by mouse models with autochthonous oral tumors.

Chemical Carcinogenesis Models

Cancer induction in animal models by exposure to carcinogens has been used extensively in cancer research for nearly 100 years, since the initial studies by Yamagiwa and Ichikawa in 1915 demonstrated that application of coal tar to the ears of rabbits induced skin squamous cell carcinomas (Yamagiwa and Ichikawa 1977). Subsequent efforts concentrated on identifying and isolating potential carcinogens that were tested for their tumorigenic properties in multiple organs in different animal models. Attempts to induce cancers of the oral cavity by treatment with chemical carcinogens in experimental models culminated in 1954 with the first report documenting squamous cell carcinoma formation in the cheek pouch of the Syrian hamster after repeated application of 9,10-dimethyl-1,2-benz(a)anthracene (DMBA) (Salley 1954). The Syrian hamster was chosen for these studies because the two cheek pouches, lined by stratified epithelia, can be readily inverted and pulled out for easy access and gross observation. Interestingly, all the animals that were treated with DMBA in this study developed oral squamous cell carcinomas with cervical lymph node metastasis. These observations predicted that the hamster cheek pouch model would be an invaluable system to study the biology of oral cancer metastasis. However, despite extensive application of this model, and meticulous search for local and distant metastases by different laboratories (Shklar 1966; Dachi et al. 1967; Levij et al. 1967), metastases were not reported again using similar carcinogenesis protocols until 1970, when a lymph node metastasis was found in one hamster from a group of ten animals that received DMBA (Rwomushana et al. 1970). This was certainly a rare case since the authors reported in the same publication that this was the only metastasis found in their laboratory out of 562 animals that had been treated with DMBA during a 4-year period.

It was reasoned that the rapid growth of the primary oral tumors that developed in the hamster cheek pouch resulted in the formation of large size tumors that compromised the life of the animals before the tumors reached metastatic potential, suggesting that efforts to increase the lifespan of tumor-bearing hamsters would allow extra time for malignant progression. In fact, excision of the largest primary oral tumors from the hamster cheek pouch increased the survival of the animals and the rates of lymph node metastasis, which reached almost 50% of the treated animals (Craig 1980). It was unclear whether the high rates of local metastasis was a direct consequence of the longer lifespan of the animals and the extended time to develop metastasis or whether the surgical procedure used to remove the tumors facilitated the spread of malignant cells. In this regard, Safour et al. demonstrated that incision of normal oral tissue with blades that had previously been used to practice incisions in hamster cheek pouch tumors induced oral cancer formation at the incision site with similar metastatic rates (Safour et al. 1984), suggesting that the surgical procedures contributed to the high rates of metastasis after removal of the primary tumors. Indeed, subsequent studies demonstrated that metastases to cervical lymph nodes were only observed in hamsters that received surgical removal of DMBA-induced oral squamous cell carcinomas, but not in control animals in which tumors were left untouched during the same period of time, again indicating that surgical excision of the primary tumors can augment the metastatic potential of oral cancer cells (Kage et al. 1987).

These studies suggested that primary tumors contain cells with potential to colonize and grow in distant organs although their dissemination may be restricted by the tumor microenvironment. Interestingly, administration of cyclosporin A after excision of DMBA-induced oral tumors increased the incidence of cervical lymph node metastasis to 90% (Yamada et al. 1992), suggesting that the immune system can control the metastatic progression of oral cancers. Later studies reported a correlation between the elevated levels of cytokines such as tumor necrosis factor alpha (TNFα) and interleukin-6 (IL-6) and suppression of the cervical lymph node metastasis of DMBA-induced oral tumors in hamsters (Nakajima et al. 1996), supporting an antimetastatic role for certain cytokines. Surgical excision of the primary tumors has been used occasionally to facilitate local metastatic spread of chemically induced oral tumors in the hamster cheek pouch, but perhaps due to the labor-intensive procedure that involves surgery for every single mouse, this procedure has not been extensively used and alternative approaches were sought.

Attempting to develop new strategies to increase the malignant potential of oral squamous cell carcinomas that develop in experimental models, several laboratories found that scratching the surface of the hamster tongue epithelium prior to the application of DMBA increased the tumor incidence, accelerated squamous cell carcinoma formation and resulted in low incidence on regional lymph node metastasis (Fujita et al. 1973; Take et al. 1999). While it is possible that the increased metastatic potential observed in the oral squamous cell carcinomas that developed in these animals reflects advanced stages of malignant progression of the primary squamous cell carcinomas generated by this protocol, it is also conceivable that the mechanical trauma induced prior to the application of the carcinogen facilitates dissemination of malignant cells as indicated above.

The limitations of the hamster cheek pouch model including the lack of hamster specific antibodies and other reagents as well as the lack of an anatomical structure similar to the cheek pouch in humans then led to search for alternative animal models for oral cancer. These included testing new chemical carcinogenesis protocols in murine models, and in this regard, it was discovered that painting the oral cavity with 4-Nitroquinoline-1-oxide (4NQO), a water soluble carcinogen, induced oral squamous cell carcinomas in both mice and rats (Fujino et al. 1965; Wallenius and Lekholm 1973). Administration of 4NQO to the oral epithelium of rats and mice results in a step-wise mechanism of tumor induction that, similar to DMBA-induced oral cancers in the hamster, follows a histologic progression model with many similarities to the human disease (Hawkins et al. 1994; Kanojia and Vaidya 2006). The observation that 4NQO administered in the drinking water also induced oral carcinomas in rats and mice expanded the use of this carcinogenesis protocol that reduces considerably the animal handling (Ohne et al. 1985; Tang et al. 2004). Nevertheless, similar to DMBA-induced oral cancers, the 4NQO-induced oral SCCs rarely metastasize, and the model has been primarily used to study early stages of oral cancer progression (Silva et al. 2007; Jiang et al. 2007; Vered et al. 2007).

Human oral cancers carry mutations that result in the activation of oncogenes or inactivation of tumor suppressor genes, which may play fundamental roles during the carcinogenesis process. Notably, chemically induced oral cancers contain alterations similar to those found in human patients, including ras and p53 muta-tions or overexpression of the EGFR (Wong 1987; Husain et al. 1989; Gimenez-Conti et al. 1992; Yuan et al. 1994; Gimenez-Conti et al. 1996; Chang et al. 2000; Muscarella et al. 2001). More complex genetic alterations such as amplification of large chromosomal regions have been found in chemically induced mouse oral tumors. For instance, mouse oral tumors induced by 4NQO exhibit gains of chro-mosome 7F4, which is homologous to human chromosome region 11q13 (Yuan et al. 1997), which has been found to be amplified in about 50% of the human head and neck squamous cell carcinomas (Williams et al. 1993; Rubin et al. 1995). Interestingly, amplification of 11q13 in humans is associated with lymph node metastasis (Muller et al. 1994) suggesting that overexpression of genes located in this chromosomal region may play an important role in malignant progression of head and neck cancers (Huang et al. 2006). Comparative analyses of the genomic and expression profiles of tumors that develop in mice and humans may help to identify changes that play a significant role in malignant progression.

In summary, the low propensity for metastasis seen in chemically induced oral cancer models, has limited the use of these types of models in studying the biology of oral cancer metastases.

Genetically Engineered Mouse Models of Metastasis

Extensive efforts to manipulate the mouse genome have resulted in the generation of transgenic mice in which oncogenes can be introduced in the mouse germline and targeted to a subset of tissues using specific promoters. This technology allows one to test the tumorigenic potential of oncogenes found in human cancers in the mouse (Stewart et al. 1984; Ruther et al. 1987; Andres et al. 1987). In addition, technological advances have permitted the introduction of germline deletions in the mouse genome to generate knockout mice that carry deletions in genes of choice. Notably, several knockout mice documented that inactivation of tumor suppressor genes dqn confers cancer susceptibility (Donehower et al. 1992) (Jacks et al. 1992; Serrano et al. 1996). Therefore, the generation of transgenic and knockout mice offers the possibility of testing the consequences of genetic alterations similar to those found in human oral cancers.

The first transgenic mice for oral cancer were generated by expressing cyclin D1 under the control of the Epstein-Barr virus ED-L2 promoter, which is expressed in the tongue, esophagus, and forestomach. These mice developed dysplasia in the oral epithelium and esophagus (Nakagawa et al. 1997). Further inactivation of the p53 gene in these mice resulted in invasive oral and esophageal tumors (Opitz et al. 2002). Similarly, inactivation of p53 accelerated oral carcinogenesis in mice that overexpress c-Myc in the stratified epithelia, which develop skin squamous cell carcinomas and a variety of oral tumors including ameloblastomas and squamous cell carcinomas (Rounbehler et al. 2001). These experiments demonstrated that combining genetic alterations in the mouse similar to those found in patients is a powerful tool to model oral cancer. However, none of the models described above developed regional or distant metastasis, suggesting that additional genetic altera-tions are required to induce metastasis. It is also possible that, since p53-null mice die from lymphomas and sarcomas within 6–12 months, the short life span of the mice did not allow sufficient time for the metastasis to develop.

To overcome these limitations, administration of chemical carcinogens to the buccal epithelium of genetically mice may be used to accelerate oral cancer forma-tion before other malignancies appear. Several mouse strains deficient in genes involved in DNA repair, genomic instability, and apoptosis have been subjected to chemical carcinogenesis protocols. For instance, inactivation of the xeroderma pigmentosum A (XPA) gene resulted in increased susceptibility to 4NQO-induced oral cancer formation (Ide et al. 2001), and further deletion of one copy of the p53 gene further accelerated oral carcinogenesis (Ide et al. 2003). Unfortunately, XPA–/–p53–/– mice died from lymphomas and sarcomas within 13 weeks, before the oral tumors progress to metastatic carcinomas. Nevertheless, these observations supported an important role for p53 mutations in oral carcinogenesis, confirming the observations outlined above.

It is worth noting that most p53 mutations found in human tumors are missense mutations that results in the change of a single amino acid, rather than gene dele-tions. Some of these mutations may confer dominant negative effects by allowing mutant p53 to bind and inactivate wild type p53. In addition, certain p53 mutants may acquire novel gain of function properties including the potential to induce oncogenic effects (Olive et al. 2004; Lang et al. 2004; Caulin et al. 2007). Interestingly, transgenic mice generated with a genomic BAC clone containing the p53 gene modified to express a $p53^{A135V}$ mutation, were highly susceptible to 4NQO-induced oral carcinogenesis with nodal invasion (Zhang et al. 2006). Although it was unclear from this study the penetrance of the regional metastatic phenotype, this report suggests that p53 mutants may be involved in local metastasis. It will be interesting to dissect the contribution of the dominant negative effects and potential gain of function properties of this mutant p53 in the metastatic phenotype observed in these mice.

Recent evidence suggest that human papillomavirus (HPV) is involved in the pathogenesis of certain head and neck cancers, including oral cancers (McKaig et al. 1998; Gillison et al. 2000). To determine the role in oral carcinogenesis of E6 and E7, the genes considered responsible for the oncogenic properties of HPV, transgenic mice expressing E6 and E7 under the control of the K14 promoter have been generated. These mice develop oral and esophageal papillomas and squamous cell carcinomas with complete penetrance after treatment with 4NQO (Strati et al. 2006). In addition, one of these mice developed metastasis to the liver. It is well documented that E6 and E7 can bind to and inactivate p53 and pRb, suggesting that pathways modulated by these tumor suppressor genes may be involved in oral cancer metastasis.

As indicated above, 4NQO is an excellent carcinogen to study early stages of oral cancer progression, but alternative carcinogenesis protocols were needed to induce metastasis of oral cancers in mice with high penetrance. Recently, it was shown that repeated applications of DMBA to the mouse oral epithelium induced oral squamous cell carcinomas that metastasized to the cervical lymph nodes 13 weeks after tumor onset with complete penetrance (Ku et al. 2007). These authors demonstrated that inactivation of one copy of the p53 gene accelerated DMBA-induced oral tumor initiation but did not have a significant effect in malignant progression and metastasis. However, the p53 gene was not detected in the majority of the metastasis that developed in p53 wild-type or p53+/− mice, suggesting that while p53 is haplosufficient in preventing local metastasis in this model, complete loss of p53 may facilitate metastatic spread of oral cancer cells (Ku et al. 2007). Interestingly, the expression profiles of the metastases that develop in p53 wild-type mice differed from those of the metastases developed in the p53 heterozygous mice, suggesting that different pathways determined the metastatic phenotype in these mice. The contribution of these pathways to the metastatic process associated with oral cancer needs further investigation, keeping in mind that the use of a chemical carcinogen such as DMBA, in addition to ras mutations may induce an array of unidentified genetic alterations, that may complicate this analysis.

Continuous efforts to improve animal models for oral cancer have focused on overcoming the major limitations of the models described above, i.e., the premature death of animals in which mutations are induced in multiple tissues or the entire animal and avoiding the use of chemical carcinogens to prevent the widespread activation of mutations. To circumvent these problems, an inducible system was developed that allows focal activation of endogenous mutations in the oral epithelium of adult mice (Caulin et al. 2004). This system is based on the generation of transgenic mice that express an inducible Cre recombinase in stratified epithelia such as the oral epithelium. Cre is a viral protein that induces deletion of DNA sequences that are flanked by loxP sites, which are 34 base pair (bp) sequences that consists of two 13 bp inverted repeats separated by an 8 bp sequence. To allow inducible activation, Cre is fused to a mutant progesterone receptor (PR) that fails to bind progesterone but binds progesterone antagonists, such as RU486 (Kellendonk et al. 1996). This fusion protein (Cre*PR1) is sequestered in the cytoplasm, and therefore inactive, until binding of RU486 induces translocation to the nucleus where it can mediate the excision of loxP-flanked sequences (Fig. 7.3a). Two lines of mice are required in this system: mice that express Cre*PR1 under the control of the Keratin 5 (K5) promoter, and mice in which the target gene has been modified by the insertion of loxP sites. After these two mouse lines are mated to generate mice that carry the K5-Cre*PR1 transgene and the loxP-modified target, focal gene deletion can be induced by application of the inducer RU486 in the oral cavity of bigenic mice.

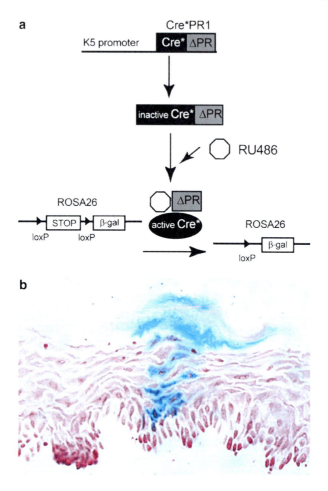

Fig. 7.3 Inducible activation of conditional alleles in the oral cavity. (**a**) Schematic representation of the inducible system for the selective expression of oncogenes in the oral epithelia. Bigenic mice were generated by crossing two different mouse lines. The first line harbors the target gene with a stop cassette flanked by loxP sites ("floxed"), whose presence blocks the expression of the gene. In this example the target gene is the ROSA26 reporter gene, in which β-galactosidase expression is prevented by the floxed stop cassette. In the second line, an inducible Cre transgene (Cre*PR1) is expressed under the transcriptional control of the K5 promoter, which drives the transgene expression into the basal layers of the stratified epithelia, where the regenerating stem cells are located. Upon RU486 binding, Cre translocates to the nucleus, where it excises the floxed stop cassette, thereby allowing expression of the target gene. (**b**) β-galactosidase activity in the oral mucosa of a bigenic mouse after activation with RU486. Note the presence of blue-stained cells in cell units through all the differentiating layers of the oral epithelium, suggesting that activation occurs in sporadic stems cells that regenerate the epithelium

Similarly, a target gene can be modified to carry an oncogenic mutation and a stop cassette that prevents the expression of the mutant allele. After Cre activation, the stop cassette is excised and the mutant allele is expressed. Therefore, this system allows activation of endogenous oncogenes and inactivation of tumor suppressor genes. The K5 promoter targets Cre*PR1 expression to the basal layer of the oral epithelium, where the stem cells that regenerate the epithelium are located (Fig. 7.3b). Therefore, once an RU486-induced mutation is activated in a stem cell in the oral epithelium, the mutation persists for the remainder of the life of the mouse (Caulin et al. 2004). Thus, this method of introducing mutations/deletions closely mimics the sporadic occurrence of somatic mutations that occurs in human cancers.

To determine whether endogenous activation of oncogenic ras can initiate oral tumor formation, the K5.Cre*PR1mice were crossed with LSL-Kras^{G12D} mice, which carry the oncogenic G12D mutation in the K-ras gene and a stop cassette that prevents the expression of the mutant allele. These mice developed oral tumors 16–20 weeks after the K-ras^{G12D} mutation was activated by topical application of RU486 in the oral epithelium (Fig. 7.4). The tumors that developed in these mice were benign papillomas that exhibited pathological and molecular features that resembled those found in human patients (Caulin et al. 2004). Notably, mice that were not treated with RU486 did not develop tumors, thereby confirming that in this model mutations are only activated after induction with RU486. Therefore, this model is ideal for generating mice that accumulate different genetic alterations following activation of Cre*PR1. Indeed, using this inducible system it was shown that deletion of the transforming growth factor-β receptor type II (TGF-βRII) in the oral epithelium in combination with ras mutations results in squamous cell carcinoma formation with complete penetrance (Lu et al. 2006). In addition, over 30% of the mice developed local lymph nodes metastasis. These experiments and the role of TGF-β signaling in oral cancer metastasis are discussed in more detail in Chap. 8 of this book.

In summary, these observations document that activating in the mouse oral epithelium mutations similar to those found in human oral cancers is a powerful tool to model oral cancer with metastatic potential. The generation of new mouse mod-

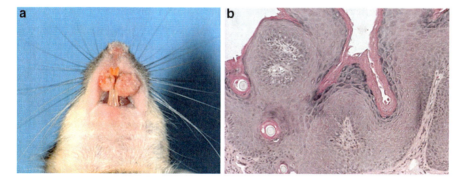

Fig. 7.4 Oral tumor formation induced by activation of endogenous oncogenic K-ras. (**a**) Gross appearance of tumors that developed in the oral cavity of bigenic K5.Cre*PR1/LSL-Kras^{G12D} mice after activation with RU486. (**b**) Hematoxylin- eosin staining showing the histology of the oral tumors that developed in these mice

els in which additional mutations are activated will help to dissect molecular mechanisms involved in oral cancer progression and metastasis. In addition, these mouse models may be used to identify novel genetic alterations that contribute to oral cancer metastasis and ultimately for testing therapeutic strategies.

Challenges to the Study of Oral Cancer Metastases and Remaining Questions

The animal models described in previous sections of this chapter document that tumors that develop in the oral epithelium in response to oncogenic mutations and/ or mutations that result in inactivation of tumor suppressor genes arise with higher latency than other common cancers. These observations strongly support the development of experimental systems that allow activation of mutations exclusively in the oral epithelium to generate models that permit full progression of the oral tumors. Inducible systems have already been used to activate endogenous mutations in oral tissues, and models developed to test the consequences of activating different combinations of genetic alteration are expected in the future. While it is possible that co-activation of few mutations may result in metastatic oral cancer formation, as illustrated above for cooperative ras and TGF-βRII mutations in local metastasis formation, it is also possible that other genetic alterations frequently found in human oral cancers contribute to metastasis only in the presence of a more complex pattern of mutations. Therefore, to fully understand the genetic requirements for oral cancer metastasis, a system that allows efficient activation of multiple mutations may be needed. The inducible system described above permits the activation of up to 4–5 mutations in a single mouse, thereby allowing the testing of multiple combinations of genetic alterations. The complexity of the breeding programs required to activate additional mutations would make this system unpractical in case additional mutations are desired to be tested. This may be particularly relevant for testing the role of cancer modifier genes, which may have small but cumulative effects during carcinogenesis. Testing the cooperative effects of these genes, or the pathways they regulate, during cancer progression will require a system that allows rapid and efficient activation of multiple mutations in oral epithelia.

Along these lines, it is worth noting that cancers that develop in the oral cavity exhibit molecular signatures consistent with the alteration of complex combinations of signaling pathways (Chung et al. 2004; Roepman et al. 2005). These analyses strongly suggest that oral cancer formation and malignant progression results from cooperation of multiple signaling pathways, which may determine the pathogenesis of the tumors, including the potential to metastasize. Therefore, modeling malignant progression of oral cancers will require a better understanding of the cooperative contribution of genetic alterations and pathways altered during the carcinogenesis process. These considerations imply that no single mouse model can recapitulate all the molecular and biological events involved in oral cancer metastasis. However, animal models in which specific combinations of mutations are activated in oral tissues will help to delineate the cooperative contributions of genetic alterations.

Comparative expression profiling of primary oral tumors and metastasis showed that molecular signatures associated with metastasis are present in the corresponding primary tumors, indicating that the metastatic potential is acquired early during tumor progression (O'Donnell et al. 2005; Roepman et al. 2006). However, only a small percentage of the cells in the primary tumors metastasize, suggesting that discrete changes critical to confer metastatic potential only occur in a subset of cells in the tumor. These genetic or epigenetic changes may vary in the context of different molecular signatures. Alternatively, it is possible that the microenvironment in the primary tumor limits the spreading of cells with full potential to metastasize, and changes in the cellular interactions in the primary tumor may allow the dissemination of metastatic cells.

Importantly, mouse models allow analysis of expression and genomic profiles of tumors at different stages of progression. Detailed characterization of molecular signatures of tumors representing different stages of tumor progression may help to identify genes or pathways involved in oral cancer metastasis. Similarly, biological processes such as cellular, invasion, evasion of apoptosis, intravasation, migration to distant organs, extravasation and colonization of the distant organ can be monitored in real time in tumors that develop in the mouse. The ability to incorporate molecular markers in transgenic and knockout vectors allows monitoring tumors cells as they leave the primary tumor and travel through the circulation to local or distant organs. Visualization of tumors cells is critical to understand molecular and biological processes involved in the metastatic process, especially to address the significance of the cellular interactions between the tumor cells and the surrounding stroma in the tumor and between tumor cells and host cells in the tissues that they colonize.

References

Andres AC, Schonenberger CA, Groner B, Hennighausen L, LeMeur M, Gerlinger P (1987) Ha-ras oncogene expression directed by a milk protein gene promoter: tissue specificity, hormonal regulation, and tumor induction in transgenic mice. Proc Natl Acad Sci USA 84:1299–1303

Baker SR (1985) An in vivo model for squamous cell carcinoma of the head and neck. Laryngoscope 95:43–56

Bibby MC (2004) Orthotopic models of cancer for preclinical drug evaluation: Advantages and disadvantages. Eur J Cancer 40:852–857

Braakhuis BJ, Sneeuwloper G, Snow GB (1984) The potential of the nude mouse xenograft model for the study of head and neck cancer. Arch Otorhinolaryngol 239:69–79

Caulin C, Nguyen T, Longley MA, Zhou Z, Wang XJ, Roop DR (2004) Inducible activation of oncogenic K-ras results in tumor formation in the oral cavity. Cancer Res 64:5054–5058

Caulin C, Nguyen T, Lang GA, Goepfert TM, Brinkley BR, Cai WW, Lozano G, Roop DR (2007) An inducible mouse model for skin cancer reveals distinct roles for gain- and loss-of-function p53 mutations. J Clin Invest 117:1893–1901

Chalfie M, Tu Y, Euskirchen G, Ward WW, Prasher DC (1994) Green fluorescent protein as a marker for gene expression. Science 263:802–805

Chang KW, Sarraj S, Lin SC, Tsai PI, Solt D (2000) P53 expression, p53 and Ha-ras mutation and telomerase activation during nitrosamine-mediated hamster pouch carcinogenesis. Carcinogenesis 21:1441–1451

Cheng L, Fu J, Tsukamoto A, Hawley RG (1996) Use of green fluorescent protein variants to monitor gene transfer and expression in mammalian cells. Nat Biotechnol 14:606–609

Chung CH, Parker JS, Karaca G, Wu J, Funkhouser WK, Moore D, Butterfoss D, Xiang D, Zanation A, Yin X, Shockley WW, Weissler MC, Dressler LG, Shores CG, Yarbrough WG, Perou CM (2004) Molecular classification of head and neck squamous cell carcinomas using patterns of gene expression. Cancer Cell 5:489–500

Clark EA, Golub TR, Lander ES, Hynes RO (2000) Genomic analysis of metastasis reveals an essential role for RhoC. Nature 406:532–535

Contag CH, Jenkins D, Contag PR, Negrin RS (2000) Use of reporter genes for optical measurements of neoplastic disease in vivo. Neoplasia 2:41–52

Craig G (1980) Metastasis from DMBA-induced carcinomas in hamster cheek pouch. In: Hillman K, Hilgard P, Eccles S (eds) Metastasis clinical and experimental aspects, developments in oncology. Martinus Nijhoff, The Hague, pp 50–54

Cui N, Nomura T, Noma H, Yokoo K, Takagi R, Hashimoto S, Okamoto M, Sato M, Yu G, Guo C, Shibahala T (2005) Effect of YM529 on a model of mandibular invasion by oral squamous cell carcinoma in mice. Clin Cancer Res 11:2713–2719

Dachi SF, Sanders JE, Urie EM (1967) Effects of dimethyl sulfoxide on dimethylbenzanthracene-induced carcinogenesis in the hamster cheek pouch. Cancer Res 27:1183–1185

Dinesman A, Haughey B, Gates GA, Aufdemorte T, Von Hoff DD (1990) Development of a new in vivo model for head and neck cancer. Otolaryngol Head Neck Surg 103:766–774

Donehower LA, Harvey M, Slagle BL, McArthur MJ, Montgomery CA Jr, Butel JS, Bradley A (1992) Mice deficient for p53 are developmentally normal but susceptible to spontaneous tumours. Nature 356:215–221

Erdem NF, Carlson ER, Gerard DA (2008) Characterization of gene expression profiles of 3 different human oral squamous cell carcinoma cell lines with different invasion and metastatic capacities. J Oral Maxillofac Surg 66:918–927

Fidler IJ (1973) Selection of successive tumour lines for metastasis. Nat New Biol 242:148–149

Fidler IJ, Kripke ML (1977) Metastasis results from preexisting variant cells within a malignant tumor. Science 197:893–895

Fidler IJ, Wilmanns C, Staroselsky A, Radinsky R, Dong Z, Fan D (1994) Modulation of tumor cell response to chemotherapy by the organ environment. Cancer Metastasis Rev 13:209–222

Fiebig HH, Berger DP (1995) Preclinical phase II trials. In: Boven E, Winograd B (eds) The nude mouse in oncology research. CRC Press, Boca Raton, pp 318–335

Fitch KA, Somers KD, Schecter GL (1988) The development of a head and neck tumor model in the nude mouse. In: Proceedings of the 2nd international head and a neck oncology research conference, Kugler Publications, Amsterdam, pp 187–190

Fujino H, Chino T, Imai T (1965) Experimental production of labial and lingual carcinoma by local application of 4-nitroquinoline N-oxide. J Natl Cancer Inst 35:907–918

Fujita K, Kaku T, Sasaki M, Onoe T (1973) Experimental production of lingual carcinomas in hamsters by local application of 9, 10-dimethyl-1, 2-benzanthracene. J Dent Res 52:327–332

Gillison ML, Koch WM, Capone RB, Spafford M, Westra WH, Wu L, Zahurak ML, Daniel RW, Viglione M, Symer DE, Shah KV, Sidransky D (2000) Evidence for a causal association between human papillomavirus and a subset of head and neck cancers. J Natl Cancer Inst 92:709–720

Gimenez-Conti IB, Bianchi AB, Stockman SL, Conti CJ, Slaga TJ (1992) Activating mutation of the Ha-ras gene in chemically induced tumors of the hamster cheek pouch. Mol Carcinog 5:259–263

Gimenez-Conti IB, LaBate M, Liu F, Osterndorff E (1996) p53 Alterations in chemically induced hamster cheek-pouch lesions. Mol Carcinog 16:197–202

Habu S, Fukui H, Shimamura K, Kasai M, Nagai Y, Okumura K, Tamaoki N (1981) In vivo effects of anti-asialo GM1. I. Reduction of NK activity and enhancement of transplanted tumor growth in nude mice. J Immunol 127:34–38

Hart IR, Fidler IJ (1980) Role of organ selectivity in the determination of metastatic patterns of B16 melanoma. Cancer Res 40:2281–2287

Hawkins BL, Heniford BW, Ackermann DM, Leonberger M, Martinez SA, Hendler FJ (1994) 4NQO carcinogenesis: A mouse model of oral cavity squamous cell carcinoma. Head Neck 16:424–432

Henson B, Li F, Coatney DD, Carey TE, Mitra RS, Kirkwood KL, D'Silva NJ (2007) An orthotopic floor-of-mouth model for locoregional growth and spread of human squamous cell carcinoma. J Oral Pathol Med 36:363–370

Hier MP, Black MJ, Shenouda G, Sadeghi N, Karp SE (1995) A murine model for the immunotherapy of head and neck squamous cell carcinoma. Laryngoscope 105:1077–1080

Hill R (2002) Tumour metastasis models. In: Alison M (ed) The cancer handbook. Nature Publishing Group, London

Hirst DG, Brown JM, Hazlehurst JL (1982) Enhancement of CCNU cytotoxicity by misonidazole: Possible therapeutic gain. Br J Cancer 46:109–116

Hoffman R (2002) Green fluorescent protein imaging of tumour growth, metastasis, and angiogenesis in mouse models. Lancet Oncol 3:546–556

Huang X, Godfrey TE, Gooding WE, McCarty KS Jr, Gollin SM (2006) Comprehensive genome and transcriptome analysis of the 11q13 amplicon in human oral cancer and synteny to the 7F5 amplicon in murine oral carcinoma. Genes Chromosomes Cancer 45:1058–1069

Husain Z, Fei YB, Roy S, Solt DB, Polverini PJ, Biswas DK (1989) Sequential expression and cooperative interaction of c-Ha-ras and c-erbB genes in in vivo chemical carcinogenesis. Proc Natl Acad Sci USA 86:1264–1268

Ide F, Oda H, Nakatsuru Y, Kusama K, Sakashita H, Tanaka K, Ishikawa T (2001) Xeroderma pigmentosum group A gene action as a protection factor against 4-nitroquinoline 1-oxide-induced tongue carcinogenesis. Carcinogenesis 22:567–572

Ide F, Kitada M, Sakashita H, Kusama K, Tanaka K, Ishikawa T (2003) p53 Haploinsufficiency profoundly accelerates the onset of tongue tumors in mice lacking the xeroderma pigmentosum group A gene. Am J Pathol 163:1729–1733

Jacks T, Fazeli A, Schmitt EM, Bronson RT, Goodell MA, Weinberg RA (1992) Effects of an Rb mutation in the mouse. Nature 359:295–300

Ji RC (2006) Lymphatic endothelial cells, tumor lymphangiogenesis and metastasis: New insights into intratumoral and peritumoral lymphatics. Cancer Metastasis Rev 25:677–694

Jiang C, Ye D, Qiu W, Zhang X, Zhang Z, He D, Zhang P, Chen W (2007) Response of lymphocyte subsets and cytokines to Shenyang prescription in Sprague-Dawley rats with tongue squamous cell carcinomas induced by 4NQO. BMC Cancer 7:40

Johnson JI, Decker S, Zaharevitz D, Rubinstein LV, Venditti JM, Schepartz S, Kalyandrug S, Christian M, Arbuck S, Hollingshead M, Sausville EA (2001) Relationships between drug activity in NCI preclinical in vitro and in vivo models and early clinical trials. Br J Cancer 84:1424–1431

Kage T, Mogi M, Katsumata Y, Chino T (1987) Regional lymph node metastasis created by partial excision of carcinomas induced in hamster cheek pouch with 9, 10-dimethyl-1, 2-benzanthracene. J Dent Res 66:1673–1679

Kanojia D, Vaidya MM (2006) 4-Nitroquinoline-1-oxide induced experimental oral carcinogenesis. Oral Oncol 42:655–667

Kasai M, Yoneda T, Habu S, Maruyama Y, Okumura K, Tokunaga T (1981) In vivo effect of anti-asialo GM1 antibody on natural killer activity. Nature 291:334–335

Kawashiri S, Kumagai S, Kojima K, Harada H, Yamamoto E (1995) Development of a new invasion and metastasis model of human oral squamous cell carcinomas. Eur J Cancer B Oral Oncol 31B:216–221

Kawashiri S, Kumagai S, Kojima K, Harada H, Nakagawa K, Yamamoto E (1999) Reproduction of occult metastasis of head and neck cancer in nude mice. Clin Exp Metastasis 17:277–282

Kellendonk C, Tronche F, Monaghan AP, Angrand PO, Stewart F, Schutz G (1996) Regulation of Cre recombinase activity by the synthetic steroid RU 486. Nucleic Acids Res 24:1404–1411

Khurana D, Martin EA, Kasperbauer JL, O'Malley BW Jr, Salomao DR, Chen L, Strome SE (2001) Characterization of a spontaneously arising murine squamous cell carcinoma (SCC VII) as a prerequisite for head and neck cancer immunotherapy. Head Neck 23:899–906

Komatsubara H, Umeda M, Oku N, Komori T (2002) Establishment of in vivo metastasis model of human adenoid cystic carcinoma: Detection of metastasis by PCR with human beta-globin gene. Kobe J Med Sci 48:145–152

Ku TK, Nguyen DC, Karaman M, Gill P, Hacia JG, Crowe DL (2007) Loss of p53 expression correlates with metastatic phenotype and transcriptional profile in a new mouse model of head and neck cancer. Mol Cancer Res 5:351–362

Kuo TH, Kubota T, Watanabe M, Furukawa T, Kase S, Tanino H, Saikawa Y, Ishibiki K, Kitajima M, Hoffman RM (1993) Site-specific chemosensitivity of human small-cell lung carcinoma growing orthotopically compared to subcutaneously in SCID mice: The importance of orthotopic models to obtain relevant drug evaluation data. Anticancer Res 13:627–630

Lang GA, Iwakuma T, Suh YA, Liu G, Rao VA, Parant JM, Valentin-Vega YA, Terzian T, Caldwell LC, Strong LC, el Naggar AK, Lozano G (2004) Gain of function of a p53 hot spot mutation in a mouse model of Li-Fraumeni syndrome. Cell 119:861–872

Lee TK, Poon RT, Wo JY, Ma S, Guan XY, Myers JN, Altevogt P, Yuen AP (2007) Lupeol suppresses cisplatin-induced nuclear factor-kappaB activation in head and neck squamous cell carcinoma and inhibits local invasion and nodal metastasis in an orthotopic nude mouse model. Cancer Res 67:8800–8809

Levij IS, Polliack A, Thorgeirsson T (1967) Correlation of cytologic smear and histologic findings during 9-10 dimethyl 1-2 benzanthracene-induced carcinogenesis in the hamster cheek pouch. Arch Oral Biol 12:859–864

Lin WC, Pretlow TP, Pretlow TG, Culp LA (1990) Bacterial lacZ gene as a highly sensitive marker to detect micrometastasis formation during tumor progression. Cancer Res 50:2808–2817

Lou E, Kellman RM, Shillitoe EJ (2002) Effect of herpes simplex virus type-1 on growth of oral cancer in an immunocompetent, orthotopic mouse model. Oral Oncol 38:349–356

Lou E, Kellman RM, Hutchison R, Shillitoe EJ (2003) Clinical and pathological features of the murine AT-84 orthotopic model of oral cancer. Oral Dis 9:305–312

Lu SL, Herrington H, Reh D, Weber S, Bornstein S, Wang D, Li AG, Tang CF, Siddiqui Y, Nord J, Andersen P, Corless CL, Wang XJ (2006) Loss of transforming growth factor-beta type II receptor promotes metastatic head-and-neck squamous cell carcinoma. Genes Dev 20:1331–1342

Maekawa K, Sato H, Furukawa M, Yoshizaki T (2002) Inhibition of cervical lymph node metastasis by marimastat (BB-2516) in an orthotopic oral squamous cell carcinoma implantation model. Clin Exp Metastasis 19:513–518

Matsui T, Ota T, Ueda Y, Tanino M, Odashima S (1998) Isolation of a highly metastatic cell line to lymph node in human oral squamous cell carcinoma by orthotopic implantation in nude mice. Oral Oncol 34:253–256

McKaig RG, Baric RS, Olshan AF (1998) Human papillomavirus and head and neck cancer: Epidemiology and molecular biology. Head Neck 20:250–265

Melancon MP, Wang Y, Wen X, Bankson JA, Stephens LC, Jasser S, Gelovani JG, Myers JN, Li C (2007) Development of a macromolecular dual-modality MR-optical imaging for sentinel lymph node mapping. Invest Radiol 42:569–578

Momose F, Araida T, Negishi A, Ichijo H, Shioda S, Sasaki S (1989) Variant sublines with different metastatic potentials selected in nude mice from human oral squamous cell carcinomas. J Oral Pathol Med 18:391–395

Morin JG, Hastings JW (1971) Energy transfer in a bioluminescent system. J Cell Physiol 77:313–318

Muller D, Millon R, Lidereau R, Engelmann A, Bronner G, Flesch H, Eber M, Methlin G, Abecassis J (1994) Frequent amplification of 11q13 DNA markers is associated with lymph node involvement in human head and neck squamous cell carcinomas. Eur J Cancer B Oral Oncol 30B:113–120

Muscarella P, Knobloch TJ, Ulrich AB, Casto BC, Moniaux N, Wittel UA, Melvin WS, Pour PM, Song H, Gold B, Batra SK, Weghorst CM (2001) Identification and sequencing of the Syrian Golden hamster (Mesocricetus auratus) p16(INK4a) and p15(INK4b) cDNAs and their homozygous gene deletion in cheek pouch and pancreatic tumor cells. Gene 278:235–243

Myers JN, Holsinger FC, Jasser SA, Bekele BN, Fidler IJ (2002) An orthotopic nude mouse model of oral tongue squamous cell carcinoma. Clin Cancer Res 8:293–298

Nakagawa H, Wang TC, Zukerberg L, Odze R, Togawa K, May GH, Wilson J, Rustgi AK (1997) The targeting of the cyclin D1 oncogene by an Epstein-Barr virus promoter in transgenic mice causes dysplasia in the tongue, esophagus and forestomach. Oncogene 14:1185–1190

Nakajima J, Mogi M, Chino T (1996) Inhibition by streptococcal immunopotentiator OK432 of lymph-node metastasis in hamster cheek-pouch carcinoma with enhancement of tumour necrosis factor-alpha and interleukin-6 in serum. Arch Oral Biol 41:513–516

Nomura T, Shibahara T, Katakura A, Matsubara S, Takano N (2007) Establishment of a murine model of bone invasion by oral squamous cell carcinoma. Oral Oncol 43:257–262

O'Donnell RK, Kupferman M, Wei SJ, Singhal S, Weber R, O'Malley B, Cheng Y, Putt M, Feldman M, Ziober B, Muschel RJ (2005) Gene expression signature predicts lymphatic metastasis in squamous cell carcinoma of the oral cavity. Oncogene 24:1244–1251

O'Malley BW Jr, Cope KA, Johnson CS, Schwartz MR (1997) A new immunocompetent murine model for oral cancer. Arch Otolaryngol Head Neck Surg 123:20–24

Ohne M, Satoh T, Yamada S, Takai H (1985) Experimental tongue carcinoma of rats induced by oral administration of 4-nitroquinoline 1-oxide (4NQO) in drinking water. Oral Surg Oral Med Oral Pathol 59:600–607

Olive KP, Tuveson DA, Ruhe ZC, Yin B, Willis NA, Bronson RT, Crowley D, Jacks T (2004) Mutant p53 gain of function in two mouse models of Li-Fraumeni syndrome. Cell 119:847–860

Opitz OG, Harada H, Suliman Y, Rhoades B, Sharpless NE, Kent R, Kopelovich L, Nakagawa H, Rustgi AK (2002) A mouse model of human oral-esophageal cancer. J Clin Invest 110:761–769

Paget S (1889) The distribution of secondary growths in cancer of the breast. Lancet 1:571–573

Patel A, Miller L, Ahmed K, Ondrey F (2004) NF-Kappa-B downregulation strategies in head and neck cancer treatment. Otolaryngol Head Neck Surg 131:288–295

Qiu C, Wu H, He H, Qiu W (2003) A cervical lymph node metastatic model of human tongue carcinoma: Serial and orthotopic transplantation of histologically intact patient specimens in nude mice. J Oral Maxillofac Surg 61:696–700

Roepman P, Wessels LF, Kettelarij N, Kemmeren P, Miles AJ, Lijnzaad P, Tilanus MG, Koole R, Hordijk GJ, van der Vliet PC, Reinders MJ, Slootweg PJ, Holstege FC (2005) An expression profile for diagnosis of lymph node metastases from primary head and neck squamous cell carcinomas. Nat Genet 37:182–186

Roepman P, de Jager A, Groot Koerkamp MJ, Kummer JA, Slootweg PJ, Holstege FC (2006) Maintenance of head and neck tumor gene expression profiles upon lymph node metastasis. Cancer Res 66:11110–11114

Rounbehler RJ, Schneider-Broussard R, Conti CJ, Johnson DG (2001) Myc lacks E2F1's ability to suppress skin carcinogenesis. Oncogene 20:5341–5349

Rubin JS, Qiu L, Etkind P (1995) Amplification of the Int-2 gene in head and neck squamous cell carcinoma. J Laryngol Otol 109:72–76

Ruther U, Garber C, Komitowski D, Muller R, Wagner EF (1987) Deregulated c-fos expression interferes with normal bone development in transgenic mice. Nature 325:412–416

Rwomushana JW, Polliack A, Levij IS (1970) Cervical lymph node metastasis of hamster cheek pouch carcinoma induced with DMBA. J Dent Res 49:184

Safour IM, Wood NK, Tsiklakis K, Doemling DB, Joseph G (1984) Incisional biopsy and seeding in hamster cheek pouch carcinoma. J Dent Res 63:1116–1120

Salley JJ (1954) Experimental carcinogenesis in the cheek pouch of the Syrian hamster. J Dent Res 33:253–262

Sano D, Myers JN (2007) Metastasis of squamous cell carcinoma of the oral tongue. Cancer Metastasis Rev 26:645–662

Serrano M, Lee H, Chin L, Cordon-Cardo C, Beach D, DePinho RA (1996) Role of the INK4a locus in tumor suppression and cell mortality. Cell 85:27–37

Shigeta T, Umeda M, Komatsubara H, Komori T (2008) Lymph node and pulmonary metastases after transplantation of oral squamous cell carcinoma cell line (HSC-3) into the subcutaneous tissue of nude mouse: Detection of metastases by genetic methods using beta-globin and mutant p53 genes. Oral Surg Oral Med Oral Pathol Oral Radiol Endod 105:486–490

Shintani S, Mihara M, Nakahara Y, Aida T, Tachikawa T, Hamakawa H (2002) Lymph node metastasis of oral cancer visualized in live tissue by green fluorescent protein expression. Oral Oncol 38:664–669

Shintani S, Li C, Mihara M, Nakashiro K, Hamakawa H (2003) Gefitinib ("Iressa"), an epidermal growth factor receptor tyrosine kinase inhibitor, mediates the inhibition of lymph node metastasis in oral cancer cells. Cancer Lett 201:149–155

Shklar G (1966) Cortisone and hamster buccal pouch carcinogenesis. Cancer Res 26:2461–2463

Silva RN, Ribeiro DA, Salvadori DM, Marques ME (2007) Placental glutathione S-transferase correlates with cellular proliferation during rat tongue carcinogenesis induced by 4-nitroquinoline 1-oxide. Exp Toxicol Pathol 59:61–68

Simon C, Nemechek AJ, Boyd D, O'Malley BW Jr, Goepfert H, Flaitz CM, Hicks MJ (1998) An orthotopic floor-of-mouth cancer model allows quantification of tumor invasion. Laryngoscope 108:1686–1691

Stewart TA, Pattengale PK, Leder P (1984) Spontaneous mammary adenocarcinomas in transgenic mice that carry and express MTV/myc fusion genes. Cell 38:627–637

Strati K, Pitot HC, Lambert PF (2006) Identification of biomarkers that distinguish human papillomavirus (HPV)-positive versus HPV-negative head and neck cancers in a mouse model. Proc Natl Acad Sci USA 103:14152–14157

Swan EA, Jasser SA, Holsinger FC, Doan D, Bucana C, Myers JN (2003) Acquisition of anoikis resistance is a critical step in the progression of oral tongue cancer. Oral Oncol 39:648–655

Take Y, Umeda M, Teranobu O, Shimada K (1999) Lymph node metastases in hamster tongue cancer induced with 9, 10-dimethyl-1, 2-benzanthracene: association between histological findings and the incidence of neck metastases, and the clinical implications for patients with tongue cancer. Br J Oral Maxillofac Surg 37:29–36

Tan MH, Holyoke ED, Goldrosen MH (1977) Murine colon adenocarcinoma: Syngeneic orthotopic transplantation and subsequent hepatic metastases. J Natl Cancer Inst 59:1537–1544

Tang XH, Knudsen B, Bemis D, Tickoo S, Gudas LJ (2004) Oral cavity and esophageal carcinogenesis modeled in carcinogen-treated mice. Clin Cancer Res 10:301–313

Varney ML, Olsen KJ, Mosley RL, Bucana CD, Talmadge JE, Singh RK (2002) Monocyte/macrophage recruitment, activation and differentiation modulate interleukin-8 production: A paracrine role of tumor-associated macrophages in tumor angiogenesis. In Vivo 16:471–477

Vered M, Allon I, Buchner A, Dayan D (2007) Stromal myofibroblasts and malignant transformation in a 4NQO rat tongue carcinogenesis model. Oral Oncol 43:999–1006

Wallenius K, Lekholm U (1973) Oral cancer in rats induced by the water-soluble carcinogen 4-nitrochinoline N-oxide. Odontol Revy 24:39–48

Weiss L (1996) Metastatic inefficiency: Intravascular and intraperitoneal implantation of cancer cells. Cancer Treat Res 82:1–11

Williams ME, Gaffey MJ, Weiss LM, Wilczynski SP, Schuuring E, Levine PA (1993) Chromosome 11Q13 amplification in head and neck squamous cell carcinoma. Arch Otolaryngol Head Neck Surg 119:1238–1243

Wong DT (1987) Amplification of the c-erb B1 oncogene in chemically-induced oral carcinomas. Carcinogenesis 8:1963–1965

Xie X, Brunner N, Jensen G, Albrectsen J, Gotthardsen B, Rygaard J (1992) Comparative studies between nude and scid mice on the growth and metastatic behavior of xenografted human tumors. Clin Exp Metastasis 10:201–210

Yamada T, Mogi M, Kage T, Ueda A, Nakajima J, Chino T (1992) Enhancement by cyclosporin A of metastasis from hamster cheek pouch carcinoma. Arch Oral Biol 37:593–596

Yamagiwa K, Ichikawa K (1977) Experimental study of the pathogenesis of carcinoma. CA Cancer J Clin 27:174–181

Yang M, Baranov E, Li XM, Wang JW, Jiang P, Li L, Moossa AR, Penman S, Hoffman RM (2001) Whole-body and intravital optical imaging of angiogenesis in orthotopically implanted tumors. Proc Natl Acad Sci USA 98:2616–2621

Yazici YD, Kim S, Jasser SA, Wang Z, Carter KB Jr, Bucana CD, Myers JN (2005) Antivascular therapy of oral tongue squamous cell carcinoma with PTK787. Laryngoscope 115:2249–2255

Yuan B, Heniford BW, Ackermann DM, Hawkins BL, Hendler FJ (1994) Harvey ras (H-ras) point mutations are induced by 4-nitroquinoline-1-oxide in murine oral squamous epithelia, while squamous cell carcinomas and loss of heterozygosity occur without additional exposure. Cancer Res 54:5310–5317

Yuan B, Oechsli MN, Hendler FJ (1997) A region within murine chromosome 7F4, syntenic to the human 11q13 amplicon, is frequently amplified in 4NQO-induced oral cavity tumors. Oncogene 15:1161–1170

Zhang L, Hellstrom KE, Chen L (1994) Luciferase activity as a marker of tumor burden and as an indicator of tumor response to antineoplastic therapy in vivo. Clin Exp Metastasis 12:87–92

Zhang Z, Wang Y, Yao R, Li J, Lubet RA, You M (2006) p53 Transgenic mice are highly susceptible to 4-nitroquinoline-1-oxide-induced oral cancer. Mol Cancer Res 4:401–410

Zucker S, Cao J, Chen WT (2000) Critical appraisal of the use of matrix metalloproteinase inhibitors in cancer treatment. Oncogene 19:6642–6650

Chapter 8
TGFβ Signaling in Head and Neck Cancer Development and Metastases

Stephen P. Malkoski, Jessyka G. Lighthall, and Xiao-Jing Wang

Abstract Transforming growth factor beta (TGFβ) signaling impacts the HSNCC development and metastases by affecting many critical processes including cell growth, proliferation, apoptosis, epithelial-to-mesenchymal transition, invasion, angiogenesis, and immune surveillance. Typically, TGFβ functions as a tumor suppressor in epithelial cells by inhibiting cell growth, promoting apoptosis, stimulating epithelial differentiation, enhancing genetic stability, and promoting cellular senescence, hence, reduced expression of TGFβ signaling components is observed in many malignancies, including HNSCC. Through a combination of genetic and epigenetic changes, TGFβ type II receptor expression is frequently reduced in HNSCC and is reduced TGFβRII expression is associated with more aggressive tumor behavior. Similarly, Smad4 expression is also commonly reduced in HNSCC and is associated with increased genomic instability. Tumor epithelial cells with TGFβ signaling defects increase TGFβ1 ligand production, which paradoxically promotes tumor growth and metastases by activating tumor-associated fibroblasts, increasing matrix degradation and angiogenesis, suppressing immune surveillance, and inducing inflammation; accordingly elevated local TGFb1 expression correlates with numerous negative clinical parameters. Given its broad role in tumor development and progression, TGFβ signaling remains an attractive therapeutic target, though the multifaceted roles of TGFβ in normal tissue homeostasis and the biphasic role of TGFβ in tumor development and progression have complicated attempts to modulate TGFβ signaling in the clinical setting.

With >45,000 new cases and >11,000 deaths per year, head and neck squamous cell carcinoma (HNSCC) is the sixth most common cancer diagnosis and the fifth most common cause of cancer mortality in the United States (Hayat et al. 2007; Jemal et al. 2007). Despite advances in surgical technique, radiation therapy, and chemotherapy, there has been minimal improvement in the 5-year survival of HNSCC patients over the past 30 years (Jemal et al. 2007). The bulk of HNSCC morbidity

X.-J. Wang (✉)
Department of Pathology, University of Colorado Denver,
12800 E 19th Ave, Box 8104, Aurora, CO, USA 80045
e-mail: xj.wang@ucdenver.edu

J. Myers (ed.), *Oral Cancer Metastasis*,
DOI 10.1007/978-1-4419-0775-2_8, © Springer Science+Business Media, LLC 2010

and mortality is related to regional tumor extension and metastases (Garavello et al. 2006). Approximately 10% of HNSCC patients have metastases at presentation, and as many as 23% develop metastases during the course of their disease (Alvi and Johnson 1997; Beer et al. 2000). Failure of local tumor control is strongly associated with subsequent development of metastases (Garavello et al. 2006).

HNSCC development, progression, and metastasis involve the accumulation of genetic mutations and epigenetic changes in the multiple pathways regulating cell growth, proliferation, and death (Hanahan and Weinberg 2000). Initiating mutations occur early in tumorigenesis and allow epithelial cells to escape growth arrest and develop a clonal population of abnormally proliferating cells. With additional mutations, these hyperproliferative cells develop a more malignant phenotype by escaping apoptosis, undergoing epithelial-to-mesenchymal transition (EMT), and invading through the basement membrane (Hanahan and Weinberg 2000). To metastasize, malignant cells must further acquire the ability to dissolve adherens junctions, activate matrix metalloproteinases (MMPs), promote angiogenesis, and evade immune surveillance (Hanahan and Weinberg 2000). Transforming growth factor beta (TGFβ) signaling impacts HSNCC development and metastases by affecting virtually all of the aforementioned biological processes.

TGFβ Signaling

The TGFβ super-family includes TGFβ, the bone morphogenic proteins (BMP), and the activins/inhibins (Shi and Massague 2003). These multifunctional cytokines regulate cell growth, differentiation, apoptosis, migration, inflammation, and angiogenesis in a tissue- and cell-context-dependent manner (Massague and Gomis 2006). To date, more than 300 transcriptional targets of the TGFβ super-family have been identified, and the list of TGFβ target genes is continuously increasing (Massague and Gomis 2006). During embryonic development, TGFβ is a key regulator of growth, vasculogenesis, and angiogenesis (Moustakas and Heldin 2007; Sporn and Roberts 1992). In adults, TGFβ mediates tissue homeostasis in epithelial tissues, endothelial cells, immune cells, and fibroblasts (Siegel and Massague 2003).

The three TGFβ ligand isoforms (TGFβ1, TGFβ2, and TGFβ3) are 70-80% homologous and have similar biological activities (Derynck et al. 1988). TGFβ ligands are secreted as inactive precursors that are proteolytically activated by extracellular metalloproteinases or membrane bound integrins (Munger et al. 1999; Yu and Stamenkovic 2000). Activated TGFβ binds a transmembrane receptor complex with intrinsic serine/threonine kinase activity (Shi and Massague 2003). There are three types of TGFβ receptors: TGFβ receptor type I (TGFβRI; also known as activin-like kinase [ALK] receptors), TGFβ receptor type II (TGFβRII), and TGFβ receptor type III (TGFβRIII, also known as betaglycan). While seven ALK isoforms and five type II receptor isoforms have been identified, TGFβ signals mainly through receptor complexes composed of ALK5 and TGFβRII (Feng and Derynck 2005; Shi and Massague 2003), though ALK1-TGFβRII complexes also mediate TGFβ signaling in endothelial cells (ten Dijke and Hill 2004). TGFβRIII binds

TGFβ with high affinity, effectively increasing TGFβ concentration at the cell surface and facilitating interactions with membrane-bound TGFβRI and TGFβRII (Lopez-Casillas et al. 1993).

TGFβRI and TGFβRII form homodimers in the endoplasmic reticulum, cytoplasm, and cell membrane that transduce a basal level of TGFβ signaling in the absence of ligand binding (Feng and Derynck 1996). TGFβ binding stimulates TGFβRII autophosphorlyation, which causes binding and transphosphorylation of TGFβRI (Feng and Derynck 2005). Activated TGFβRI then phosphorylates Smad family members, the predominant intracellular mediators of TGFβ signaling (Bierie and Moses 2006; Derynck and Zhang 2003) (Fig. 8.1). When TGFβRII interacts with ALK5, signaling is mediated through Smad2 and Smad3 (Derynck and Zhang 2003); when TGFβRII interacts with ALK1 Smad1, Smad5, and Smad8 are activated (Derynck and Zhang 2003).

The eight mammalian Smad isoforms are divided into three groups (ten Dijke and Hill 2004). TGFβ signaling is usually mediated by receptor-associated Smads (R-Smads), Smad2 and Smad3, whereas BMP signaling is typically mediated by R-Smads, Smad1, Smad5, and Smad8 (Massague 2000). Smad6 and Smad7 are inhibitory Smads (I-Smads) that block phosphorylation of R-Smads or increase

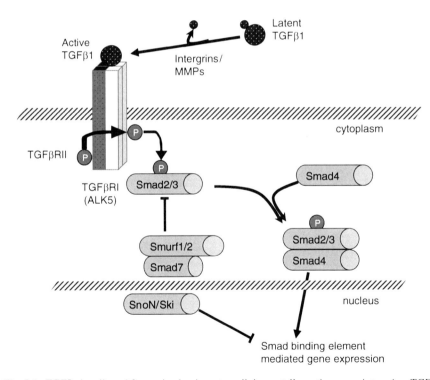

Fig. 8.1 TGFβ signaling. After activation by extracellular metalloprotinases or intergrins, TGFβ binds the TGFβ receptor complex, which then phosphorylates the R-Smads (Smad2 and Smad3). Phosphorylated R-Smads dimerize with Smad4, translocate into the nucleus, and modulate transcription via Smad binding elements (SBEs). TGFβ-Smad signaling can be negatively regulated by Smurfs, I-Smads (Smad6 and Smad7) and by Sno/Ski protooncogenes

TGFβ receptor degradation (Massague 2000). Smad4 is a coactivator that complexes with all R-Smads (Shi and Massague 2003). Phosphorylated R-Smads bind Smad4, translocate into the nucleus, and modulate gene transcription though Smad binding elements (SBEs) in the promoters of TGFβ responsive genes (Shi and Massague 2003). TGFβ effects at any particular SBE depend on the cellular context and the specific composition of Smad heterotrimers (ten Dijke and Hill 2004). TGFβ signaling can be negative regulated by Smad ubiquitination regularity factors (Smurfs) that increase proteosomal degradation of TGFb receptors and Smads (ten Dijke and Hill 2004), and by Ski family protooncogenes, such as c-Ski and SnoN, that directly interact with R-Smads and Smad4 (ten Dijke et al. 2002).

The Tumor Suppressive Role of TGFβ Signaling in Epithelia

TGFβ functions as a tumor suppressor in epithelial cells by a variety of mechanisms that include inhibiting cell growth, promoting apoptosis, stimulating epithelial differentiation, enhancing genetic stability, and promoting cellular senescence (Pardali et al. 2005; Ten Dijke et al. 2002). TGFβ causes cell cycle arrest by inducing expression of the cyclin-dependent kinase (CDK) inhibitors p15 and p21 (Massague and Wotton 2000) and by inhibiting transcription of the proto-oncogene c-myc (Chen et al. 2001a). Depending on the cellular context, TGFβ signaling can induce apoptosis and epithelial differentiation through Smad-dependent and Smad-independent mechanisms (Klopcic et al. 2007; Perlman et al. 2001; Rodius et al. 2007; Yanagisawa et al. 1998). TGFβ is induced after radiation-induced DNA damage (Ewan et al. 2002), and defective TGFβ signaling in keratinocytes causes the accumulation of chromosomal defects prior to malignant transformation (Glick et al. 1999). In sum, these studies are consistent with the function of TGFβ as an epithelial tumor suppressor; accordingly, a reduced expression of the TGFβ signaling components is frequently observed in many malignancies, including HNSCC (Levy and Hill 2006).

Role of TGF-β Receptors in HNSCC

Alterations in TGFβ receptor expression have been reported in a variety of malignancies, including HNSCC (Muro-Cacho et al. 1999; Wang et al. 1997). Though TGFβRI mutations are reported in 19% of HNSCC metastases (Chen et al. 2001b), and reduced TGFβRI immunostaining correlates with increased depth of invasion and increased metastases in esophageal squamous cell carcinoma (SCC) (Fukai et al. 2003), associations between TGFβRI defects and HNSCC clinical parameters have not been examined. In comparison, TGFβRII loss can be identified by array comparative genomic hybridization in 40-50% of oral squamous cell carcinoma (SCC) (Snijders et al. 2005; Sparano et al. 2006), and TGFβRII mutations have been identified in 21% of HNSCC

(Wang et al. 1997). In addition, promoter hypermethylation and promoter mutations can reduce TGFβRII expression in HNSCC cell lines (Garrigue-Antar et al. 1995; Worsham et al. 2006). Through a combination of genetic and epigenetic changes, TGFβRII expression is reduced in as many as 70% of HNSCCs (Lu et al. 2006).

Although reduced TGFβRII expression is associated with reduced tumor differentiation and a more aggressive tumor behavior in HNSCC (Fukai et al. 2003; Muro-Cacho et al. 1999), TGFβRII is not reduced in nonmalignant mucosa adjacent to HNSCC (Lu et al. 2006), raising the question of whether TGFβRII loss is a cause or a consequence of HNSCC development. To address this issue, we developed inducible, head and neck-specific, knockout systems and found that TGFβRII deletion in head and neck epithelium does not cause spontaneous HNSCC in mice, which implies that TGFβRII loss cannot initiate HNSCC formation (Lu et al. 2006). However, with the addition of an activating K-ras or H-ras mutation, head and neck TGFβRII deletion resulted in HSNCC formation and metastasis, suggesting that TGFβRII loss promotes the malignant progression of initiated tumor cells (Fig. 8.2, Lu et al. 2006). These tumors not only have a reduced expression of p15 and p21 and an increased expression of c-myc as would be expected from TGFβ signaling disruption, but also an increased cyclin D1 expression, epidermal growth factor receptor (EGFR) expression, and Stat3 activation, all of which are common in human HNSCC (Lu et al. 2006). The tumors also appear pathologically similar to human HNSCC and frequently metastasize to cervical lymph nodes; hence, this represents the first genetically engineered, full penetrance HSNCC mouse model with clinical, pathological, and molecular similarities to human HNSCC (Lu et al. 2006). Another report shows that malignant oral keratinocytes expressing a dominant negative TGFβRII demonstrate increased metastatic potential when injected into the floor of the mouth of athymic mice (Huntley et al. 2004). Taken together, these results show that TGFβRII appears to function as a tumor suppressor in HNSCC and that TGFβRII loss promotes tumor growth, malignant conversion, and metastases in HNSCC.

Role of Smads in HNSCC

Alterations in Smad expression and function can also disrupt TGFβ signaling and facilitate escape from TGFβ-mediated growth arrest and apoptosis (Riggins et al. 1997). Genetic mutation of the common Smad, Smad4, occurs frequently in pancreatic and colon cancer and is associated with both increased nodal involvement and metastases (Levy and Hill 2006). While genetic mutation of Smad4 occurs infrequently in HNSCC (Qiu et al. 2007), loss of heterozygocity (LOH) at the Smad4 locus is observed in both human HNSCC (Kim et al. 1996; Papadimitrakopoulou et al. 1998) and HNSCC cell lines Takebayashi et al. 2000, (2004). Accordingly, we found that approximately 70% of HNSCCs also demonstrate a reduced Smad4 mRNA expression (unpublished data). Loss of Smad4 protein by immunostaining has been reported in 20-50% of HNSCCs (Iamaroon et al. 2006; Muro-Cacho et al.

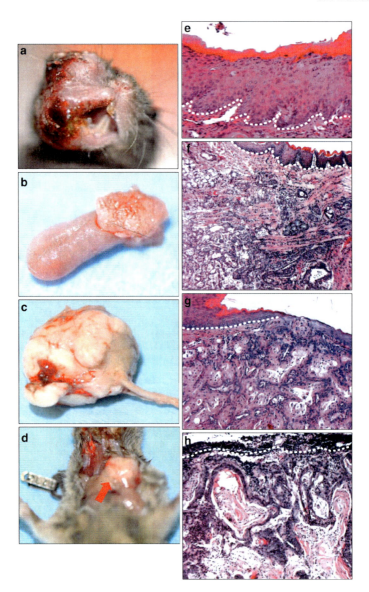

Fig. 8.2 Genetically engineered mouse model with full penetrance of HNSCC (modified from Lu et al. (2006) with permission of CSHL press). Gross appearance of HNSCC arising from the buccal mucosa (**a**), tongue (**b**), lower esophagus (**c**) in mice with TGFβRII deletion and Ras activation in the head and neck epithelium. Ras activation was produced by knock-in of oncogenic K-ras^{G12D} mutation (**a**) or by treatment with 7, 12-dimethylbenz (**a**) anthracene (DMBA), which causes activating Ha-ras mutations (**b** and **c**). A jugular lymph node metastasis from a DMBA-treated mouse with head and neck epithelial TGFβRII deletion (**d**). Buccal dysplasia (**e**), tongue SCC (panel **f**), and buccal SCC (panel **g**) in an animal with head and neck epithelial TGFβRII deletion and a K-ras^{G12D} mutation and a lymph note metastasis (**h**) of the oral tumor developed from the above mice

2001; Xie et al. 2003) and is probably the result of LOH, but may also be mediated by increased activity of Smad ubiquitin-E3 ligases (ten Dijke and Hill 2004). While associations between Smad4 loss and clinical outcomes in HNSCC have not been evaluated, Smad4 loss is correlated with increased tumor invasion and more frequent nodal metastases in esophageal SCC (Fukuchi et al. 2002b; Natsugoe et al. 2002).

Studies from animal models support the role of Smad4 as a tumor suppressor in HNSCC and highlight differences in the way TGFβ signaling defects promote HNSCC. Whereas TGFβRII deletion in the oral epithelium does not cause HSNCC formation in the absence of an initiating event (Lu et al. 2006), Smad4 deletion in the oral epithelium results in the development of HNSCC with metastases (our unpublished data). This is the first example of HNSCC development caused by a single gene deletion and suggests that Smad4 is a more potent tumor suppressor than TGFβRII, perhaps because it transduces signals from both TGFβ and BMP pathways. Further analysis revealed that these tumors have an increased chromosomal instability, which also likely contributes to both HNSCC formation and progression. These observations are consistent with the role of Smad4 in other epithelial layers, as conditional deletion of Smad4 in the epidermis or mammary gland also causes spontaneous SCC development (Qiao et al. 2006; Yang et al. 2005).

Data regarding the role of Smad2 are more limited. Loss of Smad2 protein is reported in 15-40% of HNSCC and is associated with a worse prognosis (Muro-Cacho et al. 2001; Xie et al. 2003). In esophageal SCC, reduced phospho-Smad2 (activated Smad2) is correlated with increased pathologic stage, increased lymph node involvement, more frequent distant metastasis, and decreased patient survival. However, it is unclear if this represents a specific reduction of Smad2 expression or a generalized loss of TGFβ signaling competency (Fukuchi et al. 2006; Muro-Cacho et al. 2001). While mechanisms of Smad2 loss in HNSCC have not been evaluated, Smad2 is located close to Smad4 on chromosome 18 and is frequently deleted with Smad4 in colon and pancreatic cancers (Jonson et al. 1999). Hence, it is possible that HNSCCs also have simultaneous Smad2 and Smad4 deletion.

To date, no animal models have evaluated the role of Smad2 in HNSCC, though some insight can be gleaned from animal models of other epithelial malignancies. While epidermal deletion of Smad2 does not cause the development of spontaneous skin SCC, it does increase susceptibility to chemical skin carcinogenesis (our unpublished data). Interestingly, skin SCCs arising in this background are more poorly differentiated and undergo earlier EMT than chemically induced skin SCC in wild-type mice, suggesting a specific role for Smad2 in mediating EMT and tumor dedifferentiation. It remains to be seen whether deletion of Smad2 in oral epithelium causes either spontaneous HNSCC or an increased susceptibility to oral carcinogens.

In contrast to Smad2 and Smad4, the studies do not support a role of Smad3 as a tumor suppressor in HNSCC. While Smad2 and Smad4 expression are frequently reduced in human HNSCC, Smad3 is generally retained in HNSCC, skin SCC, and lung SCC (unpublished data), and germline Smad3 deletion confers resistance to chemical skin carcinogenesis in a gene-dosage dependent manner (Li et al. 2004a; Tannehill-Gregg et al. 2004). Smad3 knockout mice exhibit reduced numbers of tumor-associated macrophages and also have reduced keratinocyte hyperproliferation as a result of reduced AP1 family member expression (Li et al. 2004a). In addition, Smad3 transcriptionally upregulates Gli1, a sonic hedgehog signaling component often activated in cancer (Dennler et al. 2007). Given that mice expressing a dominant negative TGFβRII exclusively in T cells are protected against tumors induced by injection of melanoma cells (Gorelik and Flavell 2001), it is possible that impaired TGFβ signaling in immunocytes contributes to the resistance to chemical skin carcinogenesis seen with germline Smad3 deletion. These observations highlight the tissue and tumor-specificity of both TGFβ signaling and TGFβ signaling defects.

Role of TGFβ Signaling Inhibitors in HNSCC

An increased expression of molecules that block TGFβ signaling can also promote tumor growth and development. Smad7 blocks Smad2 phosphorylation (Nakao et al. 1997) and targets TGFβRI and Smad2 for proteosomal degradation mediated by Smurf1 and Smurf2 (Ebisawa et al. 2001; Kavsak et al. 2000; Zhang et al. 2001), while c-Ski and SnoN negatively regulate Smad2, Smad3, and Smad4 (He et al. 2003). Increased expression of Smad7, Smurf2, and c-Ski in esophageal SCC has been associated with increased depth of tumor invasion, increased nodal involvement, and shorter survival (Fukuchi et al. 2002a, 2004b; Osawa et al. 2004). Smad7 overexpression has been observed in HNSCC cell lines (Pring et al. 2006), and we have observed Smad7 overexpression in human HNSCC tumor samples (unpublished data). However, the precise role of Smad7 in HNSCC is unknown. Smad7 overexpression in vivo causes epithelial hyperproliferation and decreased apoptosis (Han et al. 2006; He et al. 2002), and Smad7 overexpression in keratinocytes causes conversion of Ha-ras initiated papillomas to SCC in a skin graft model (Liu et al. 2003). These studies point to an oncogenic effect of Smad7. On the other hand, Smad7 overexpression directly inhibits Wnt/β-catenin signaling independent of TGFβ receptor and R-Smad degradation (Han et al. 2006), and Smad7 also has potent anti-inflammatory properties through blockade of tumor necrosis factor-α (TNFα) signaling (Hong et al. 2007). Given the importance of chronic inflammation in cancer progression and metastasis, and the potent oncogenic role of Wnt/β-catenin signaling, the net effect of Smad7 on HNSCC development and progression remains to be determined.

Tumor Promoting Role of the TGFβ1 Ligand in HNSCC

As described above, TGFβ signaling has a tumor-suppressive effect. However, TGFβ1 is often overexpressed in cancer (Bierie and Moses 2006). During early stage carcinogenesis TGFβ is tumor suppressive (Cui et al. 1996; Weeks et al. 2001). However, in response to defective TGFβ signaling, tumor epithelial cells increase TGFβ1 production, which can paradoxically <u>promote</u> tumor growth and metastases via its paracrine effects on tumor stroma (Bierie and Moses 2006). An elevated local TGFβ1 expression correlates with increased nodal involvement, more advanced disease at presentation, and reduced survival (Levy and Hill 2006; Lu et al. 2004). Elevated local TGFβ1 can frequently be detected in normal tissue adjacent to HNSCC, suggesting that TGFβ1 overexpression occurs at the early stage of HNSCC development (Lu et al. 2004).

Chemical skin carcinogenesis models illustrate the stage-dependent tumor promoting actions of TGFβ (Cui et al. 1996; Han et al. 2005; Weeks et al. 2001). While constitutive epidermal TGFβ1 expression reduces the formation of benign papillomas during early disease, TGFβ1 promotes malignant conversion of papillomas to highly dysplastic spindle cell carcinomas (Cui et al. 1996). Similarly, when TGFβ1 expression is induced in benign papillomas, it increases malignant conversion and metastases (Weeks et al. 2001). Local TGFβ1 overexpression plays a critical tumor promoting role in the setting of TGFβRII deletion: When forced TGFβ1 overexpression is coupled with the expression of a dominant negative TGFβRII, metastases increase two-fold in a skin chemical carcinogenesis model (Han et al. 2005).

Mechanisms of TGFβ1-Mediated Tumor Promotion

TGFβ1 produced by tumor epithelial cells promotes tumor growth and metastases through a variety of mechanisms that include promoting tumor epithelial cells to develop a more fibroblastoid and migratory phenotype, activating tumor-associated fibroblasts, increasing matrix degradation and angiogenesis, suppressing immune surveillance, and inducing inflammation (Bierie and Moses 2006).

TGFβ1 stimulates a variety of epithelial cells to assume a mesenchymal phenotype characterized by loss of E-cadherin, upregulation of mesenchymal markers, fibroblastoid morphology, and increased motility (Grunert et al. 2003). This appears to require interactions between TGFβ signaling and the components of other signaling pathways including the Ras/Raf and Rho/Rac pathways (Han et al. 2005; Zavadil and Bottinger 2005). Earlier studies suggested that TGFβ1-mediated EMT in H-ras transformed mammary epithelial cells (Oft et al. 1996). Similarly, K-ras or H-ras initiated epithelial cells stimulated by TGFβ demonstrate an increased invasive potential, particularly at the leading edge of the tumor (Grunert et al. 2003). However, we observed that while TGFβ1 mediated increased angiogenesis through activation of the mitogen-activated protein kinase (MAPK) pathway, EMT appears to be mediated through Smad-dependent activation of the Notch pathway (Han et al. 2005). Further, blocking TGFβ signaling abrogates TGFβ1-mediated EMT, but not metastasis, indicating that EMT and metastasis can be uncoupled (Han et al. 2005). These observations help explain how TGFβ1 promotes malignant conversion of H-ras initiated papillomas to highly dysplastic spindle cell carcinomas in vivo (Cui et al. 1996).

MMPs secreted from tumor epithelia or stroma cells degradate the basement membrane, facilitating migration of tumor cells through the extracellular matrix.

TGFβ1 stimulates the secretion of MMP1, MMP9, and MMP10 in HNSCC cell lines (Leivonen et al. 2006; Wilkins-Port and Higgins 2007). In vivo expression of TGFβ1 in chemically induced papillomas or orthotopically transplanted prostate cancer cells is associated with an increased elaboration of MMP2 and MMP9 (Stearns et al. 1999; Weeks et al. 2001), and TGFβ1 treatment increases MMP production and motility in orthotopically transplanted gastric carcinoma cells (Wang et al. 2006). In addition, a TGFβ signaling disruption in mammary carcinoma cells causes recruitment of myeloid cells at the invading tumor edge; these cells secrete MMP2, MMP13, and MMP14 and increase the metastatic potential of the mammary tumor cells (Yang et al. 2008). Of particular interest, is the fact that MMP1 can also activate latent TGFβ1 (Iida and McCarthy 2007), demonstrating the complex paracrine interactions that occur between tumor epithelial cells, fibroblasts, and the extracellular matrix to regulate tumor cell migration and invasion.

TGFβ1 is a key regulator of vascular development and maintenance and stimulates both vasculogenesis and angiogenesis by increasing the production of angiogenic factors such as the vascular endothelial growth factor (VEGF) and the hepatocyte growth factor (HGF) and by directly regulating endothelial cells (Bertolino et al. 2005). Secreted TGFβ1 into the tumor stroma stimulates endothelial cell proliferation through ALK1 receptor complexes on endothelial cells and Smad1/5/8 signaling (Bertolino et al. 2005). Forced TGFβ1 overexpression in mouse head and neck epithelia induces angiogenesis through a similar mechanism (Lu et al. 2004). In addition to directly stimulating endothelial cells, TGFβ1 treatment of human lung cancer cells stimulates the production of VEGF (Pertovaara et al. 1994), and TGFβ1 treatment of oral myofibroblasts stimulates the secretion of HGF (Lewis et al. 2004), both of which can promote tumor growth as well as angiogenesis. In vivo, TGFβ1 expression in chemically induced papillomas reduces the expression of the angiogenic inhibitors thrombospondin 1 and 2 with an associated increase in angiogenesis (Weeks et al. 2001).

Because TGFβ1 is overexpressed in pathologically normal appearing mucosa adjacent to HNSCC, we developed an inducible transgenic system to examine the effect of TGFβ1 in normal head and neck epithelia (Lu et al. 2004). Surprisingly, TGFβ1 overexpression in head and neck epithelia did not inhibit growth but instead induced massive inflammation and angiogenesis with resultant epithelial hyperproliferation (Lu et al. 2004). A similar phenotype is also observed when TGFβ1 is overexpressed in the epidermis (Li et al. 2004b). TGFβ1 overexpression causes the infiltration of macrophages, neutrophils, and mast cells, all of which secrete numerous inflammatory cytokines, chemokines, and angiogenic factors (Li et al. 2004b; Lu et al. 2004). In addition, the proinflammatory Th17 cells also require TGFβ1 for maturation and activation (Korn et al. 2007; Li et al. 2007). However, when the epidermal keratinocytes are separated from the inflammatory cells and stromal cells, TGFβ1-induced growth inhibition is restored (Li et al. 2004b), suggesting that TGFβ1-induced inflammation, angiogenesis, and fibroblast proliferation can completely override the TGFβ1-dependent growth inhibition of epithelial cells. Given the impact of chronic inflammation on cancer formation and progression (Balkwill and Coussens 2004; Coussens and Werb

2002), it is possible that TGFβ1-mediated inflammation represents an additional mechanism by which TGFβ1 creates a tumor-promoting microenvironment. Interestingly, TGFβ1 can also be a potent immune suppressor. TGFβ1 suppresses the production of cytotoxic gene products by T cells (Thomas and Massague 2005), and blockade of TGFβ signaling in T cells improves the immune response to tumor cells (Gorelik and Flavell 2001; Zhang et al. 2005), demonstrating that despite a robust infiltration of immune cells into a tumor, TGFβ1 can blunt the functional antitumor immune response.

As mentioned, HNSCCs often demonstrate both an increased TGFβ1 production and a reduced TGFβ signaling (Lu et al. 2006). The increased TGFβ1 production may be a result of a negative feedback for reduced functional TGFβ signaling in tumor epithelia. Indeed, the deletion of either TGFβRII or Smad4 in head and neck epithelia causes increased TGFβ1 mRNA and protein (Lu et al. 2006, and our unpublished data). In this situation, not only have tumor epithelial cells lost the ability to respond to TGFβ1 growth inhibition, but the excess TGFβ1 secreted into the tumor stroma creates a tumor-promoting microenvironment through its effects on endothelial cells, inflammatory cells, and fibroblasts. Supporting this notion, we found increased inflammatory cytokines/chemokines in TGFβRII-deleted head and neck mouse tumors, such as interleukin-1β; macrophage inflammatory protein-2; and stromal derived factor-1 and its receptor, CXCR4 (Lu et al. 2006). Elevated levels of these molecules are also seen in skin or oral tissue with TGFβ1 transgene expression alone (Li et al. 2004b; Lu et al. 2004). Further, several known TGFβ target genes that promote tumor invasion, such as connective tissue growth factor, α-smooth muscle actin, and tenascin-C, are also elevated in the tumor stroma of TGFβRII-deleted head and neck mouse tumors. Taken together, our studies suggest that inflammation and the associated increase in inflammatory cytokines/chemokines are the result of the increased TGFβ1 paracrine effect in head and neck cancer with TGFβRII loss, which further contributes to the malignant progression of these tumors.

Contribution of TGFβ Signaling in Tumor-Associated Stroma to HNSCC

The understanding of the role that stromal cells play in supporting epithelial carcinogenesis continues to evolve, and reports of TGFβ signaling defects in tumor stromal cells are beginning to emerge. HNSCC tumor-associated fibroblasts demonstrate both increased TGFβ1 expression (Rosenthal et al. 2004) and LOH at the TGFβRII locus (Weber et al. 2007). Reduced TGFβRII expression in tumor-associated macrophages has been observed in colon cancer and is associated with increased incidence of lymph node metastases (Bacman et al. 2007). Most provocatively, TGFβRII deletion specifically in fibroblasts, causes spontaneous forestomach SCC and prostate intraepithelial hyperplasia (Bhowmick et al. 2004). Further analysis reveals that TGFβRII deletion in fibroblasts increases

HGF expression, which activates its receptor, c-Met, in tumor epithelia, resulting, at least in part, in promoting tumor invasion and growth (Cheng et al. 2005). Similarly, Smad4 deletion, specifically in T lymphocytes, causes a dense inflammatory infiltrate in the gastrointestinal tract stroma with the subsequent development of epithelial cancers, including oral SCC (Kim et al. 2006). In sum, these studies directly demonstrate the ability of the stromal cells to regulate tumor formation in the adjacent epithelial layers as well as the complex paracrine signaling that occurs between the tumor epithelial cells and the infiltrating tumor stroma cells within the tumor microenvironment.

Serum TGFβ1 as a Marker of Disease Burden in Cancer Patients

Elevated TGFβ1 can also be detected in the serum of patients with breast, gastric, colorectal, esophageal, and lung cancer (Barthelemy-Brichant et al. 2002; Fukuchi et al. 2004a; Ivanovic et al. 2006; Saito et al. 2000; Sun et al. 2007; Tsushima et al. 1996). In gastric cancer, an elevated serum TGFβ1 correlates with lymph node metastases, peritoneal involvement, and a poor prognosis (Saito et al. 2000). Elevated serum TGFβ1 correlates with more frequent liver metastasis in colorectal carcinoma (Tsushima et al. 2001) and is associated with higher-stage, more frequent metastases, and a decreased 2-year survival in breast cancer (Ivanovic et al. 2006). Similarly, an elevated serum TGFβ1 is an independent marker of decreased survival in esophageal cancer (Fukuchi et al. 2004a). These observations have spurred an interest in using serum TGFβ1 to predict response to therapy and the development of recurrent or metastatic disease. Serum TGFβ1 levels decrease after therapy in esophageal, colorectal, and nasopharyngeal carcinoma (Chen et al. 2005; Sun et al. 2007; Tsushima et al. 2001), and patients with higher post-treatment serum TGFβ1 are at an increased risk of developing metastasis (Tsushima et al. 2001). Interestingly, in an orthotopic murine model of metastatic HNSCC, serum TGFβ1 elevations temporally coincided with the development of metastasis (Dasgupta et al. 2006). At this point, although serum TGFβ1 may be a marker for overall disease burden and potentially for recurrent or metastatic disease, it is unclear whether the sensitivity, specificity, and predictive value of TGFβ1 levels are great enough to be of clinical utility.

TGFβ Signaling as a Potential Pharmacological Target for Cancer Therapy

Given its broad role in tumor development and progression, TGFβ signaling is a logical therapeutic target.. However, the multifaceted roles of TGFβ in normal tissue homeostasis coupled with the biphasic role of TGFβ in tumor development and progression have complicated attempts to modulate TGFβ signaling. Successful therapeutic manipulation of TGFβ signaling will require blockade of the pro-oncogenic TGFβ actions (i.e., increased EMT, invasion, metastases, angiogenesis, and immune suppression) without adversely affecting the TGFβ-stimulated growth arrest or apoptosis; however, most epithelial tumors have probably escaped TGFβ-mediated growth inhibition by clinical presentation. Several potential strategies have emerged; the most promising are inhibition or sequestration of soluble TGFβ, blockade of TGFβ signaling with small molecule kinase inhibitors or anti-sense oligonucleotides, and adoptive transfer of immune cells that have been rendered insensitive to TGFβ (Pennison and Pasche 2007; Yingling et al. 2004). Although no clinical or preclinical studies in HNSCC have been reported, other cancer models demonstrate the potential feasibility and efficacy of manipulating TGFβ signaling.

Treatment with an Fc-TGFβRII fusion protein did not prevent the development of primary tumors in a mouse model of mammary cancer; it did, however, decrease tumor cell motility with a commensurate reduction in metastases (Muraoka et al. 2002). In an analogous genetic model, constitutive expression of the soluble Fc-TGFβRII fusion protein reduced the formation of metastases without a reduction in primary tumor frequency – but also without any observable side effects (Yang et al. 2002). Similarly, blockade of all the three TGFβ isoforms reduced the development of metastases after thoracic radiation or chemotherapy in a mouse model of breast cancer (Biswas et al. 2007). Importantly, in all these models, the severe inflammatory phenotype observed with germline TGFβ1 disruption was not observed (Kulkarni et al. 1993; Shull et al. 1992), nor was there an increase in primary tumor size or multiplicity, although a nonstatistical increase in metastases was observed with anti-TGFβ antibody in the absence of radiation (Biswas et al. 2007). Alternatively, reduction in serum TGFβ by immunoabsorption increases immune cell function and decreases tumor growth in a xenograft hepatocellular cancer rat model (Yamamoto et al. 2006). In sum, these reports suggest that systemic TGFβ1 blockade may be a safe and effective strategy to reduce metastases in human malignancy.

Small molecule inhibitors, predominantly targeting the intracellular kinase domain of TGFβRI, are also being developed. SD-208 suppresses TGFβ-mediated EMT and migration in cultured pancreatic carcinoma cells, mammary tumor cells, and glioma cells as well as in an analogous orthotopic transplant models (Gaspar et al. 2007; Ge et al. 2006; Uhl et al. 2004). LY364947 increased the tumor delivery of doxorubicin-laden nanoparticles by inhibiting tumor endothelial cells in a pancreatic tumor cell xenograft model (Kano et al. 2007). Another TGFβRI kinase inhibitor, SB-4361542, appears to have similar activity in a variety of cancer cell lines (Inman et al. 2002; Tojo et al. 2005); however, none of these molecules has reached clinical trials. In contrast, after showing preclinical efficacy, oligonucleotides targeting TGFβRII have reached phase IIb trials for high-grade glioma (Schlingensiepen et al. 2006, 2008).

Another interesting approach is to enhance the antitumor immune response by blocking TGFβ signaling in T cells. Mice expressing a dominant negative TGFβRII in T cells are almost completely protected against tumors induced by injection of B16-F10 melanoma cells, and adoptively transferred T cells from these animals exhibit potent antitumor activity in preexisting tumors developed in Rag1 mice (Gorelik and Flavell 2001). Likewise, both specific tumor immunity and antitumor activity were observed after tumor-sensitized T cells transfected with retrovirus expressing a dominant negative TGFβRII were adoptively transferred introduced into recipient mice harboring tumors derived from the same cell line (Zhang et al. 2005). These studies not only provide compelling proof of concept data but also highlight the immune-suppressive potency of TGFβ. However, the level of TGFβ signaling targeted for antitumor approaches involving the immune system will be critical: while blockade of TGFβRII in T cells is tumor protective (Gorelik and Flavell 2001), Smad4 deletion in T cells causes stromal inflammation and gastrointestinal tumors (Kim et al. 2006).

Summary and Future Perspectives

Defective TGFβ signaling in the head and neck epithelia occurs through a variety of genetic, epigenetic, and post-translational mechanisms and involves multiple members of the TGFβ-Smad signaling cascade; however, defects involving loss of TGFβRII and Smad4 have been best characterized in HNSCC. TGFβ signaling defects allow epithelial cells to escape TGFβ-mediated growth inhibition and cause increased local and systemic TGFβ production, which then promotes metastases by stimulating tumor cell invasion, angiogenesis, and inflammation. Both loss of TGFβ-dependent tumor suppression and the pro-metastatic effects of TGFβ1 involve crosstalk between TGFβ signaling and other signaling pathways critical to tumor growth and metastases. For example, in our HNSCC mouse model, it was necessary to combine Ras initiation with TGFβRII deletion to generate tumors (Lu et al. 2006). That these tumors harbor molecular alterations commonly observed in human HNSCC, such as increased expression of EGFR and Stat3 activation (Lu et al. 2006), suggests that therapies targeting other pathways (e.g., EGFR kinase inhibitors) may be active against HNSCC with defective TGFβ signaling and that combination therapies targeting both tumor epithelia cells and stromal TGFβ signaling may be even more efficacious. While it is currently unknown whether systemic TGFβ levels correlate with the disease burden, the presence of local or distant metastases, or the response to therapy in HNSCC, it is possible that serum TGFβ will eventually be used as a staging tool or to monitor therapeutic responses. At least initially, specific targeting of the TGFβ pathway is likely to be reserved for HNSCC with regional or distant metastases because of concerns about a TGFβ pathway blockade increasing primary tumor growth. Given the available preclinical data, it appears that at least a short-term systemic TGFβ blockade is safe; however, the long-term effects of this strategy as well as the optimal situations for targeting TGFβ signaling remain active areas of research.

References

Alazzouzi H, Alhopuro P, Salovaara R, Sammalkorpi H, Jarvinen H, Mecklin JP, Hemminki A, Schwartz S Jr, Aaltonen LA, Arango D (2005) SMAD4 as a prognostic markeNoar in colorectal cancer. Clin Cancer Res 11:2606–2611

Alvi A, Johnson JT (1997) Development of distant metastasis after treatment of advanced-stage head and neck cancer. Head Neck 19:500–505

Bacman D, Merkel S, Croner R, Papadopoulos T, Brueckl W, Dimmler A (2007) TGF-beta receptor 2 downregulation in tumour-associated stroma worsens prognosis and high-grade tumours show more tumour-associated macrophages and lower TGF-beta1 expression in colon carcinoma: a retrospective study. BMC Cancer 7:156

Balkwill F, Coussens LM (2004) Cancer: an inflammatory link. Nature 431:405–406

Barthelemy-Brichant N, David JL, Bosquee L, Bury T, Seidel L, Albert A, Bartsch P, Baugnet-Mahieu L, Deneufbourg JM (2002) Increased TGFbeta1 plasma level in patients with lung cancer: potential mechanisms. Eur J Clin Invest 32:193–198

Beer KT, Greiner RH, Aebersold DM, Zbaren P (2000) Carcinoma of the oropharynx: local failure as the decisive parameter for distant metastases and survival. Strahlenther Onkol 176:16–21

Bertolino P, Deckers M, Lebrin F, ten Dijke P (2005) Transforming growth factor-beta signal transduction in angiogenesis and vascular disorders. Chest 128:585S–590S

Bhowmick NA, Chytil A, Plieth D, Gorska AE, Dumont N, Shappell S, Washington MK, Neilson EG, Moses HL (2004) TGF-beta signaling in fibroblasts modulates the oncogenic potential of adjacent epithelia. Science 303:848–851

Bierie B, Moses HL (2006) Tumour microenvironment: TGFbeta: the molecular Jekyll and Hyde of cancer. Nat Rev Cancer 6:506–520

Biswas S, Guix M, Rinehart C, Dugger TC, Chytil A, Moses HL, Freeman ML, Arteaga CL (2007) Inhibition of TGF-beta with neutralizing antibodies prevents radiation-induced acceleration of metastatic cancer progression. J Clin Invest 117:1305–1313

Chen CR, Kang Y, Massague J (2001a) Defective repression of c-myc in breast cancer cells: A loss at the core of the transforming growth factor beta growth arrest program. Proc Natl Acad Sci U S A 98:992–999

Chen T, Yan W, Wells RG, Rimm DL, McNiff J, Leffell D, Reiss M (2001b) Novel inactivating mutations of transforming growth factor-beta type I receptor gene in head-and-neck cancer metastases. Int J Cancer 93:653–661

Chen HW, Chang YC, Lai YL, Chen YJ, Huang MJ, Leu YS, Fu YK, Wang LW, Hwang JJ (2005) Change of plasma transforming growth factor-beta1 levels in nasopharyngeal carcinoma patients treated with concurrent chemo-radiotherapy. Jpn J Clin Oncol Vol 35:427–432

Cheng N, Bhowmick NA, Chytil A, Gorksa AE, Brown KA, Muraoka R, Arteaga CL, Neilson EG, Hayward SW, Moses HL (2005) Loss of TGF-beta type II receptor in fibroblasts promotes mammary carcinoma growth and invasion through upregulation of TGF-alpha-, MSP- and HGF-mediated signaling networks. Oncogene 24:5053–5068

Coussens LM, Werb Z (2002) Inflammation and cancer. Nature 420:860–867

Cui W, Fowlis DJ, Bryson S, Duffie E, Ireland H, Balmain A, Akhurst RJ (1996) TGFbeta1 inhibits the formation of benign skin tumors, but enhances progression to invasive spindle carcinomas in transgenic mice. Cell 86:531–542

Dasgupta S, Bhattacharya-Chatterjee M, O'Malley BW Jr, Chatterjee SK (2006) Tumor metastasis in an orthotopic murine model of head and neck cancer: possible role of TGF-beta 1 secreted by the tumor cells. J Cell Biochem 97:1036–1051

Dennler S, Andre J, Alexaki I, Li A, Magnaldo T, ten Dijke P, Wang XJ, Verrecchia F, Mauviel A (2007) Induction of sonic hedgehog mediators by transforming growth factor-beta: Smad3-dependent activation of Gli2 and Gli1 expression in vitro and in vivo. Cancer Res 67:6981–6986

Derynck R, Zhang YE (2003) Smad-dependent and Smad-independent pathways in TGF-beta family signalling. Nature 425:577–584

Derynck R, Lindquist PB, Lee A, Wen D, Tamm J, Graycar JL, Rhee L, Mason AJ, Miller DA, Coffey, RJ et al (1988) A new type of transforming growth factor-beta, TGF-beta 3. Embo J 7:3737–3743

Ebisawa T, Fukuchi M, Murakami G, Chiba T, Tanaka K, Imamura T, Miyazono K (2001) Smurf1 interacts with transforming growth factor-beta type I receptor through Smad7 and induces receptor degradation. J Biol Chem 276:12477–12480

Ewan KB, Henshall-Powell RL, Ravani SA, Pajares MJ, Arteaga C, Warters R, Akhurst RJ, Barcellos-Hoff MH (2002) Transforming growth factor-beta1 mediates cellular response to DNA damage in situ. Cancer Res 62:5627–5631

Feng XH, Derynck R (1996) Ligand-independent activation of transforming growth factor (TGF) beta signaling pathways by heteromeric cytoplasmic domains of TGF-beta receptors. J Biol Chem 271:13123–13129

Feng XH, Derynck R (2005) Specificity and versatility in tgf-beta signaling through Smads. Annu Rev Cell Dev Biol 21:659–693

Fukai Y, Fukuchi M, Masuda N, Osawa H, Kato H, Nakajima T, Kuwano H (2003) Reduced expression of transforming growth factor-beta receptors is an unfavorable prognostic factor in human esophageal squamous cell carcinoma. Int J Cancer 104:161–166

Fukuchi M, Fukai Y, Masuda N, Miyazaki T, Nakajima M, Sohda M, Manda R, Tsukada K, Kato H, Kuwano H (2002a) High-level expression of the Smad ubiquitin ligase Smurf2 correlates with poor prognosis in patients with esophageal squamous cell carcinoma. Cancer Res 62:7162–7165

Fukuchi M, Masuda N, Miyazaki T, Nakajima M, Osawa H, Kato H, Kuwano H (2002b) Decreased Smad4 expression in the transforming growth factor-beta signaling pathway during progression of esophageal squamous cell carcinoma. Cancer 95:737–743

Fukuchi M, Miyazaki T, Fukai Y, Nakajima M, Sohda M, Masuda N, Manda R, Tsukada K, Kato H, Kuwano H (2004a) Plasma level of transforming growth factor beta1 measured from the azygos vein predicts prognosis in patients with esophageal cancer. Clin Cancer Res 10:2738–2741

Fukuchi M, Nakajima M, Fukai Y, Miyazaki T, Masuda N, Sohda M, Manda R, Tsukada K, Kato H, Kuwano H (2004b) Increased expression of c-Ski as a co-repressor in transforming growth factor-beta signaling correlates with progression of esophageal squamous cell carcinoma. Int J Cancer 108:818–824

Fukuchi M, Nakajima M, Miyazaki T, Masuda N, Osawa H, Manda R, Tsukada K, Kato H, Kuwano H (2006) Lack of activated Smad2 in transforming growth factor-beta signaling is an unfavorable prognostic factor in patients with esophageal squamous cell carcinoma. J Surg Oncol 94:51–56

Garavello W, Ciardo A, Spreafico R, Gaini RM (2006) Risk factors for distant metastases in head and neck squamous cell carcinoma. Arch Otolaryngol Head Neck Surg 132:762–766

Garrigue-Antar L, Munoz-Antonia T, Antonia SJ, Gesmonde J, Vellucci VF, Reiss M (1995) Missense mutations of the transforming growth factor beta type II receptor in human head and neck squamous carcinoma cells. Cancer Res 55:3982–3987

Gaspar NJ, Li L, Kapoun AM, Medicherla S, Reddy M, Li G, O'Young G, Quon D, Henson M, Damm DL, Muiru GT, Murphy A, Higgins LS, Chakravarty S, Wong DH (2007) Inhibition of transforming growth factor beta signaling reduces pancreatic adenocarcinoma growth and invasiveness. Mol Pharmacol 72:152–161

Ge R, Rajeev V, Ray P, Lattime E, Rittling S, Medicherla S, Protter A, Murphy A, Chakravarty J, Dugar S, Schreiner G, Barnard N, Reiss M (2006) Inhibition of growth and metastasis of mouse mammary carcinoma by selective inhibitor of transforming growth factor-beta type I receptor kinase in vivo. Clin Cancer Res 12:4315–4330

Glick A, Popescu N, Alexander V, Ueno H, Bottinger E, Yuspa SH (1999) Defects in transforming growth factor-beta signaling cooperate with a Ras oncogene to cause rapid aneuploidy and malignant transformation of mouse keratinocytes. Proc Natl Acad Sci U S A 96:14949–14954

Gorelik L, Flavell RA (2001) Immune-mediated eradication of tumors through the blockade of transforming growth factor-beta signaling in T cells. Nat Med 7:1118–1122

Grunert S, Jechlinger M, Beug H (2003) Diverse cellular and molecular mechanisms contribute to epithelial plasticity and metastasis. Nat Rev Mol Cell Biol 4:657–665

Han G, Lu SL, Li AG, He W, Corless CL, Kulesz-Martin M, Wang XJ (2005) Distinct mechanisms of TGF-beta1-mediated epithelial-to-mesenchymal transition and metastasis during skin carcinogenesis. J Clin Invest 115:1714–1723

Han G, Li AG, Liang YY, Owens P, He W, Lu S, Yoshimatsu Y, Wang D, Ten Dijke P, Lin X, Wang XJ (2006) Smad7-induced beta-catenin degradation alters epidermal appendage development. Dev Cell 11:301–312

Hanahan D, Weinberg RA (2000) The hallmarks of cancer. Cell 100:57–70

Hayat MJ, Howlader N, Reichman ME, Edwards BK (2007) Cancer statistics, trends, and multiple primary cancer analyses from the Surveillance, Epidemiology, and End Results (SEER) Program. Oncologist 12:20–37

He W, Li AG, Wang D, Han S, Zheng B, Goumans MJ, Ten Dijke P, Wang XJ (2002) Overexpression of Smad7 results in severe pathological alterations in multiple epithelial tissues. Embo J 21:2580–2590

He J, Tegen SB, Krawitz AR, Martin GS, Luo K (2003) The transforming activity of Ski and SnoN is dependent on their ability to repress the activity of Smad proteins. J Biol Chem 278:30540–30547

Hong S, Lim S, Li AG, Lee C, Lee YS, Lee EK, Park SH, Wang XJ, Kim SJ (2007) Smad7 binds to the adaptors TAB2 and TAB3 to block recruitment of the kinase TAK1 to the adaptor TRAF2. Nat Immunol 8:504–513

Huntley SP, Davies M, Matthews JB, Thomas G, Marshall J, Robinson CM, Eveson JW, Paterson IC, Prime SS (2004) Attenuated type II TGF-beta receptor signalling in human malignant oral keratinocytes induces a less differentiated and more aggressive phenotype that is associated with metastatic dissemination. Int J Cancer 110:170–176

Iamaroon A, Pattamapun K, Piboonniyom SO (2006) Aberrant expression of Smad4, a TGF-beta signaling molecule, in oral squamous cell carcinoma. J Oral Sci 48:105–109

Iida J, McCarthy JB (2007) Expression of collagenase-1 (MMP-1) promotes melanoma growth through the generation of active transforming growth factor-beta. Melanoma Res 17:205–213

Inman GJ, Nicolas FJ, Callahan JF, Harling JD, Gaster LM, Reith AD, Laping NJ, Hill CS (2002) SB-431542 is a potent and specific inhibitor of transforming growth factor-beta superfamily type I activin receptor-like kinase (ALK) receptors ALK4, ALK5, and ALK7. Mol Pharmacol 62:65–74

Ivanovic V, Demajo M, Krtolica K, Krajnovic M, Konstantinovic M, Baltic V, Prtenjak G, Stojiljkovic B, Breberina M, Neskovic-Konstantinovic Z, Nikolic-Vukosavljevic D, Dimitrijevic B (2006) Elevated plasma TGF-beta1 levels correlate with decreased survival of metastatic breast cancer patients. Clin Chim Acta 371:191–193

Jemal A, Siegel R, Ward E, Murray T, Xu J, Thun MJ (2007) Cancer statistics, 2007. CA Cancer J Clin 57:43–66

Jonson T, Gorunova L, Dawiskiba S, Andren-Sandberg A, Stenman G, ten Dijke P, Johansson B, Hoglund M (1999) Molecular analyses of the 15q and 18q SMAD genes in pancreatic cancer. Genes Chromosomes Cancer 24:62–71

Kano MR, Bae Y, Iwata C, Morishita Y, Yashiro M, Oka M, Fujii T, Komuro A, Kiyono K, Kaminishi M, Hirakawa K, Ouchi Y, Nishiyama N, Kataoka K, Miyazono K (2007) Improvement of cancer-targeting therapy, using nanocarriers for intractable solid tumors by inhibition of TGF-beta signaling. Proc Natl Acad Sci U S A 104:3460–3465

Kavsak P, Rasmussen RK, Causing CG, Bonni S, Zhu H, Thomsen GH, Wrana JL (2000) Smad7 binds to Smurf2 to form an E3 ubiquitin ligase that targets the TGF beta receptor for degradation. Mol Cell 6:1365–1375

Kim SK, Fan Y, Papadimitrakopoulou V, Clayman G, Hittelman WN, Hong WK, Lotan R, Mao L (1996) DPC4, a candidate tumor suppressor gene, is altered infrequently in head and neck squamous cell carcinoma. Cancer Res 56:2519–2521

Kim BG, Li C, Qiao W, Mamura M, Kasprzak B, Anver M, Wolfraim L, Hong S, Mushinski E, Potter M, Kim SJ, Fu XY, Deng C, Letterio JJ (2006) Smad4 signalling in T cells is required for suppression of gastrointestinal cancer. Nature 441:1015–1019

Klopcic B, Maass T, Meyer E, Lehr HA, Metzger D, Chambon P, Mann A, Blessing M (2007) TGF-beta superfamily signaling is essential for tooth and hair morphogenesis and differentiation. Eur J Cell Biol 86:781–799

Korn T, Oukka M, Bettelli E (2007) Th17 cells: Effector T cells with inflammatory properties. Semin Immunol 19:362–371

Kulkarni AB, Huh CG, Becker D, Geiser A, Lyght M, Flanders KC, Roberts AB, Sporn MB, Ward, JM, Karlsson S (1993) Transforming growth factor beta 1 null mutation in mice causes excessive inflammatory response and early death. Proc Natl Acad Sci U S A 90:770–774

Leivonen SK, Ala-Aho R, Koli K, Grenman R, Peltonen J, Kahari VM (2006) Activation of Smad signaling enhances collagenase-3 (MMP-13) expression and invasion of head and neck squamous carcinoma cells. Oncogene 25:2588–2600

Levy L, Hill CS (2006) Alterations in components of the TGF-beta superfamily signaling pathways in human cancer. Cytokine Growth Factor Rev 17:41–58

Lewis MP, Lygoe KA, Nystrom ML, Anderson WP, Speight PM, Marshall JF, Thomas GJ (2004) Tumour-derived TGF-beta1 modulates myofibroblast differentiation and promotes HGF/SF-dependent invasion of squamous carcinoma cells. Br J Cancer 90:822–832

Li AG, Lu SL, Zhang MX, Deng C, Wang XJ (2004a) Smad3 knockout mice exhibit a resistance to skin chemical carcinogenesis. Cancer Res 64:7836–7845

Li AG, Wang D, Feng XH, Wang XJ (2004b) Latent TGFbeta1 overexpression in keratinocytes results in a severe psoriasis-like skin disorder. Embo J 23:1770–1781

Li MO, Wan YY, Flavell RA (2007) T cell-produced transforming growth factor-beta1 controls T cell tolerance and regulates Th1- and Th17-cell differentiation. Immunity 26:579–591

Liu X, Lee J, Cooley M, Bhogte E, Hartley S, Glick A (2003) Smad7 but not Smad6 cooperates with oncogenic ras to cause malignant conversion in a mouse model for squamous cell carcinoma. Cancer Res 63:7760–7768

Lopez-Casillas F, Wrana JL, Massague J (1993) Betaglycan presents ligand to the TGF beta signaling receptor. Cell 73:1435–1444

Lu SL, Reh D, Li AG, Woods J, Corless CL, Kulesz-Martin M, Wang XJ (2004) Overexpression of transforming growth factor beta1 in head and neck epithelia results in inflammation, angiogenesis, and epithelial hyperproliferation. Cancer Res 64:4405–4410

Lu SL, Herrington H, Reh D, Weber S, Bornstein S, Wang D, Li AG, Tang CF, Siddiqui Y, Nord J, Andersen P, Corless CL, Wang XJ (2006) Loss of transforming growth factor-beta type II receptor promotes metastatic head-and-neck squamous cell carcinoma. Genes Dev 20:1331–1342

Massague J (2000) How cells read TGF-beta signals. Nat Rev Mol Cell Biol 1:169–178

Massague J, Gomis RR (2006) The logic of TGFbeta signaling. FEBS Lett 580:2811–2820

Massague J, Wotton D (2000) Transcriptional control by the TGF-beta/Smad signaling system. Embo J 19:1745–1754

Moustakas A, Heldin CH (2007) Signaling networks guiding epithelial-mesenchymal transitions during embryogenesis and cancer progression. Cancer Sci 98:1512–1520

Munger JS, Huang X, Kawakatsu H, Griffiths MJ, Dalton SL, Wu J, Pittet JF, Kaminski N, Garat C, Matthay MA, Rifkin DB, Sheppard D (1999) The integrin alpha v beta 6 binds and activates latent TGF beta 1: a mechanism for regulating pulmonary inflammation and fibrosis. Cell 96:319–328

Muraoka RS, Dumont N, Ritter CA, Dugger TC, Brantley DM, Chen J, Easterly E, Roebuck LR, Ryan S, Gotwals PJ, Koteliansky V, Arteaga CL (2002) Blockade of TGF-beta inhibits mammary tumor cell viability, migration, and metastases. J Clin Invest 109:1551–1559

Muro-Cacho CA, Anderson M, Cordero J, Munoz-Antonia T (1999) Expression of transforming growth factor beta type II receptors in head and neck squamous cell carcinoma. Clin Cancer Res 5:1243–1248

Muro-Cacho CA, Rosario-Ortiz K, Livingston S, Munoz-Antonia T (2001) Defective transforming growth factor beta signaling pathway in head and neck squamous cell carcinoma as evidenced by the lack of expression of activated Smad2. Clin Cancer Res 7:1618–1626

Nakao A, Afrakhte M, Moren A, Nakayama T, Christian JL, Heuchel R, Itoh S, Kawabata M, Heldin NE, Heldin CH, ten Dijke P (1997) Identification of Smad7, a TGFbeta-inducible antagonist of TGF-beta signalling. Nature 389:631–635

Natsugoe S, Xiangming C, Matsumoto M, Okumura H, Nakashima S, Sakita H, Ishigami S, Baba M, Takao S, Aikou T (2002) Smad4 and transforming growth factor beta1 expression in patients with squamous cell carcinoma of the esophagus. Clin Cancer Res 8:1838–1842

Oft M, Peli J, Rudaz C, Schwarz H, Beug H, Reichmann E (1996) TGF-beta1 and Ha-Ras collaborate in modulating the phenotypic plasticity and invasiveness of epithelial tumor cells. Genes Dev 10:2462–2477

Osawa H, Nakajima M, Kato H, Fukuchi M, Kuwano H (2004) Prognostic value of the expression of Smad6 and Smad7, as inhibitory Smads of the TGF-beta superfamily, in esophageal squamous cell carcinoma. Anticancer Res 24:3703–3709

Papadimitrakopoulou VA, Oh Y, El-Naggar A, Izzo J, Clayman G, Mao L (1998) Presence of multiple incontiguous deleted regions at the long arm of chromosome 18 in head and neck cancer. Clin Cancer Res 4:539–544

Pardali K, Kowanetz M, Heldin CH, Moustakas A (2005) Smad pathway-specific transcriptional regulation of the cell cycle inhibitor p21(WAF1/Cip1). J Cell Physiol 204:260–272

Pennison M, Pasche B (2007) Targeting transforming growth factor-beta signaling. Curr Opin Oncol 19:579–585

Perlman R, Schiemann WP, Brooks MW, Lodish HF, Weinberg RA (2001) TGF-beta-induced apoptosis is mediated by the adapter protein Daxx that facilitates JNK activation. Nat Cell Biol 3:708–714

Pertovaara L, Kaipainen A, Mustonen T, Orpana A, Ferrara N, Saksela O, Alitalo K (1994) Vascular endothelial growth factor is induced in response to transforming growth factor-beta in fibroblastic and epithelial cells. J Biol Chem 269:6271–6274

Pring M, Prime S, Parkinson EK, Paterson I (2006) Dysregulated TGF-beta1-induced Smad signalling occurs as a result of defects in multiple components of the TGF-beta signalling pathway in human head and neck carcinoma cell lines. Int J Oncol 28:1279–1285

Qiao W, Li AG, Owens P, Xu X, Wang XJ, Deng CX (2006) Hair follicle defects and squamous cell carcinoma formation in Smad4 conditional knockout mouse skin. Oncogene 25:207–217

Qiu W, Schonleben F, Li X, Su GH (2007) Disruption of transforming growth factor beta-Smad signaling pathway in head and neck squamous cell carcinoma as evidenced by mutations of SMAD2 and SMAD4. Cancer Lett 245:163–170

Riggins GJ, Kinzler KW, Vogelstein B, Thiagalingam S (1997) Frequency of Smad gene mutations in human cancers. Cancer Res 57:2578–2580

Rodius S, Indra G, Thibault C, Pfister V, Georges-Labouesse E (2007) Loss of alpha6 integrins in keratinocytes leads to an increase in TGFbeta and AP1 signaling and in expression of differentiation genes. J Cell Physiol 212:439–449

Rosenthal E, McCrory A, Talbert M, Young G, Murphy-Ullrich J, Gladson C (2004) Elevated expression of TGF-beta1 in head and neck cancer-associated fibroblasts. Mol Carcinog 40:116–121

Saito H, Tsujitani S, Oka S, Kondo A, Ikeguchi M, Maeta M, Kaibara N (2000) An elevated serum level of transforming growth factor-beta 1 (TGF-beta 1) significantly correlated with lymph node metastasis and poor prognosis in patients with gastric carcinoma. Anticancer Res 20:4489–4493

Schlingensiepen KH, Schlingensiepen R, Steinbrecher A, Hau P, Bogdahn U, Fischer-Blass B, Jachimczak P (2006) Targeted tumor therapy with the TGF-beta2 antisense compound AP 12009. Cytokine Growth Factor Rev 17:129–139

Schlingensiepen KH, Fischer-Blass B, Schmaus S, Ludwig S (2008) Antisense therapeutics for tumor treatment: the TGF-beta2 inhibitor AP 12009 in clinical development against malignant tumors. Recent Results Cancer Res 177:137–150

Shi Y, Massague J (2003) Mechanisms of TGF-beta signaling from cell membrane to the nucleus. Cell 113:685–700

Shull MM, Ormsby I, Kier AB, Pawlowski S, Diebold RJ, Yin M, Allen R, Sidman C, Proetzel G, Calvin D et al (1992) Targeted disruption of the mouse transforming growth factor-beta 1 gene results in multifocal inflammatory disease. Nature 359:693–699

Siegel PM, Massague J (2003) Cytostatic and apoptotic actions of TGF-beta in homeostasis and cancer. Nat Rev Cancer 3:807–821

Snijders AM, Schmidt BL, Fridlyand J, Dekker N, Pinkel D, Jordan RC, Albertson DG (2005) Rare amplicons implicate frequent deregulation of cell fate specification pathways in oral squamous cell carcinoma. Oncogene 24:4232–4242

Sparano A, Quesnelle KM, Kumar MS, Wang Y, Sylvester AJ, Feldman M, Sewell DA, Weinstein GS, Brose MS (2006) Genome-wide profiling of oral squamous cell carcinoma by array-based comparative genomic hybridization. Laryngoscope 116:735–741

Sporn MB, Roberts AB (1992) Transforming growth factor-beta: recent progress and new challenges. J Cell Biol 119:1017–1021

Stearns ME, Garcia FU, Fudge K, Rhim J, Wang M (1999) Role of interleukin 10 and transforming growth factor beta1 in the angiogenesis and metastasis of human prostate primary tumor lines from orthotopic implants in severe combined immunodeficiency mice. Clin Cancer Res 5:711–720

Sun SP, Jin YN, Yang HP, Wei Y, Dong Z (2007) Serum transforming growth factor-beta1 level reflects disease status in patients with esophageal carcinoma after radiotherapy. World J Gastroenterol 13:5267–5272

Takebayashi S, Ogawa T, Jung KY, Muallem A, Mineta H, Fisher SG, Grenman R, Carey TE (2000) Identification of new minimally lost regions on 18q in head and neck squamous cell carcinoma. Cancer Res 60:3397–3403

Takebayashi S, Hickson A, Ogawa T, Jung KY, Mineta H, Ueda Y, Grenman R, Fisher SG, Carey TE (2004) Loss of chromosome arm 18q with tumor progression in head and neck squamous cancer. Genes Chromosomes Cancer 41:145–154

Tannehill-Gregg SH, Kusewitt DF, Rosol TJ, Weinstein M (2004) The roles of Smad2 and Smad3 in the development of chemically induced skin tumors in mice. Vet Pathol 41:278–282

ten Dijke P, Hill CS (2004) New insights into TGF-beta-Smad signalling. Trends Biochem Sci 29:265–273

Ten Dijke P, Goumans MJ, Itoh F, Itoh S (2002) Regulation of cell proliferation by Smad proteins. J Cell Physiol 191:1–16

Thomas DA, Massague J (2005) TGF-beta directly targets cytotoxic T cell functions during tumor evasion of immune surveillance. Cancer Cell 8:369–380

Tojo M, Hamashima Y, Hanyu A, Kajimoto T, Saitoh M, Miyazono K, Node M, Imamura T (2005) The ALK-5 inhibitor A-83–01 inhibits Smad signaling and epithelial-to-mesenchymal transition by transforming growth factor-beta. Cancer Sci 96:791–800

Tsushima H, Kawata S, Tamura S, Ito N, Shirai Y, Kiso S, Imai Y, Shimomukai H, Nomura Y, Matsuda Y, Matsuzawa Y (1996) High levels of transforming growth factor beta 1 in patients with colorectal cancer: association with disease progression. Gastroenterology 110:375–382

Tsushima H, Ito N, Tamura S, Matsuda Y, Inada M, Yabuuchi I, Imai Y, Nagashima R, Misawa H, Takeda H, Matsuzawa Y, Kawata S (2001) Circulating transforming growth factor beta 1 as a predictor of liver metastasis after resection in colorectal cancer. Clin Cancer Res 7:1258–1262

Uhl M, Aulwurm S, Wischhusen J, Weiler M, Ma JY, Almirez R, Mangadu R, Liu YW, Platten M, Herrlinger U, Murphy A, Wong DH, Wick W, Higgins LS, Weller M (2004) SD-208, a novel transforming growth factor beta receptor I kinase inhibitor, inhibits growth and invasiveness and enhances immunogenicity of murine and human glioma cells in vitro and in vivo. Cancer Res 64:7954–7961

Wang D, Song H, Evans JA, Lang JC, Schuller DE, Weghorst CM (1997) Mutation and downregulation of the transforming growth factor beta type II receptor gene in primary squamous cell carcinomas of the head and neck. Carcinogenesis 18:2285–2290

Wang KS, Hu ZL, Li JH, Xiao DS, Wen JF (2006) Enhancement of metastatic and invasive capacity of gastric cancer cells by transforming growth factor-beta1. Acta Biochim Biophys Sin (Shanghai) 38:179–186

Weber F, Xu Y, Zhang L, Patocs A, Shen L, Platzer P, Eng C (2007) Microenvironmental genomic alterations and clinicopathological behavior in head and neck squamous cell carcinoma. JAMA 297:187–195

Weeks BH, He W, Olson KL, Wang XJ (2001) Inducible expression of transforming growth factor beta1 in papillomas causes rapid metastasis. Cancer Res 61:7435–7443

Wilkins-Port CE, Higgins PJ (2007) Regulation of extracellular matrix remodeling following transforming growth factor-beta1/epidermal growth factor-stimulated epithelial-mesenchymal transition in human premalignant keratinocytes. Cells Tissues Organs 185:116–122

Worsham MJ, Chen KM, Meduri V, Nygren AO, Errami A, Schouten JP, Benninger MS (2006) Epigenetic events of disease progression in head and neck squamous cell carcinoma. Arch Otolaryngol Head Neck Surg 132:668–677

Xie W, Bharathy S, Kim D, Haffty BG, Rimm DL, Reiss M (2003) Frequent alterations of Smad signaling in human head and neck squamous cell carcinomas: a tissue microarray analysis. Oncol Res 14:61–73

Yamamoto Y, Ueda Y, Itoh T, Iwamoto A, Yamagishi H, Shimagaki M, Teramoto K (2006) A novel immunotherapeutic modality with direct hemoperfusion targeting transforming growth factor-beta prolongs the survival of tumor-bearing rats. Oncol Rep 16:1277–1284

Yanagisawa K, Osada H, Masuda A, Kondo M, Saito T, Yatabe Y, Takagi K, Takahashi T (1998) Induction of apoptosis by Smad3 and down-regulation of Smad3 expression in response to TGF-beta in human normal lung epithelial cells. Oncogene 17:1743–1747

Yang YA, Dukhanina O, Tang B, Mamura M, Letterio JJ, MacGregor J, Patel SC, Khozin S, Liu ZY, Green J, Anver MR, Merlino G, Wakefield LM (2002) Lifetime exposure to a soluble TGF-beta antagonist protects mice against metastasis without adverse side effects. J Clin Invest 109:1607–1615

Yang L, Mao C, Teng Y, Li W, Zhang J, Cheng X, Li X, Han X, Xia Z, Deng H, Yang X (2005) Targeted disruption of Smad4 in mouse epidermis results in failure of hair follicle cycling and formation of skin tumors. Cancer Res 65:8671–8678

Yang L, Huang J, Ren X, Gorska AE, Chytil A, Aakre M, Carbone DP, Matrisian LM, Richmond A, Lin PC, Moses HL (2008) Abrogation of TGFbeta signaling in mammary carcinomas recruits Gr-1 + CD11b + myeloid cells that promote metastasis. Cancer Cell 13:23–35

Yingling JM, Blanchard KL, Sawyer JS (2004) Development of TGF-beta signalling inhibitors for cancer therapy. Nat Rev Drug Discov 3:1011–1022

Yu Q, Stamenkovic I (2000) Cell surface-localized matrix metalloproteinase-9 proteolytically activates TGF-beta and promotes tumor invasion and angiogenesis. Genes Dev 14:163–176

Zavadil J, Bottinger EP (2005) TGF-beta and epithelial-to-mesenchymal transitions. Oncogene 24:5764–5774

Zhang Y, Chang C, Gehling DJ, Hemmati-Brivanlou A, Derynck R (2001) Regulation of Smad degradation and activity by Smurf2, an E3 ubiquitin ligase. Proc Natl Acad Sci U S A 98:974–979

Zhang Q, Yang X, Pins M, Javonovic B, Kuzel T, Kim SJ, Parijs LV, Greenberg NM, Liu V, Guo Y, Lee C (2005) Adoptive transfer of tumor-reactive transforming growth factor-beta-insensitive CD8+ T cells: eradication of autologous mouse prostate cancer. Cancer Res 65:1761–1769

Chapter 9
Growth Factor Receptor Signaling and Metastasis of Oral Cancer

Ali Razfar and Jennifer R. Grandis

Abstract Growth factor receptor signaling activates a number of pathways involved in cellular proliferation and survival. Overexpression and activation of various growth factor receptors have been implicated in a number of cancers. The progression of tumor cells to an invasive phenotype requires a number of important steps, including the loss of cellular adhesion complexes and the migration of tumor cells to distant sites. These steps are regulated by growth factor receptors such as epidermal growth factor receptor (EGFR) and c-Met leading to metastasis. Overexpression and activation of EGFR lead to loss of intercellular adhesions through the downregulation of E-cadherins, desmosomes, and focal adhesion kinase. Furthermore, EGFR signaling can upregulate matrix metalloproteases (MMPs), leading to the degradation of the extracellular matrix and increased motility. Hepatocyte growth factor (HGF)/c-Met signaling can also disrupt E-cadherin expression and upregulate MMP expression, resulting in a more invasive phenotype. Thus, growth factor receptors play a major role in tumor metastasis through the regulation of key intermediary steps.

Introduction

Tumor metastasis is the leading determinant of cancer progression and patient survival. In head and neck squamous cell carcinoma (HNSCC), cervical lymph node metastasis is the most important prognostic factor in predicting the clinical outcome. HNSCC patients with lymph node metastases have a survival rate that is half of that found for patients with no evidence of lymph nodes metastases (Zhang et al. 2002). The ability of primary tumor cells to invade regional tissue and seed distant organs requires a series of sequential steps. Tumor cells must dissociate from their adhesive interactions with surrounding tissue, migrate through the extracellular matrix (ECM) and basement membrane, invade lymphatic and/or blood vessels,

J.R. Grandis (✉)
The Eye and Ear Institute, Room 105, 200 Lothrop Street, Pittsburgh, PA, 15213, USA
e-mail: jgrandis@pitt.edu

and finally enter and take residence in the target organ. Growth factor signaling regulates cell growth, survival, and proliferation. Alterations in growth factor signaling pathways play a major role in cancer progression and metastasis. Growth factor receptors such as the epidermal growth factor receptor (EGFR) and c-Met are often upregulated and/or constitutively activated in a number of different cancers. In this chapter, we will review the pivotal role that growth factor receptors play in HNSCC metastasis.

Expression of Epidermal Growth Factor Receptor in Squamous Cell Carcinoma of the Head and Neck

EGFR is a member of the erbB family of transmembrane cell-surface receptor tyrosine kinases. Activation of EGFR through ligand binding to the extracellular domain, leads receptor dimerization and activation of its kinase and subsequent activation of a several downstream signaling pathways including the signal transducers and activators of transcription (STATs), mitogen-activated protein kinase (MAPK), AKT, and phospholipase C (PLC) pathways. These pathways mediate various cellular responses, including cell proliferation, survival, cell motility, invasion, and adhesion (Yarden and Sliwkowski 2001). These cellular functions play crucial roles in the process of tumor cell invasion. It is widely accepted that EGFR and its ligands are overexpressed in a number of epithelial tumors (Hynes and Lane 2005). The EGFR ligand, transforming growth factor-α (TGF-α), EGFR mRNA, and protein have been shown to be highly overexpressed in tumor specimens of patients with HNSCC when compared with normal controls (Grandis et al. 1998) (Fig. 9.1). This finding confirmed the earlier report of elevated expression of TGF-α and EGFR in HNSCC primary tumors and cervical metastases (Christensen et al. 1993). Cases of HNSCC with nodal involvement have been shown to have a significantly higher gene copy number of EGFR than HNSCC tumors without nodal involvement (Todd et al. 1989). Elevated levels of another EGFR activating ligand, amphiregulin, have also been implicated in HNSCC. An increase in the level of amphiregulin expression was correlated with clinical progression of HNSCC (Tsai et al. 2006). Recombinant amphiregulin can increase the growth, invasive capacity, and migration of oral cancer cells, at least in part, via induction of the inflammatory mediator COX-2 (Tsai et al. 2006).

Data from Hiraishi et al. showed that 92.3% of HNSCC tumors expressed EGFR and 98.0% expressed p-EGFR (Hiraishi et al. 2006). In the same study, 63.4% and 69.2% of patients showed high expression levels of EGFR and p-EGFR, respectively. High EGFR expression was correlated with tumor invasiveness. However, expression of EGFR and p-EGFR did not correlate with clinical factors such as tumor stage, lymph node metastasis, distant metastasis, or differentiation. Differences between these findings and previous reports might have resulted from technical considerations in performing immunohistochemical (IHC) evaluation of EGFR expression or from alternate ways in which the EGFR pathway can become activated.

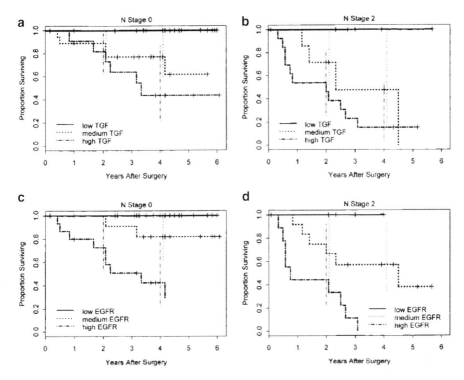

Fig. 9.1 Kaplan–Meier analysis showing the overall cause-specific survival among 49 patients with N0 (**a, c**) and 27 patients with N2 (**b, d**) head and neck cancer, according to the levels of transforming growth factor-α (TGF) (**a, b**) or epidermal growth factor receptor (EGFR) (**c, d**) in the primary tumor. Vertical lines denote 95% confidence intervals at 2 and 4 years

For example, in glioblastoma cells, a mutation leading to the deletion of exons 2–7 results in a truncated EGFR protein known as EGFRvIII that has contituitive tyrosine kinase activity and promotes aggressive tumor growth in vivo (Lorimer 2002). EGFRvIII has now been detected in HNSCC where expression correlates with resistance to chemotherapy and EGFR targeting using an EGFR-specific antibody (Sok et al. 2006). Activating point mutations have also been identified in the EGFR tyroisine kinase domain in some cases of nonsmall cell lung cancer and have been linked to increased response rates to EGFR tyrosine kinase inhibitors. However, these types of mutations are exceedingly rare in HNSCC.

Role of EGFR Signaling in Intercellular Adhesion

Dissociation of cell–cell adhesion plays an important role in tumor metastasis. Two major mechanisms of cell–cell adhesion are adherens junctions and desmosomes. Adherens junctions are adhesive complexes that utilize cadherins and catenins to bind to microfilament networks within the cell (Perez-Moreno et al. 2003). Desmosomes are adhesive structures that anchor to intracellular intermediate filament networks through the interaction of various adaptors proteins such as desmoplakins, plakoglobins, and cadherins (Yin and Green 2004). Disruption of adherens junctions through the reduced expression of E-cadherin, α-catenin, and β-catenin is associated with regional lymph node metstasis in HNSCC (Tanaka et al. 2003). Examination of the distribution of desmosomes using electron microscopy and immunohistochemistry in HNSCC specimens reveals that specimens from patients with cervical metastasis have fewer desmosomes than do specimens from patients with no metastasis (Tanaka et al. 2002). EGFR signaling pathways play a critical role in the regulation of these adhesive complexes. Thus, the interplay between EGFR signaling and intercellular adhesion is probably a major component of tumor metastasis and cancer progression.

E-cadherin has proven to be an important molecule in the progression of cancer and can serve as an indicator of the metastatic potential of a primary tumor. Expression of E-cadherin negatively correlates with histologic grade, tumor size, clinical staging, lymph node metastasis, and tumor invasion and correlates with a poor prognosis in esophageal SCC (Zhao et al. 2003). Loss of E-cadherin expression in the primary tumor correlates with development of nodal metastasis, tumor progression, and poor prognosis for patients with HNSCC (Bankfalvi et al. 2002; Lee et al. 2002). In three-dimensional organotypic models, suppression of E-cadherin leads to a more invasive phenotype of squamous cell carcinoma cell lines, whereas maintenance of E-cadherin expression can prevent invasion both in vitro and in vivo (Margulis et al. 2005). EGFR and its ligands have been shown to be the key regulators of E-cadherin expression. EGF treatment of a human breast cancer cell line induced the dissociation of actin, alpha-actin, and vinculin from the E-cadherin complex. Furthermore, antibodies blocking the function of EGFR resulted in cellular aggregation and the formation of E-cadherin adhesion complexes with actin and vinculin in the same cell line (Hazan and Norton 1998). In lung cancer cell lines, anti-EGFR antibodies were shown to upregulate the expression of E-cadherin, resulting in cells differentiating to a more epithelial than mesenchymal phenotype. Thus, EGFR modulation of E-cadherin is not only important for tumor metastasis but also likely involved in the epithelial-to-mesenchymal transition (EMT).

The underlying mechanisms of EGFR regulation of E-cadherin are only partially understood. EGFR signaling was shown to induce caveolin-dependent endocytosis of E-cadherin, subsequently leading to disruption of cell–cell adhesion and initiating EMT of tumor cells (Lu et al. 2003). In the same study, prolonged EGF treatment resulted in a downregulation of caveolin-1 and subsequent upregulation of transcriptional repressor SNAIL, inhibiting E-cadherin expression. A common downstream target of EGFR is the phosphoinositide 3 kinase (PI3K)/Akt pathway. Phosphorylated-Akt has been shown to be inversely correlated with E-cadherin expression in HNSCC (Lim et al. 2005). Akt activation represses E-cadherin expression through upregulation of the repressors SNAIL and SIP1 (Grille et al. 2003). Thus, it can be postulated that EGFR overexpression leads to increased activation of the PI3K-Akt pathway resulting in upregulation of the E-cadherin SNAIL and SIP1 (see Fig. 9.2).

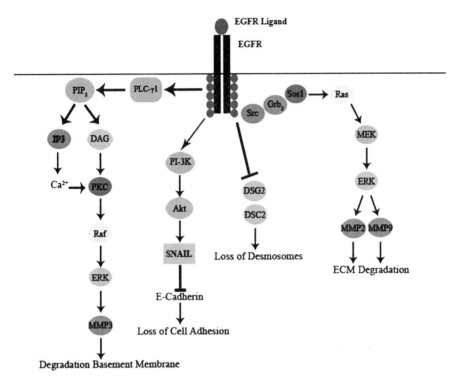

Fig. 9.2 EGFR signaling pathway in metastasis of squamous cell carcinoma of the head and neck (HNSCC). EGFR ligand binds to EGFR, leading to autophosphorylation of five sites and the phosphorylation of PLC-γ1. This leads to the hydrolysis of PIP2 to IP3 and DAG. Ultimately, both these pathways can activate the PKC/Raf/Erk pathway. This activates MMP3, which is able to degrade the basement membrane. EGFR signaling also induces the PI3K/Akt pathway, leading to the upregulation of SNAIL, a suppressor of E-cadherin. This results in the loss of cell adhesion and invasive phenotype. EGFR also downregulates DSG2 and DSC2, leading to loss of desmosome assembly and reduced cell adhesion. EGFR can activate the MAPK/ERKpathway, leading to the activation of MMP2 and MMP9. This results in ECM degradation and enhanced motility. *PLCg-1* phospholipase C gamma 1; *PIP2* phosphatidylinositol (4,5) bisphosphate; *IP3* inositol-triphosphate; *DAG* diacylglycerol; *PKC* protein kinase C; *ERK* extracellular signal-regulated kinase; *MAPK* mitogen-activated protein kinase; *MMP* matrix metalloproteinase; *EGFR* epidermal growth factor receptor; *PI-3K* phosphoinositide kinase 3

Furthermore, E-cadherin is likely endocytosed through the EGFR/caveolin-1 dependent pathway leading to cell–cell detachment and increased invasive capacity.

Desmosomes are important structures involved in cell–cell adhesion as well as intracellular signaling. There is accumulating evidence implicating desmosomes in the progression of cancer. A number of cancers have shown either loss of expression or overexpression of desmosomal cadherins (Chidgey and Dawson 2007). This is most likely due to the multiple roles desmosomes can play in the cell. In HNSCC, the desmosomal adaptor protein plakoglobin was downregulated in all tumors compared with normal epithelium, and 87.1% of tumors displayed an abnormal cytoplasmic localization of this protein (Papagerakis et al. 2004). Plakophilins are a member of the *armadillo* family of proteins which are required for desmosomal function. In HNSCC, expression levels of plakophilin-1 and -3 have been inversely correlated with tumor grade, and there is no expression of plakophilin-2, a ubiquitous desmosomal protein (Schwarz et al. 2006).

Desmosomes have also been implicated in the metastatic ability of tumors. Downregulation of plakophilin-1 leads to decreased desmosome assembly, increased cell motility, and increased invasion in HNSCC (Sobolik-Delmaire et al. 2007). EGFR signaling plays a significant role in the regulation of adherens junctions (see Fig. 9.2). Studies to date suggest a role for EGFR signaling in desmosome assembly and function. In the conditions of reduced cell–cell adhesion, inhibition of EGFR led to a transition from mesenchymal to epithelial morphology of HNSCC (Ghosh et al. 2002). Furthermore, the levels of desmosomal components such as desmoglein 2 and desmocollin 2 increased and were recruited to cell–cell borders. Tyrosine kinase inhibition can lead to decreased phosphorylation of desmoglein 2 and plakoglobin (Ghosh et al. 2002). Thus, EGFR inhibition may increase cell–cell adhesion and desmosome function in HNSCC and prevent metastasis.

Epidermal Growth Factor Receptor and Focal Adhesion Kinase

Focal adhesion kinase (FAK) has been shown to be overexpressed in a number of tumors, particularly those with high invasive potential (Owens et al. 1995). FAK is a tyrosine kinase that helps mediate integrin signaling at focal adhesion complexes and is involved in cellular adhesion, growth, and differentiation. There is growing evidence implicating FAK in HNSCC invasion and metastasis. FAK has been found to be overexpressed in highly invasive HNSCC compared with normal oral mucosa (Kornberg 1998). In a study comparing two different oral carcinoma cell lines, FAK was expressed at higher levels in the cell line with more invasive properties. Furthermore, the overexpression of FAK in the less invasive cell line led to a 4.5-fold increase in invasion compared with control cells (Schneider et al. 2002). EGFR signaling has been implicated in modulating the function of FAK, although the exact mechanism has yet to be identified. In another study, EGFR inhibition by gefitinib led to the downregulation of integrins and phosphorylation of FAK leading to decreased adhesion to ECM and a reduction in metastasis (Shintani et al. 2003).

Epidermal Growth Factor Receptor Signaling and Cell Motility

One of the major steps in tumor metastasis is degradation of the ECM. This enables primary cancer cells to move through the matrix and target distant sites. MMPs are a group of zinc endopeptidases that degrade the components of the ECM such as collagen, fibronectin, glycoproteins, and proteoglycans. These enzymes have been widely implicated in a number of invasive tumors. In HNSCC, activation of MMP-2 and MMP-9 is significantly higher in cancer cells than in normal oral mucosa (Patel et al. 2005). In another study of HNSCC, MMP-9 overexpression was found to be significantly correlated with metastatic tumors (Hong et al. 2000). MMP-3 is involved in the degradation of the basement membrane, a necessary step of tumor metastasis, and one study identified a positive correlation between the expression of EGFR and MMP-3 in HNSCC (Kusukawa et al. 1996). Furthermore, MMP-3 was expressed at the advancing front of the cancer and was associated with advanced pathological stage, diffuse invasive mode, and neck metastasis (Kusukawa et al. 1996). There is a high correlation between the invasive phenotype of HNSCC and the expression levels of EGFR and MMP-9 (O-Charoenrat et al. 2000b). The relationship between EGFR signaling and MMP activation has been elucidated in a number of studies (See Fig. 9.2). In HNSCC, EGFR signaling led to an upregulation and activation of MMP-9 causing a more invasive phenotype (O-Charoenrat et al. 2000a). Subsequently, blocking EGFR signaling with the tyrosine kinase inhibitor gefinitib led to a reduction of MMP-2 and MMP-9 activity and reduced the invasion of HNSCC in vitro (Lee et al. 2007b). There is evidence that the MAPK pathway may be important for mediating EGFR's regulation of MMPs, as blockade of the MAPK pathway with a MAPK extracellular signal-regulated kinase (MEK) inhibitor leads to marked reduction in MMP-2 activity and decreased invasion of HNSCC (Lin et al. 2006). The MAPK/ERK and PI3K/Akt pathways have also been shown to activate MMP-9 (Cooper et al. 2004; Lee et al. 2007a). Thus, EGFR signaling can modulate the expression and activation of various MMPs, which are critical in HNSCC metastasis.

PLC-γ1 is a downstream target of EGFR signaling and is a major pathway involved in cell motility. EGFR signaling mediates cell motility through the activation of PLC-γ1 and subsequent hydrolysis of phosphoinsotide 4,5-bisphosphate (PIP$_2$) releasing gelsolin, which modifies the actin cytoskeleton (Chou et al. 2002). Due to the importance of cell motility in tumor metastasis, the relationship between EGFR signaling and the promigratory effects of PLC-γ1 has been studied in a number of human tumors. Both EGFR and PLC-γ1 have been shown to be overexpressed in mammary carcinoma cells when compared with normal breast tissue (Arteaga et al. 1991). In HNSCC, both PLC-γ1 and phosphorylated PLC-γ1, the active form of PLC-γ1, were found to be overexpressed when compared with normal epithelial tissue (Thomas et al. 2003). Upon stimulation of EGFR, PLC-γ1 was activated in HNSCC cell lines and mediated tumor invasion in vitro (Thomas et al. 2003). HNSCC invasion was blocked following either EGFR inhibition or PLC-γ1 inhibition, suggesting that EGFR activation of PLC-γ1 directly mediates tumor invasion (Thomas et al. 2003). Furthermore, PLC-γ1 can activate transcription of MMP-3 through the protein kinase C/Raf/ERK pathway and further aid in cell motility and invasion (Zhang et al. 2007). EGFR signaling modulates PLC-γ1 activation and plays an important role in tumor cell migration and invasion.

Hepatocyte Growth Factor/c-Met signaling in Head and Neck Squamous Cell Carcinoma Metastasis

The c-Met receptor is a tyrosine kinase that regulates a number of pathways involved in cell growth and differentiation. HGF binds to c-Met, leading to auto-phosphorylation on two tyrosine residues and the activation of multiple signaling pathways. The HGF/c-Met signaling pathways can activate cell growth, survival, and mitogenesis in a number of different cells, including epithelial cells (Peruzzi and Bottaro 2006). HGF signaling has also been implicated in several human cancers where it contributes to cancer progression and tumor metastasis. The c-Met protein was found to be overexpressed in 12 HNSCC cell lines when compared with the levels in normal epithelial cells (Morello et al. 2001). HGF serum concentrations were elevated in HNSCC patients compared with healthy control subjects (Uchida et al. 2001). In the same study, HGF serum concentrations were found to be decreased in the HNSCC cohort following curative therapy. Both mRNA and proteins levels of HGF and c-Met have been found to be overexpressed in HNSCC tumors when compared with normal mucosa (Kim et al. 2006). The expression of c-Met has been correlated with increased regional and distant metastasis and decreased HNSCC disease-free survival (Endo et al. 2006). In a type I collagen matrix, HGF was shown to significantly enhance the invasive growth of HNSCC cell lines (Uchida et al. 2001).

HGF/c-Met signaling may mediate tumor progression and metastasis by a variety of mechanisms. One of the crucial steps in tumor metastasis is the loss of cellular adhesion. In cell lines of HNSCC, the absence of HGF led to epithelial cells forming tightly packed monolayers. Upon activation of c-Met by HGF, those inter-cellular adhesion complexes were disrupted and cells displayed a migratory pheno-type (Morello et al. 2001). HGF stimulation of c-Met led to the downregulation of E-cadherin and translocation of E-cadherin to the cytoplasm leading to enhanced invasion in HNSCC (Lynch et al. 2007). HGF induced the phosphorylation of β-catenin, leading to a dissociation of E-cadherin and β-catenin (Hiscox et al. 2006). In HNSCC, HGF induced the upregulation of unbound β-catenin and disrup-tion of E-cadherin junctions (Murai et al. 2004). HGF signaling can also upregulate expression of Snail, a repressor protein involved in EMT, via the MAPK/Egr-1 pathway (Grotegut et al. 2006). Increased Snail leads to enhanced cell scattering, migration, and invasion of tumor cells. HGF was also shown to induce migration through the phosphorylation of FAK leading to the recruitment of integrins, cytoskeletal proteins, and FAK into focal adhesions (Matsumoto et al. 1994).

Matrix Metalloproteases in HNSCC Migration and Invasion

The role of MMPs in tumor invasion and metastasis has been elucidated in a number of human cancers. Levels of MMP-2 and MMP-9 were shown to be higher in cancer cells than in normal cells, and MMP-9 levels correlated with tumor metastasis (Hong et al. 2000; Patel et al. 2005). MMPs may be activated downstream of several receptor tyrosine kinases including EGFR and c-Met. HGF-induced invasion of cancer cells corresponded with an increase in MMP-9 expression (Fridman et al. 2007). In the same study, inhibiting the kinase activity of c-Met led to the suppression of downstream Akt phosphorylation and nuclear factor kappa B (NF-κB) deactivation, resulting in inhibition of MMP-9. Another ligand for c-Met, scatter factor (SF), was found to induce expression of MMP-9 and MMP-2 in HNSCC cell lines (Bennett et al. 2000). E1AF is a transcription factor of the Ets-oncogene family that regulates the expression of MMPs (Higashino et al. 1995). HGF stimulated the transcription of the E1AF gene and resulted in the upregulation of MMP-1, MMP-3, and MMP-9 mRNA levels (Hanzawa et al. 2000). Furthermore, these HGF-activated cells were able to degrade collagen gels, displaying their invasive phenotype. Thus, HGF/c-Met signaling appears to modulate MMP expression and activity through a number of pathways, resulting in increased invasion of HNSCC.

Conclusion

Metastasis is a major prognostic factor in HNSCC. Growth factor receptor signaling plays a major role in tumor progression and invasion. The EGFR and HGF/c-Met signaling pathways regulate a number of important steps in tumor invasion, including loss of intercellular adhesion and degradation of ECM. Both EGFR and c-Met signaling disrupt cellular adhesion complexes by acting on E-cadherins through the PI3K-Akt and MAPK/Egr-1 pathways, respectively. In addition, EGFR signaling can also downregulate desmosome assembly, aiding in tumor metastasis. Growth factor receptor signaling is also involved in degradation of ECM through the action of MMPs. Activation of the EGFR and c-Met pathways leads to the upregulation of MMP-2 and MMP-9 enhancing tumor cell motility and invasion. Furthermore, EGFR activation of PLC-γ1 stimulates MMP-3 expression through the protein kinase C/Raf/ERK pathway, leading to degradation of basement membrane. Understanding the role of growth factor signaling in the steps of invasion in HNSCC will aid in the development of targeted therapies to prevent metastasis and increase survival.

References

Arteaga CL, Johnson MD, Todderud G, Coffey RJ, Carpenter G, Page DL (1991) Elevated Content of the Tyrosine Kinase Substrate Phospholipase C-1 in Primary Human Breast Carcinomas. Proc Am Assoc Cancer Res 88:10435–10439
Bankfalvi A, Krassort M et al (2002) Gains and losses of adhesion molecules (CD44, E-cadherin, and beta-catenin) during oral carcinogenesis and tumour progression. J Pathol 198:343–351
Bennett JH, Morgan MJ et al (2000) Metalloproteinase expression in normal and malignant oral keratinocytes: stimulation of MMP-2 and -9 by scatter factor. Eur J Oral Sci 108:281–291
Chidgey M, Dawson C (2007) Desmosomes: a role in cancer? Br J Cancer 96:1783–1787

Chou JD, Stolz B et al (2002) Distribution of gelsolin and phosphoinositol 4, 5-bisphosphate in lamellipodia during EGF-induced motility. Int J Biochem Cell Biol 34:776–790

Christensen ME, Therkildsen MH et al (1993) Immunoreactive transforming growth factor alpha and epidermal growth factor in oral squamous cell carcinomas. J Pathol 169:323–328

Cooper JS, Pajak TF et al (2004) Postoperative concurrent radiotherapy and chemotherapy for high-risk squamous-cell carcinoma of the head and neck. N Engl J Med 350(19):1937–1944

Endo K, Shirai A et al (2006) Prognostic value of cell motility activation factors in patients with tongue squamous cell carcinoma. Hum Pathol 37(8):1111–1116

Fridman JS, Caulder E et al (2007) Selective inhibition of ADAM metalloproteases as a novel approach for modulating ErbB pathways in cancer. Clin Cancer Res 13(6):1892–1902

Ghosh S, Munshi HG et al (2002) Loss of adhesion-regulated proteinase production is correlated with invasive activity in oral squamous cell carcinoma. Cancer 95(12):2524–2533

Grandis JR, Chakraborty A et al (1998) Downmodulation of TGF-alpha protein expression with antisense oligonucleotides inhibits proliferation of head and neck squamous carcinoma but not normal mucosal epithelial cells. J Cell Biochem 69:55–62

Grille SJ, Bellacosa A et al (2003) The protein kinase Akt induces epithelial mesenchymal transition and promotes enhanced motility and invasiveness of squamous cell carcinoma lines. Cancer Res 63(9):2172–2178

Grotegut S, von Schweinitz D et al (2006) Hepatocyte growth factor induces cell scattering through MAPK/Egr-1-mediated upregulation of Snail. EMBO J 25(15):3534–3545

Hanzawa M, Shindoh M et al (2000) Hepatocyte growth factor upregulates E1AF that induces oral squamous cell carcinoma cell invasion by activating matrix metalloproteinase genes. Carcinogenesis 21(6):1079–1085

Hazan RB, Norton L (1998) The epidermal growth factor receptor modulates the interaction of E-cadherin with the actin cytoskeleton. J Biol Chem 273(15):9078–9084

Higashino F, Yoshida K et al (1995) Ets-related protein E1A-F can activate three different matrix metalloproteinase gene promoters. Oncogene 10(7):1461–1463

Hiraishi Y, Wada T et al (2006) Immunohistochemical expression of EGFR and p-EGFR in oral squamous cell carcinomas. Pathol Oncol Res 12:87–91

Hiscox S, Morgan L et al (2006) Elevated Src activity promotes cellular invasion and motility in tamoxifen resistant breast cancer cells. Breast Cancer Res Treat 97:263–274

Hong SD, Hong SP et al (2000) Expression of matrix metalloproteinase-2 and -9 in oral squamous cell carcinomas with regard to the metastatic potential. Oral Oncol 36(2):207–213

Hynes NE, Lane HA (2005) ERBB receptors and cancer: the complexity of targeted inhibitors. Nat Rev Cancer 5:341–354

Kim CH, Moon SK et al (2006) Expression of hepatocyte growth factor and c-Met in hypopharyngeal squamous cell carcinoma. Acta Otolaryngol 126(1):88–94

Kornberg LJ (1998) Focal adhesion kinase expression in oral cancers. Head Neck 20(7):634–639

Kusukawa J, Harada H et al (1996) The significance of epidermal growth factor receptor and matrix metalloproteinase-3 in squamous cell carcinoma of the oral cavity. Eur J Cancer B Oral Oncol 32B(4):217–221

Lee CK, Raz R et al (2002) STAT3 is a negative regulator of granulopoiesis but is not required for G-CSF-dependent differentiation. Immunity 17(1):63–72

Lee CW, Lin CC et al (2007a) TNF-alpha induces MMP-9 expression via activation of Src/EGFR, PDGFR/PI3K/Akt cascade and promotion of NF-kappaB/p300 binding in human tracheal smooth muscle cells. Am J Physiol Lung Cell Mol Physiol 292(3):L799–L812

Lee EJ, Whang JH et al (2007b) The epidermal growth factor receptor tyrosine kinase inhibitor ZD1839 (Iressa) suppresses proliferation and invasion of human oral squamous carcinoma cells via p53 independent and MMP, uPAR dependent mechanism. Ann N Y Acad Sci 1095:113–128

Lim J, Kim JH et al (2005) Prognostic value of activated Akt expression in oral squamous cell carcinoma. J Clin Pathol 58(11):1199–1205

Lin CS, Jen YM et al (2006) Squamous cell carcinoma of the buccal mucosa: an aggressive cancer requiring multimodality treatment. Head Neck 28(2):150–157

Lorimer IA (2002) Mutant epidermal growth factor receptors as targets for cancer therapy. Curr Cancer Drug Targets 2:91–102

Lu Z, Ghosh S et al (2003) Downregulation of caveolin-1 function by EGF leads to the loss of E-cadherin, increased transcriptional activity of beta-catenin, and enhanced tumor cell invasion. Cancer Cell 4(6):499–515

Lynch TJ Jr, Kim ES et al (2007) Epidermal growth factor receptor inhibitor-associated cutaneous toxicities: an evolving paradigm in clinical management. Oncologist 12(5):610–621

Margulis A, Zhang W et al (2005) E-cadherin suppression accelerates squamous cell carcinoma progression in three-dimensional, human tissue constructs. Cancer Res 65(5):1783–1791

Matsumoto K, Matsumoto K et al (1994) Hepatocyte growth factor/scatter factor induces tyrosine phosphorylation of focal adhesion kinase (p125FAK) and promotes migration and invasion by oral squamous cell carcinoma cells. J Biol Chem 269(50):31807–31813

Morello S, Olivero M et al (2001) MET receptor is overexpressed but not mutated in oral squamous cell carcinomas. J Cell Physiol 189(3):285–290

Murai M, Shen X et al (2004) Overexpression of c-met in oral SCC promotes hepatocyte growth factor-induced disruption of cadherin junctions and invasion. Int J Oncol 25(4):831–840

Owens LV, Xu L et al (1995) Overexpression of the focal adhesion kinase (p125FAK) in invasive human tumors. Cancer Res 55(13):2752–2755

O-Charoenrat PH, Modjtahedi H et al (2000a) Epidermal growth factor-like ligands differentially up-regulate matrix metalloproteinase 9 in head and neck squamous carcinoma cells. Cancer Res 60(4):1121–1128

O-Charoenrat P Rhys-Evans et al (2000b) Overexpression of epidermal growth factor receptor in human head and neck squamous carcinoma cell lines correlates with matrix metalloproteinase-9 expression and in vitro invasion. Int J Cancer 86(3):307–317

Papagerakis S, Shabana AH et al (2004) Altered plakoglobin expression at mRNA and protein levels correlates with clinical outcome in patients with oropharynx squamous carcinomas. Hum Pathol 35(1):75–85

Patel BP, Shah PM et al (2005) Activation of MMP-2 and MMP-9 in patients with oral squamous cell carcinoma. J Surg Oncol 90(2):81–88

Perez-Moreno M, Jamora C et al (2003) Sticky business: orchestrating cellular signals at adherens junctions. Cell 112(4):535–548

Peruzzi B, Bottaro DP (2006) Targeting the c-Met signaling pathway in cancer. Clin Cancer Res 12(12):3657–3660

Schneider GB, Kurago Z et al (2002) Elevated focal adhesion kinase expression facilitates oral tumor cell invasion. Cancer 95(12):2508–2515

Schwarz J, Ayim A et al (2006) Differential expression of desmosomal plakophilins in various types of carcinomas: correlation with cell type and differentiation. Hum Pathol 37(5):613–622

Shintani S, Li C et al (2003) Gefitinib ("Iressa"), an epidermal growth factor receptor tyrosine kinase inhibitor, mediates the inhibition of lymph node metastasis in oral cancer cells. Cancer Lett 201(2):149–155

Sobolik-Delmaire T, Katafiasz D et al (2007) Decreased plakophilin-1 expression promotes increased motility in head and neck squamous cell carcinoma cells. Cell Commun Adhes 14(2):99–109

Sok JC, Coppelli FM et al (2006) Mutant epidermal growth factor receptor (EGFRvIII) contributes to head and neck cancer growth and resistance to EGFR targeting. Clin Cancer Res 12(17):5064–5073

Tanaka M, Kitajima Y et al (2002) Abnormal expression of E-cadherin and beta-catenin may be a molecular marker of submucosal invasion and lymph node metastasis in early gastric cancer. Br J Surg 89(2):236–244

Tanaka N, Odajima T et al (2003) Expression of E-cadherin, alpha-catenin, and beta-catenin in the process of lymph node metastasis in oral squamous cell carcinoma. Br J Cancer 89(3):557–563

Thomas SM, Coppelli FM et al (2003) Epidermal growth factor receptor-stimulated activation of phospholipase Cgamma-1 promotes invasion of head and neck squamous cell carcinoma. Cancer Res 63(17):5629–5635

Todd R, Donoff BR et al (1989) TGF-alpha and EGF-receptor mRNAs in human oral cancers. Carcinogenesis 10(8):1553–1556

Tsai ST, Yang KY et al (2006) Amphiregulin as a tumor promoter for oral squamous cell carcinoma: involvement of cyclooxygenase 2. Oral Oncol 42:381–390

Uchida D, Kawamata H et al (2001) Role of HGF/c-met system in invasion and metastasis of oral squamous cell carcinoma cells in vitro and its clinical significance. Int J Cancer 93(4):489–496

Yarden Y, Sliwkowski MX (2001) Untangling the ErbB signalling network. Nat Rev Mol Cell Biol 2:127–137

Yin T, Green KJ (2004) Regulation of desmosome assembly and adhesion. Semin Cell Dev Biol 15(6):665–677

Zhang Q, Bhola NE et al (2007) Antitumor mechanisms of combined gastrin-releasing peptide receptor and epidermal growth factor receptor targeting in head and neck cancer. Mol Cancer Ther 6(4):1414–1424

Zhang X, Liu Y et al (2002) A lymph node metastatic mouse model reveals alterations of metastasis-related gene expression in metastatic human oral carcinoma sublines selected from a poorly metastatic parental cell line. Cancer 95(8):1663–1672

Zhao XJ, Li H et al (2003) Expression of e-cadherin and beta-catenin in human esophageal squamous cell carcinoma: relationships with prognosis. World J Gastroenterol 9(2):225–232

Chapter 10
Nuclear Transcription Factors and Signaling Pathways in Oral Cancer Metastasis

Zhong Chen, Reza Ehsanian, and Carter Van Waes

Abstract Tumor progression of oral and other head and neck squamous cell carcinomas (HNSCCs) from dysplasia to metastasis involves a series of pathologic phenotypic changes considered to be the hallmarks of cancer, and these have been associated with a number of genetic, epigenetic, and molecular alterations (Fig. 10.1). Pathologic phenotypic changes precede metastasis and include increased cell proliferation, survival, and horizontal spread, which require certain molecular changes that together with later events contribute to the metastatic phenotype. These steps commonly include altered expression of molecules regulating the cell cycle and death (e.g., p53), growth factor response (epidermal growth factor receptor, EGFR), protein synthesis and metabolism (mammalian targets of rapamycin, mTOR), and cell immortality (telomerase). The subsequent steps of invasion and metastasis involve penetration and breakdown of the extracellular matrix (ECM) comprising the basement membrane and interstitial connective tissue; formation and invasion of a new stroma of host inflammatory and mesenchymal cells; neoangiogenesis and lymphangiogenesis; and distant spread via these lymphatics and blood vessels to secondary regional and distant sites. The molecular events accompanying the metastatic stage commonly include loss of expression or function of tumor suppressor genes or increased expression or function of oncogenes including numerous growth factors, cytokines, cell adhesion molecules and proteases, signal kinases, and nuclear transcription factors. Nuclear transcription factors appear to play a central role in malignant transformation and metastasis, since direct overexpression, mutation or activation of these molecules, or components of various upstream signaling pathways that modulate their function (Chaps. 8, 9, 11, 13) result in altered

C.V. Waes (✉)
Head and Neck Surgery Branch, National Institute on Deafness and Other Communication Disorders, National Institutes of Health, 10 Center Drive, CRC Room 4-2732, Bethesda, MD, 20892, USA
e-mail: vanwaesc@nidcd.nih.gov

J. Myers (ed.), *Oral Cancer Metastasis*,
DOI 10.1007/978-1-4419-0775-2_10, © Springer Science+Business Media, LLC 2010

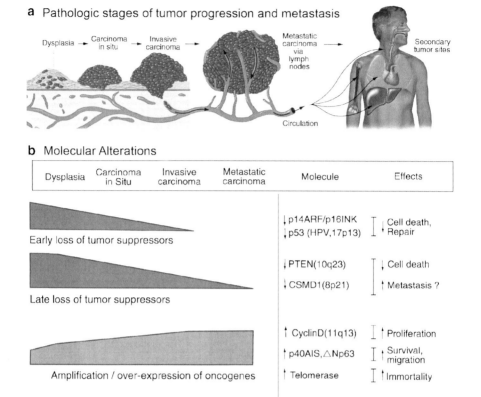

a Pathologic stages of tumor progression and metastasis

b Molecular Alterations

Fig. 10.1 Model of histopathologic and molecular changes with progression and metastasis of HNSCC. (**a**) Histopathologic changes during tumor progression and metastasis of HNSCC. (**b**) Molecular alterations with tumor progression and metastasis. *p14/16* protein 14 and 16 kDa, *p53* protein 53 kDa, *PTEN* phosphatase and tensin homolog deleted on chromosome 10, *CSMD1* Cub Sushi Multiple Domains1, *p40AIS* activated in squamous carcinoma, *ΔNp63* deltaNp63, *IL* interleukin, *TNF* tumor necrosis factor, *NF-κB* nuclear factor-kappa B, *TGF* transforming growth factor, *EGFR* epidermal growth factor receptor, *AP* activator protein, *STAT* signal transducers and activators of transcription, *BCL-XL* BCL2-related protein, long isoform, *GRO1* growth regulated oncogene1, *MMP* matrix metalloproteinase, *PDGF* platelet-derived growth factor, *VEGF* vascular endothelial growth factor, *eIFs* eukaryotic translation initiation factors, *EGR1* early growth response 1, *AKT* protein kinase B-alpha, *mTOR* mammalian targets of rapamycin

regulation of expression of diverse gene programs that produce the phenotypic changes characteristic of cancer and metastasis (Chaps. 4, 5, 12–14).

Background and Overview

Nuclear transcription factors are proteins or protein complexes that function to promote transcription of genomic DNA to messenger RNA by binding to their specific short DNA recognition sequences (referred to as binding motifs or sites) in the 5' promoter region of target genes. Their binding to DNA may be induced or constitutive, and modulated between inactive, repressive, or activated states by extracellular or intracellular signals. Transcription factor binding motifs are present in multiple genes and most transcription factors regulate multiple target genes to coordinate necessary molecular changes for a phenotypic response. For example, transcription factors can regulate several genes important for phenotypic changes in cancer, such as those related to the cell cycle, DNA repair and synthesis, and cell death (e.g., p53 and E2F), or wider sets of genes involved in cell proliferation, survival, inflammation, angiogenesis, adhesion and migration (e.g., activator protein-1 [AP-1], nuclear factor-kappaB [NF-κB], signal transducer and transcription factor [STAT]-3, early growth response-1 [EGR-1], and deltaNp63 [ΔNp63]). In addition, gene promoters often contain more than one transcription factor binding site for several of these transcription factors, so that a part or the whole gene program can be repressed, induced, or amplified by a variety of signals. Several nuclear transcription factors have been found to be commonly activated or suppressed in head and neck and other cancers and contribute to the malignant phenotype.

The TP53 or p53 gene encodes a 53 kDa protein that forms a tetrameric DNA binding complex. It is mutated in approximately 50% of HNSCCs, resulting in loss of function or altered function of the p53 protein. In some head and neck tumors, inactivation of p53 expression has been shown to result from protein degradation by the human papillomavirus (HPV) E6 gene expression, or increased expression and complex formation with its inactivating protein HDM2 induced by other transcription factors, such as NF-κB. p53 may also be inactivated at the transcriptional level itself by loss of signal activation or by genetic or epigenetic alteration of the ATM or p14ARF/p16INK4a loci, which encode proteins involved in the p53 pathway mediated damage response. After DNA damage or mutation, intact p53 functions to regulate genes that cause cell cycle arrest, promote DNA repair, or lead to cell death. Loss of this function can lead to proliferation and further loss of genomic stability, additional genetic changes, and progression to metastasis. Thus, p53, p14ARF/p16INK4a, and ATM are considered as important tumor suppressor genes in HNSCC and other cancers.

ΔNp63 is another member of the p53 family, whose function is distinguished from p53 as a prosurvival transcription factor. ΔNp63 is overexpressed in a subset of HNSCCs and can promote cell proliferation by repression of expression of p53 and its cell cycle regulatory target p21. It has also been shown to promote survival, through binding and inhibition of another proapoptotic p53 family member, p73. ΔNp63 inhibits the ability of p73 to promote expression of the genes encoding NOXA and PUMA, which promote cell death. ΔNp63 has been shown to activate a different gene program than p53 in breast cancer, including a cell adhesion and protease gene program associated with metastasis. This gene program includes integrin α6β4, previously shown to be overexpressed in HNSCC with poorer prognosis.

The AP-1 transcription factor is composed of cJUN and FOS family proteins. JUN was originally described as a viral oncogene that promotes proliferation and cell survival. The cellular proto-oncogenes cJUN and FRA-1 are family members shown to be activated and to bind and regulate target genes in HNSCC. JUN and FOS family proteins are primarily activated by mitogen-activated protein kinase (MAPK) pathways, which in turn mediate signals of a number of upstream cytokines, growth factors, receptors, and kinases whose expression or function is commonly altered in HNSCC. These include the epidermal growth factor (EGF) ligand and receptor family, kinases RAS, and SRC, themselves regarded as oncogenes in HNSCC and other cancers. AP-1 and these upstream signal activators help to activate cell cycle and survival proteins such as cyclin D and the BCL family of proteins, as well as genes encoding for proteins involved in matrix remodeling through matrix metalloproteinases (MMPs), cell adhesion and motility, and angiogenesis and inflammation through production of vascular endothelial growth factor (VEGF) and interleukin (IL)-8, which mediate important events in metastasis. However, blockade of these pathways or AP-1 usually only partially rather than completely inhibits these target genes and phenotypic changes, consistent with important contributory role of other transcription factors.

The NF-κB family of transcription factors is made up of 5 subunits, NF-κB1 (p50), NF-κB2 (p52), RELA, RELB, and cREL, that combine in different ways to make heterodimeric NF-κB protein complexes that are bound in inactivated state to inhibitor-κBs (IκBs) in the cell cytoplasm. Signal activation of NF-κBs involves phosphorylation of IκB by IκB kinases (IKKs), whereupon NF-κB/REL complexes are translocated to the cell nucleus where they can activate diverse transcriptional programs.

NF-κB was first implicated as an oncogenic transcription factor through discovery of a viral form of REL which causes avian lymphomas. NF-κB1/RELA has been found to play an important role in aberrant gene expression and the malignant phenotype of HNSCC. Nuclear activation of all 5 NF-κB members has been demonstrated. NF-κB is inducible by nicotine and chemicals contained in tobacco and betel nut, two of the most important carcinogenic agents that promote the development of HNSCC. Constitutive nuclear activation of NF-κB has been shown to occur in premalignant dysplastic lesions and approximately 85% of HNSCC, indicating aberrant activation is an early event, and strong nuclear immunostaining is associated with an increased rate of malignant progression of dysplasia and decreased survival in patients with HNSCC. NF-κB has been found to be constitutively activated in HNSCC cell lines and tumors, suggesting that further events contribute to sustained activation. Thus far, expression and autocrine activation by IL-1α and TNF have been implicated in activation of NF-κB in HNSCC. Overexpression and aberrant EGFR signaling appear to contribute to constitutive activation of NF-κB pathway. Activation of NF-κB via the PI3K, AKT, and CK2 kinases also appears to be important in signal activation of these pathways in HNSCC. NF-κB regulates or coregulates key genes involved in cell proliferation (cyclin D1), survival (BCL-XL), migration and invasion (MMP9), and angiogenesis (IL-8, growth regulated oncogene 1 [GRO1, previously called KC or GRO-α]) in cancer (Fig. 10.2). Recently, NF-κB-mediated activation of one of the cytokines, Interleukin-6 (IL-6), has been shown in turn to be an important activator of STAT3, another transcription factor that controls the expression of genes that are important in cell survival.

STAT3 is an activating transcription factor implicated in HNSCC. STAT3 may be activated by EGFR and/or IL-6R and their ligands, transforming growth factor-α (TGF-α) and IL-6. Activation via EGFR can involve SRC and via IL-6 can involve JAK and/or MEK kinases. STAT3 phosphorylation and dimerization result in DNA binding. Target genes of STAT3 include *BCL-XL*, a key antiapoptotic gene involved in cell survival of HNSCC cells as well as transcription factor c-*MYC* and G1 phase cyclin *cyclinD*.

EGR-1 is another mitogen inducible transcription factor, activated in HNSCC by hepatocyte growth factor/scatter factor (HGF/SF) and c-MET, which encodes the HGF receptor. Overexpression of HGF by tumor stroma and increased responsiveness to c-MET activation have been implicated in lymph node metastasis of HNSCC. HGF and c-MET signaling induce activation of EGR1 through protein kinase C (PKC) and MAPK pathways. EGR1 promotes the expression of the angiogenesis factors, VEGF and platelet-derived growth factor (PDGF), which are important in tumor progression and metastasis.

The cross talk in signaling that leads to comodulation of these transcription factors and the presence of different combinations of binding site cassettes for these factors in target genes result in the formation of a network that can potentially mediate carcinogenesis and metastatic progression from a variety of molecular events. Alteration of expression of one or more cytokines and growth factors leading to coactivation of signal transcription factors such as NF-κB, AP-1, and STAT-3 has been shown to alter the balance between cell survival and death and angiogenesis factor expression by HNSCC. For example, increased expression of NF-κB and STAT3-regulated proteins such as BCL-2 and BCL-XL, together with decreased expression of the p53 regulated proteins p21 and BAX, has been shown to be important in preventing programmed cell death of HNSCC cells. Similarly, coactivation of NF-κB and AP-1 has been shown to upregulate expression of the proangiogenic factors IL-8, GRO-1, and VEGF, which have been implicated in both tumorigenesis and metastasis.

In this chapter, we will discuss some of the experimental evidence from animal and human studies which have enabled the determination of the modes of activation, gene targets, and functional roles of these signal-activated nuclear transcription factors, as well as their contributions to the metastatic processes in HNSCC.

Molecular Changes During Development of Head and Neck Squamous Cell Carcinoma

Tumor Suppressor Genes Encoding Transcription Factors in HNSCC

Chromosome 17p13 encodes the p53 gene, which is altered with relatively low frequency in dysplasia and carcinoma in situ (CIS), but with increased frequency in about 50% of primary carcinomas (Califano et al. 1996). Alternatively, HPV infection and E6 expression have been shown to inactivate p53, presumably at an earlier stage, particularly in oropharyngeal squamous cell carcinoma (SCC) (Gillison et al. 2000). As described above, a variety of functions have been attributed to the p53 gene, which is thought to mediate tumor suppression by cell-cycle arrest and DNA repair or induction of cell death when DNA damage is irreversible (Sidransky and Hollstein 1996). Tumor suppressor p53 may also repress the activation of prosurvival genes by NF-κB (Lee et al. 2007) by competing for a transcriptional cofactor called CBP/p300 (Webster and Perkins 1999). Thus loss of p53 can lead to dysfunction of mechanisms by which cancer cells undergo repair or cell death, as well as potentially promote activation of prosurvival pathways (Friedman et al. 2007).

A locus on the short (p) arm of chromosome 9 located at 9p21 has been found to exhibit loss of heterozygosity (LOH) at an early stage during development of hyperplasia (Califano et al. 1996). The 9p21 locus has been found to encode overlapping genes that encode proteins called p14ARF and p16INK4a, and this locus is found to be inactivated in the majority of HNSCC by homozygous deletion, mutation, or methylation of the regulatory promoter region (Reed et al. 1996). The p14ARF protein is an important activator of the p53 pathway and repressor of the NF-κB pathway during programmed cell death (Rocha et al. 2005), so its loss may be an important early event in dysregulation of both the p53 and NF-κB pathways, which are altered in dysplastic and malignant squamous epithelia (Gorgoulis et al. 1994; Zhang et al. 2005). The p16INK4a protein is a cyclin-dependent kinase called CDKN2/MTS-1/INK4A that normally inhibits cell-cycle progression. Thus, genetic or epigenetic alteration of this locus can result in the loss of p14ARF protein causing decreased programmed cell death, and the loss of p16INK4a causing increased proliferation. Consistent with this, re-expression of p16 in HNSCC cells by gene transfer suppresses cell growth in vitro (Liggett et al. 1996). Re-expression of p14ARF has been shown to repress NF-κB-mediated prosurvival gene expression and promote cell death in other cell types (Rocha et al. 2005).

Loss of heterozygosity involving chromosome 8p is observed later, in association with invasive HNSCC, and a locus on chromosome 8p23 is associated with poor prognosis (Scholnick et al. 1996). The putative tumor suppressor gene at the chromosome 8p23 locus has been identified and is a large transmembrane protein called CSMD1 (Scholnick and Richter 2003). Another gene that infrequently undergoes mutations that result in loss of function maps to the chromosome 8p21 region in HNSCC, and is a p53 regulated growth inhibitory gene that is a member of the TNF–related apoptosis-inducing ligand (TRAIL) family (Pai et al. 1998).

Loss of heterozygosity at chromosome 10q23 is detected with intermediate frequency in primary HNSCC and has been found to reflect deletion or inactivation of a gene called phosphatase and tensin homolog deleted on chromosome 10 (PTEN) (Okami et al. 1998). PTEN suppresses the activation of AKT, also known as protein kinase B. AKT plays an important role in the activation of transcription factor NF-κB and coactivator CBP/p300, and transcription of prosurvival genes (Madrid et al. 2001), and activation of molecular target of rapamycin (mTOR), important in translation of proteins, such as the angiogenesis factor, VEGF (Amornphimoltham et al. 2005). Early activation of AKT by autocrine stimuli such as EGFR and cytokine receptors (Pernas et al. 2008; Bancroft et al. 2002), and later by loss of PTEN, could lead to increased survival and growth of HNSCC and other cancers.

Tumor Oncogenes and Transcriptional Regulation in HNSCC

A locus on the long (q) arm of chromosome 11 located at 11q13 is amplified with increasing frequency during the CIS stage (Califano et al. 1996) and is associated with increased expression of a cell-cycle regulatory protein called cyclin D1 (Fu et al. 2004). Alternatively, cyclin D1 may be overexpressed as a result of tran-scriptional activation by NF-κB or STAT-3 (Chang and Van Waes 2005; Lee et al. 2007). Cyclin D1 is required for progression of cells through the cell cycle, thereby stimulating squamous cells to proliferate. Inhibition of cyclin D1 results in inhibition of growth of HNSCC in vitro.

On chromosome 3q, amplification of a homologue of p53 was identified, and the protein encoded by this region, designated p40AIS (amplified in SCC), was found to be expressed at high levels with high frequency in HNSCC and lung squamous cell carcinoma (Hibi et al. 2000). p40AIS is a short splice variant of the related p53 family member called ΔNp63, and both lack the tumor suppressor function of p53. Expression of AIS has been found to promote the growth of rat cells in soft agar and in mice, indicating that it may play an early role in transformation as an onco-gene. Increased p40 expression appears to be correlated with the loss of p53, and p40 may interact and inhibit normal p53 function. Subsequently, ΔNp63 has recently been shown to promote survival of a subset of HNSCC by binding and inhibiting p73, another proapoptotic p53 family member (Rocco et al. 2006). ΔNp63 also upregulates expression of integrin α6β4 and the ECM protein laminin 5 (Carroll et al. 2006), both shown to be important markers of poor prognosis and mediators of cell adhesion of HNSCC (Van Waes et al. 1991).

In summary, HNSCCs have been found to accumulate a series of genetic or epigenetic changes during tumor development. The functions of the affected genes identified to date are consistent with the changes required for the development of cancer, namely regulating cell-cycle progression and proliferation, cell death, and lifespan. Other altered genes are involved in cell adhesion, migration, matrix remodeling, and angiogenesis. The occurrence of multiple events at different stages in individual cancers of different patients suggest that different combinations of several key genes affecting these phenotypic changes can contribute to the common histopathologic stages of tumor development observed in HNSCC.

Aberrant Activation of Signaling, Gene Transcription, and Protein Translation in HNSCC

The genetic or epigenetic changes in HNSCC can lead to altered activation of several signaling and transcription factor pathways that in turn regulate many of the several hundred genes and proteins whose expression is altered in cancer. These common pathways explain why most cancers show aberrant activation of certain gene programs involved in cell proliferation, survival, migration, angiogenesis, and metastasis. As important common pathways, they may also prove to be useful markers for molecular diagnosis and targets for therapy. The accumulation of molecular changes in expression or activation of several key growth factors, cytokines, receptors, or their downstream signaling and transcription factors with cytopathologic changes that occur during the stages of tumor development of HNSCC are summarized in Fig. 10.1, 10.2.

Aberrant Activation of the NF-κB Pathway in HNSCC

NF-κB is a signal transcription factor found to play an important role in aberrant gene expression and the malignant phenotype of SCC and other cancers (Van Waes 2007). NF-κB is inducible by nicotine and chemicals contained in tobacco and betel nut, two of the most important carcinogenic agents that promote the development of HNSCC (Tsurutani et al. 2005; Ni et al. 2007; Allen et al. 2007b). Increased nuclear activation of NF-κB has been shown to occur in premalignant dysplastic lesions and approximately 85% of HNSCCs, indicating it is an early event, and strong immunostaining is associated with increased rate of malignant progression of dysplasia and decreased survival in patients with HNSCC (Zhang et al. 2005; Allen et al. 2008). NF-κB was found to be constitutively activated in HNSCC cell lines and tumor, suggesting that further events contribute to sustained activation (Zhang et al. 2005; Chang and Van Waes 2005; Duffey et al. 1999; Ondrey et al. 1999). Thus far, expression and autocrine activation by IL-1α and TNF have been implicated in the activation of NF-κB in HNSCC (Wolf et al. 2001; Jackson-Bernitsas et al. 2007; Duffey et al. 2000). EGFR appears also to contribute weakly to constitutive activation of NF-κB pathway (Bancroft et al. 2002). Activation of NF-κB via the PI3K, AKT, and CK2 kinases appears to be important in signal activation of these pathways in HNSCC (Bancroft et al. 2002; Yu et al. 2006).

By cDNA microarray profiling, NF-κB was found to directly or indirectly regulate approximately 60% of the genes aberrantly expressed with malignant progression in a murine SCC model (Loercher et al. 2004). Consistent with this model, among approximately1260 differentially expressed genes identified from 10 HNSCC cell lines by a 24K cDNA microarray, 60% of the genes were identified as NF-κB regulated genes by bioinformatics analysis (Yan et al. 2007a). Independently, in microarray gene profiles of HNSCC specimens from patients at high risk for malignant progression, Chung et al identified a 75-gene list predictive of disease recurrence as the most prominent molecular characteristics of the high-risk tumors. Further evaluation of this gene set showed that many of these genes were involved in the epithelial-to-mesenchymal transition (EMT) and deregulation of NF-κB signals (Chung et al. 2006). NF-κB regulates key genes involved in cell proliferation (cyclin D1), survival (BCL-XL) (Duan et al. 2007; Lee et al. 2008), migration and invasion (MMP9), and angiogenesis (IL-8, GRO1) (Duffey et al. 1999; Dong et al. 1999) in HNSCC (Fig. 10.3). This has been further confirmed by blocking NF-κB activation and seeing decreased expression of these genes with concomitant inhibition of cell proliferation, survival, migration, angiogenesis, and tumorigenesis in SCC (Loercher et al. 2004; Duffey et al. 1999; Dong et al. 1999). Recently, NF-κB-mediated activation of one of the cytokines, IL-6, has been shown to be an important activator of STAT3, also important in cell survival (Lee et al. 2006, 2008; Squarize et al. 2006).

Overexpression of TGF-α/EGFR and IL-6/IL-6R and Activation of the MAPK/AP-1 and JAK/STAT3 Pathways in HNSCC

Another of the early alterations in signaling identified in the development of HNSCC is overexpression of EGFR and one of its stimulatory factors, TGF-α (Bancroft et al. 2002; Grandis et al. 1998b; Pernas et al. 2008) (see Fig. 10.2). More than 90% of HNSCCs overexpress EGFR and TGF-α (Grandis et al. 1998b). Increased expression of TGF-α and EGFR has been detected in tumor cells and normal mucosa of patients with HNSCC compared with normal mucosa from controls, indicating that TGF-α and EGFR expression may be an early event in carcinogenesis of HNSCC (Grandis et al. 1998b). Increased expression of both TGF-α and EGFR occurs with progression to carcinoma. EGFR and TGF-α appear to be overexpressed owing to transcriptional activation of the genes for this receptor and ligand in most HNSCCs. Patients with carcinomas expressing higher levels of these factors have been shown to have a shortened disease-free survival, independent of cervical lymph node stage.

Production of TGF-α and expression of EGFR establish a potential autocrine signal pathway for continuous stimulation of proliferation of squamous cells, and the importance of TGF-α and EGFR expression in the growth of HNSCC has been established (Bancroft et al. 2002; Grandis et al. 1998b; Pernas et al. 2008).

Inhibition of either TGF-α or EGFR expression or function using antisense oligonucleotides or pharmacologic inhibitors in combination with radiation was found to decrease proliferation and growth of HNSCC cells in vitro and of xenografts in mice in vivo (Bancroft et al. 2002; Grandis et al. 1998a; He et al. 1998; Bonner et al. 2000; Milas et al. 2000; Pernas et al. 2008). The effects of EGFR activation are in part mediated through the RAS signal transcription factor pathway, wherein RAS activation of the MAPK or extracellular signal-regulated kinase (ERK) leads to the activation of the transcription factor, AP-1 (Bancroft et al. 2002). EGFR signaling can also activate the signal transducer and activator of transcription 3 (STAT3) (Grandis et al. 2000; Lee et al. 2006). EGFR activation of STAT3 helps inhibit HNSCC cells from undergoing cell death (apoptosis) and stimulates proliferation. The cytokine, IL-6 is regulated by NF-κB and is another important factor that activates STAT3 through JAK pathway signaling (Squarize et al. 2006; Lee et al. 2006). Thus, overexpression of the EGFR appears to be one of several factors contributing to MAPK and STAT3 activation, which leads to increased proliferation and decreased cell death, and contribute to HNSCC tumorigenesis.

Aberrant Activation of PI3K/AKT/mTOR Pathway

Aberrant activation of the PI3K/AKT signaling pathway has been implicated in promoting the survival of cells that constitute many malignancies, including HNSCC (Dong et al. 2001a; Madrid et al. 2001; Pernas et al. 2008; Bancroft et al. 2002). Our laboratory has previously shown that overexpression and autocrine activation of EGFR activated PI3K and ERK/MAPK pathways promote the expression of proinflammatory and proangiogeneic cytokines including IL-8 and VEGF, through the activation of NF-κB and AP-1 transcription factors (Bancroft et al. 2002; Lee et al. 2006). In addition, we have shown that the proangiogenic activity of HGF/SF in HNSCC is correlated with higher levels of the angiogenic factors IL-8 and VEGF in the serum of patients with HNSCC (Dong et al. 2001a). HGF induces a significant increase of IL-8 and VEGF cytokine production through phosphorylation of PI3K and ERK/MAPK (Dong et al. 2001a). The cytokine and growth factor-induced activation of the PI3K and AKT kinases activates another important target, mTOR, that is important in activating kinases and proteins that enhance protein translation in HNSCC (Nathan et al. 2004). Activation of eIF4E (elongation initiating factor) has been associated with activation of AKT and mTOR in HNSCC. This protein has been implicated in enhancing the translation of angiogenesis factors such as VEGF (Nathan et al. 1999). Although inhibition of mTOR by rapamycin has little effect on HNSCC lines in vitro, this inhibition sensitizes HNSCC cells to apoptosis and reduces angiogenesis in vivo in animal models (Amornphimoltham et al. 2005).

Transcriptional Regulation and Signal Pathways Promote Invasion, Migration, and Metastasis of HNSCC and Other Cancers

Molecular Mediators of Tumor Progression and Metastasis

The progression of cancer to invasion and metastasis leads to significant morbidity and mortality. Figures 10.1 and 10.3 highlight some of the intermediate and late histopathologic and molecular events associated with tumor progression and metastasis. Development of invasive carcinoma is associated with focal dissolution of the basement membrane and ECM and the detachment and migration of cells into the submucosal tissue. HNSCC that exhibits a streaming pattern of small clusters of cells through the ECM are associated with more aggressive behavior and poor prognosis (Truelson et al. 1992). Tumor progression to a size that becomes visible and has an effect on adjacent structures requires an increase in the supply of oxygen and nutrients and removal of waste. Folkman established the concept that new blood vessel formation is critical in cancer (Folkman 1996). Enlargement of tumors to a size beyond 0.5 cm exceeds the range for diffusion of oxygen from existing vessels and necessitates new blood vessel formation, called neoangiogenesis. Such new vessel formation has been demonstrated in all cancers and is commonly associated with an increase in inflammatory cells. Increased vessel density and inflammation within tumors have been associated with more rapid growth, metastasis, and a decrease in survival, suggesting that the increase in vessels may relate to the increased access for metastasizing cancer cells. Invasion of the lymphatics and blood vessels and circulation of cells are necessary for regional and distant spread of HNSCC.

Growth of the tumor epithelia and angiogenesis is also accompanied by increased infiltration of inflammatory cells and proliferation of fibrous stroma. Several studies have suggested that tumor cells that induce host inflammatory and stromal cell responses grow, invade, and metastasize more rapidly. Chen et al. have shown that during progression, SCCs undergo additional changes needed for growth and metastasis that depend on the host (Chen et al. 1997). Young and colleagues have shown that inflammatory cells infiltrating human and murine SCCs are one of the host components that promote growth and metastasis (Young et al. 1997). These inflammatory cells bear a stem cell marker called CD34 and appear to differentiate into granulocytes and the endothelial cells that form new blood vessels. Young (2000) and Pekarek et al. (1995) have shown that the granulocytes promote increased growth and metastasis. Granulocytes from the host can release growth factors (Pekarek et al. 1995) and proteases (Itoh et al. 1999) that stimulate growth and invasion of tumor cells. Squamous cell carcinomas induce proliferation of stromal fibroblasts. Fibroblasts also secrete factors, such as HGF, and ECM substances that can promote growth (Tamura et al. 1993). The establishment of metastases requires cell arrest and vessel formation in a new location. HNSCC shows a predilection for metastases to the lymphatics, lungs, liver, and bone marrow, suggesting that the cells and substrates of the reticuloendothelial system provide a favorable environment for arrest and formation of SCC metastases (Fig. 10.1, 10.2).

Molecules Involved in Cell Adhesion, Migration, and Invasion

HNSCCs exhibit alterations in expression of a repertoire of cell adhesion molecules and ECM substances that function in attachment and migration. Increased expression of cell adhesion molecules called integrins has been detected in HNSCC (Van Waes et al. 1995). The integrins are heterodimers composed of α and β subunits that form a superfamily of cell surface receptors involved in cell–cell and cell–ECM adhesions and recognition. The integrin $\alpha6\beta4$, $\alpha2\beta1$, and $\alpha3\beta1$ heterodimers are normally expressed among proliferating layers of squamous cell epithelium but are expressed in suprabasilar layers of many SCCs in association with the increased proliferation and immortalization that occur during early tumor development (Van Waes et al. 1995). Increased suprabasilar expression of $\alpha6\beta4$, as detected by monoclonal antibody A9, was found to be correlated with a poorer prognosis in a prospective study of 80 patients with HNSCC (Wolf et al. 1990). Expression of integrin $\alpha6\beta4$ has been shown to promote aggressive tumor behavior (Rabinovitz and Mercurio 1996). The $\alpha6\beta4$, $\alpha2\beta1$, and $\alpha3\beta1$ integrins have been found to be receptors for the ECM protein laminin, and $\alpha2\beta1$ and $\alpha3\beta1$ integrins also bind to collagen. HNSCCs secrete the basement membrane component laminin in vitro and in situ, and the blockade of $\alpha6\beta4$, $\alpha2\beta1$, and $\alpha3\beta1$ completely inhibits attachment of HNSCC to laminin and collagen. Monoclonal antibody to the $\alpha6$ integrin also has been shown to reduce binding to activated endothelial cells. Thus, HNSCC exhibits constitutive alterations in expression of a repertoire of integrin cell adhesion molecules, and expression of integrin $\alpha6\beta4$ in particular is linked with aggressive tumor behavior. Recently, integrin $\alpha6\beta4$ expression has been shown to be upregulated by transcription factor ΔNp63 in breast (Carroll et al. 2006; Leong et al. 2007) and head and neck cancers (Yang et al. 2009).

Increased expression and activation of enzymes involved in remodeling of the ECM have been detected in HNSCC and are associated with increased invasiveness. The MMPs comprise a family of proteases that digest the ECM and are upregulated in HNSCC (see Figs. 10.1 and 10.2). HNSCC exhibits increased expression of urokinase-type plasminogen activator (uPA) and uPA receptor, as well as the membrane-type MMP-1, collagenase 1, stromelysin 1, and gelatinase B (Rosenthal et al. 1998). Expression of these factors and invasiveness appear to be inducible by EGF or HGF (Rosenthal et al. 1998; Hanzawa et al. 2000; O-charoenrat et al. 2000). Invasion of EGF- or HGF-stimulated cells is completely suppressed by recombinant and synthetic MMP inhibitors (Rosenthal et al. 1998). These studies suggest that MMPs may be more important than the plasminogen activator-plasmin system in mediating EGF- or HGF-induced tumor cell invasion of interstitial matrix barriers. Inflammatory cells infiltrating tumors also can express MMPs. MMP-9 may be expressed by host-derived neutrophils, macrophages, and mast cells attracted to the tumor site. MMP-9 expressed by bone marrowderived cells appears to promote malignant tumor progression of squamous cell carcinoma in vivo (Coussens et al. 2000).

Cytokine and Growth Factors Involved in Inflammation and Angiogenesis

The demonstration of the role of host inflammatory and angiogenesis responses in development and progression of SCC has led to efforts to identify the molecules involved. HNSCCs have been found to express a number of cytokines and growth factors that mediate inflammatory and angiogenesis responses (see Figs. 10.1 and 10.2).

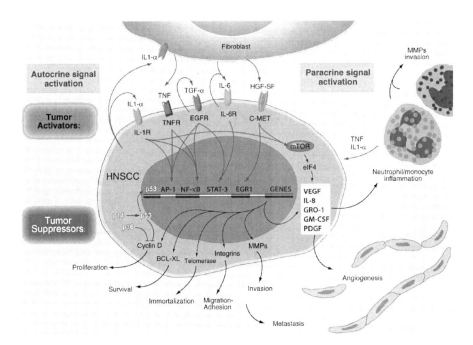

Fig. 10.2 Modulation of nuclear transcription factors in response to autocrine and paracrine factors mediated signals that activate or suppress tumor progression and metastasis of HNSCC. Factors produced by tumor and host cells provide autocrine and paracrine stimuli that activate signal receptors, transcription factors, and genes. Genes activated by transcription factors effect cellular changes in HNSCC that lead to tumor progression and host inflammatory and angiogenesis responses that promote malignant tumor invasion and metastasis. *IL* interleukin, *TNF* tumor necrosis factor, *TGF* transforming growth factor, *EGFR* epidermal growth factor receptor, *HGF/SF* hepatocyte growth factor/scatter factor, *AP* activator protein, *NF-κB* nuclear factor-kappa B, *STAT* signal transducers and activators of transcription, *EGR* early growth response, *p14/16* protein 14 and 16 kDa, *p53* protein 53 kDa, *BCL-XL* BCL2-related protein, long isoform, *MMP* matrix metalloproteinase, *GRO* growth-regulated oncogene, *VEGF* vascular endothelial growth factor, *GM-CSF* granulocyte-macrophage colony-stimulating factor, *PDGF* platelet-derived growth factor

SCC produces a repertoire of factors in vitro and in situ that includes IL-1α, IL-6, IL-8, granulocyte-macrophage colony-stimulating factor (GM-CSF), GRO-1, and VEGF (Chen et al. 1998, 1999; Loukinova et al. 2000). Tumor fibroblasts have been shown to produce HGF (Tamura et al. 1993). IL-6, IL-8, GRO-1, VEGF, and HGF are of sufficient stability and are produced at high enough concentrations that they have been detected in the serum of patients (Dong et al. 2001a; Druzgal et al. 2005; Chen et al. 1999; Allen et al. 2007a). Decreasing cytokine levels were associated with response, while increasing levels were related to progression of recurrence (Druzgal et al. 2005).

IL-1 is a cytokine that can regulate NF-κB activation and expression of several of the other factors detected in squamous cell carcinoma (Chen et al. 1998). IL-1 can serve as an autocrine factor to stimulate HNSCC to produce IL-6, IL-8, GM-CSF, and VEGF, and as a paracrine factor to stimulate production of HGF by stromal fibroblasts (Fig. 10.2). In addition, IL-1 has important systemic regulatory effects as an important mediator of acute-phase reactions, increased catabolic state, and cachexia, often observed in patients with aggressive HNSCC (Chen et al. 1998; Chen et al. 1999). IL-1 and IL-6 both can have direct effects as autocrine or paracrine factors that can stimulate proliferation of HNSCC cells (Hong et al. 2000; Lee et al. 2006; Wolf et al. 2001; Squarize et al. 2006).

IL-8 and GRO-1 are both members of a related family of chemoattractant and proliferative factors that contain a cysteine-X-cysteine (C-X-C) amino acid motif. IL-8 and GRO-1 have been shown to serve as chemoattractants for neutrophils, monocytes, and endothelial cells, which are major constituents of the inflammatory response in HNSCC (Fig. 10.2). Loukinova et al. have shown that expression of Gro-1, the murine homologue of GRO-1 and IL-8, promotes aggressive growth and metastases, angiogenesis, and inflammatory cell infiltration in SCC (Loukinova et al. 2000). The aggressive pattern of growth is reversed in knockout mice deficient in CXC receptor 2, the receptor for the chemokine. These results provide direct evidence that tumor factors and the host response induced by them are critical in tumor progression and metastasis of squamous cell carcinoma. Kitadai et al. have shown that IL-8 has similar effects on growth of other histologic types of human tumors as xenografts in mice (Kitadai et al. 1999). Young et al have shown that GM-CSF produced by squamous cell carcinoma may also play a role in the

Fig. 10.3 (continued) After 1–2 weeks incubation, colonies of adherent cells with epithelial morphology surrounding the tumor nodules could be visualized. When monolayers reached confluency and were devoid of any visible fibroblasts, the cells were trypsinized for passage and expansion as cell lines in tissue culture flasks. The cell lines re-isolated from lymph nodes were designated as Pam-LY lines, and the cell lines re-isolated from lung nodules were designated as Pam-LU lines. The pictures on the right panels show gross and macroscopic appearance of Pam 212 primary tumor, as well as the lymph node and pulmonary metastases in BALB/c mice. The gross picture shows the primary Pam 212 tumor located in the inguinal region (P) with inguinal and axillary lymph nodes (LY) enlarged by metastases. The lung metastases (LU) are shown after staining lung with India ink. Histology of Pam 212 primary tumor (P), inguinal lymph node (LY), and pulmonary metastases (LU) were examined by light microscopy, and photomicrographs were taken at original magnification X200

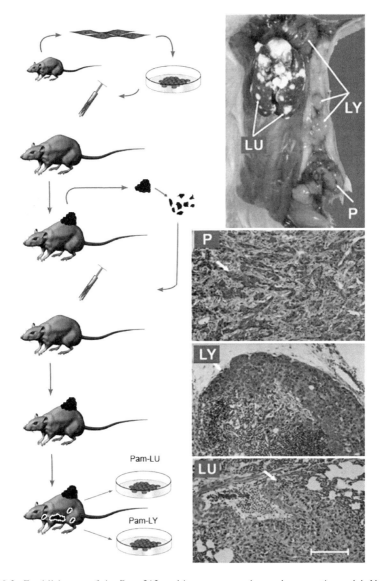

Fig. 10.3 Establishment of the Pam 212 multistage progression and metastatic model. Neonatal keratinocytes of male BALB/c mice was isolated and cultured in vitro. After long-term culture, a spontaneously transformed cell line were derived and named as Pam 212. Subcutaneous injection of Pam 212 cells forms local SCC in syngeneic BALB/c mice. The metastatic Pam tumor model was established by inoculating Pam 212 cells into athymic nude BALB/c congenic mice, the resulting tumors were cut into 1 mm² fragments, and ~5–6 fragments were transplanted to normal BALB/c mice by injecting back into the flank. Two months after tumor transplantation, the tumor size reached or exceeded 1.5 cm in diameter, the mice were euthanized and the lymph nodes, lungs, and other organs were carefully examined and harvested for the histologic examination and lung staining. To establish the metastatic cell lines, Pam tumor metastases to the lymph nodes and lungs were excised and cut into pieces of 1–2 mm diameter and cultured in 24-well tissue culture plates.

activity of CD34 progenitors of granulocytes and endothelium, which they reported as associated with metastasis (Young et al. 1997). VEGF also promotes angiogenesis and stimulates expression of $\alpha v \beta 3$ and $\alpha v \beta 5$ integrin heterodimers that are involved in migration of endothelial cells during angiogenesis. Inhibition of αv integrins inhibits tumorigenesis of SCC in mice (Van Waes et al. 2000).

Activation of the HGF/c-MET-Mediated Signal Pathway and Transcriptional Regulation

HGF and its receptor c-MET, a proto-oncogene product which is a transmembrane tyrosine kinase (Bottaro et al. 1991), have been shown to promote mitogenic, motogenic, morphogenic and antiapoptotic effects in normal and malignant cells (Birchmeier et al. 2003; Matsumoto and Nakamura 1997; Birchmeier and Gherardi 1998). Aberrant c-MET signaling through *c-MET* gene amplification, mutations, and autocrine or paracrine activation of c-MET receptor has been reported in a variety of human tumors, including breast, prostate, lung, pancreatic, bladder, and head and neck cancers (Jiang et al. 1999). HGF binds to the c-MET receptor and induces the activation of multiple signaling cascades which alter cellular adhesion, migration, and ECM integrity, ultimately leading to tumor invasion and metastatic behaviors (Jiang et al. 2005; Birchmeier et al. 2003; Matsumoto and Nakamura 2006). Among the signal molecules downstream from c-MET receptor, GAB1 is a crucial scaffolding adaptor protein in responding to extracellular stimuli, through direct interaction with tyrosine phosphorylation sites (mainly pY1349) of c-MET receptor (Sachs et al. 2000; Maroun et al. 1999). The binding leads to a prolonged phosphorylation of GAB1, which mediates additional interactions and phosphorylations of multiple molecules, such as SHP2, PI3K, phospholipase C, and CRK through their SH2 domains (Gu and Neel 2003; Rosario and Birchmeier 2003). The activation cascades of the intermediate kinases and phosphotases lead to the activation of the RAS, RAF, and ERK/MAPK pathways. The GAB1–SHP2–ERK/MAPK cascade regulates ETS/AP1 transcription factors and adhesion molecules, which control cell proliferation, junction formation, and cell migration (Maroun et al. 1999; Potempa and Ridley 1998; Ridley et al. 1995; Birchmeier et al. 2003). Both ERK/MAPK and the PI3K pathways contribute to c-Met-mediated cell adhesion, spreading, and motility (Potempa and Ridley 1998), and PI3K-activated AKT primarily controls cell survival (Fan et al. 2001; Xiao et al. 2001). Other molecules downstream from the c-Met receptor, such as RAS, RAC1, and PAK, control cytoskeletal rearrangement and cell adhesion (Ridley et al. 1995; Royal et al. 2000). RAP1 regulates cell motility (Sakkab et al. 2000; Lamorte et al. 2000), and JNK, STAT3, and NF-κB participate in c-MET signaling pathways directly or indirectly, leading to cell transformation, anchorage-independent growth, and branched endothelial tubule formation (Boccaccio et al. 1998; Zhang et al. 2002; Schaper et al. 1997; Muller et al. 2002).

HGF/c-MET signaling promotes vascular endothelial cell migration and angio-genesis in tumors such as papillary carcinoma, breast and prostate cancers, and head and neck cancers (Grant et al. 1993; Scarpino et al. 2003; Davies et al. 2003; Di Renzo et al. 1991; Dong et al. 2001a; Dong et al. 2001b). The mechanisms of action have been shown to be direct activation of the PI3K/AKT and ERK/MAPK pathways in endothelial cells (Sengupta et al. 2003), with induction of VEGF or IL-8 (Dong et al. 2001a) and inhibition of thrombospondin-1 (Zhang et al. 2003). Activation of the HGF/c-MET signaling cascade also results in the phosphoryla-tion, ubiquitylation, and degradation of the E-cadherin and cadherin-associated proteins (Matteucci et al. 2006). The loss of E-cadherins disrupts tight junctions leading to detachment of malignant cells from the primary site of tumor formation (Hiscox and Jiang 1997). In addition, HGF has been shown to induce phosphoryla-tion of focal adhesion kinase (FAK) (Beviglia and Kramer 1999; Liu et al. 2002; Lai et al. 2000), which is involved in integrin-mediated signal transduction and aids in cell motility. HGF/c-MET signaling stimulates detachment and increases mobil-ity of tumor cells, which is coupled with the induction of tumor cell's binding to and degradation of the basement membrane and ECM. HGF/c-MET signaling has also been found to increase the localization of mechanical linkers of the cytoskel-eton, termed paxillins, to integrins (Liu et al. 2002) and to increase the expression of the α2 and α3 subunits of the integrin receptor (Beviglia and Kramer 1999; Lai et al. 2000). The increase in attachment is followed by the breakdown of the barrier by proteolytic enzymes. HGF/c-MET signaling has been reported to stimu-late production of uPA-dependant proteolytic network (Nishimura et al. 2003), MMPs, and tissue inhibitors of matrix metalloproteinases (TIMPs) (Gong et al. 2003). Once the tumor cell has broken the barrier formed by the basement mem-brane and the ECM, HGF/c-MET signaling promotes the interaction of tumor cells with endothelial cells in the organs that the tumor spreads to by increasing the expression of adhesion molecules such as CD44 (Hiscox and Jiang 1997) on the endothelium and the tumor cell (Mine et al. 2003). This increase in the interaction of the tumor cells with the endothelium of blood vessels ultimately enables tumor cell invasion and the resulting metastasis to distant tissues.

In cancers of epithelial origin, HGF is expressed predominately by stromal cells, whereas the c-MET receptor is mainly expressed by cancer cells (Kolatsi-Joannou et al. 1997). Activation of c-MET in HNSCC occurs often through HGF-dependent paracrine mechanisms (Dong et al. 2001a; Dong et al. 2004). HGF has been impli-cated as an important factor produced by stroma and contributes to the malignant phenotypes (Matsumoto and Nakamura 1997; Matsumoto et al. 1996). In vivo, tumor cells modify their microenviornment by producing factors that stimulate production of HGF by stromal cells. IL-1, IL-6, EGF, basic fibroblast growth factor (FGF), PDGF, and TGF-α are a few of the signaling molecules produced by tumor cells that induce HGF production by stromal cells (Nakamura et al. 1997; Gohda et al. 1994; Seslar et al. 1995). Activation of c-MET receptor in cancers has also been identified through activating mutations in both sporadic and inherited forms of human renal papillary carcinomas (Danilkovitch-Miagkova and Zbar 2002), as well as in HNSCC and other metastatic lesions (Di Renzo et al. 1991). Such mutations alter sequences within the kinase domain, leading to ligand-independent activation of the receptor's tyrosine kinase (Liang et al. 1996). In addition, other oncogenes such as activated RAS can induce c-MET overexpression through transcriptional mechanisms (Furge et al. 2001; Ivan et al. 1997), and mouse models reveal that tumor cells achieve increased signaling by overexpression of HGF or c-MET receptor (Takayama et al. 1997; Stabile et al. 2006; Patane et al. 2006; Dong et al. 2004).

Human HNSCCs have been shown to express, with activated c-MET, an increased responsiveness to HGF, leading to increased angiogenesis and metasta-sis, directly through the promotion of scattering and migration and indirectly through the induction of proinflammatory and proangiogenic factors, including IL-8, VEGF, and PDGF (Dong et al. 2001a; Worden et al. 2005). The invasion and metastasis mediated by HGF-dependant c-MET activation have been demon-strated with in vitro models in which invasion of collagen gel (a model of the ECM) by oral squamous cancer cells is enhanced with stromal cells or stromal-derived conditioned media (Matsumoto et al. 1989). In vivo animal models also support the importance of stromal cells in accelerating growth, invasiveness, and metastasis of epithelial malignancies (Camps et al. 1990; Jiang et al. 1999; Weidner et al. 1990; Nakamura et al. 1997; Dong et al. 2004). Such experimental evidence is supported by clinical investigations showing that elevated HGF level has been found in HNSCC patients' serum, which is correlated with increased serum levels of IL-8 and VEGF, as well as the poor prognosis (Dong et al. 2001a). HGF-induced c-MET activation in HNSCC leads to activation of the PI3K/Akt, ERK/MAPK, and PKC pathways (Dong et al. 2001a; Worden et al. 2005) and also activates another transcription factor, EGR-1 (Worden et al. 2005). EGR-1 in turn can increase the levels of PDGF and VEGF contributing to HNSCC angio-genesis (Worden et al. 2005).

EGR1 is a less studied transcription factor, which belongs to a family of related zinc finger transcription factors including EGR-2, EGR-3, and EGR-4 (Mages et al. 1993; Sukhatme et al. 1988). Activation of EGR-1 is mainly through rapid and transiently induced expression in response to diverse environmental stimuli including mitogens, tissue injury, irradiation, neuronal excitation, and differentia-tion signals (Wright et al. 1990; Cao et al. 1992; Gashler and Sukhatme 1995). Mitogens activate ERK pathway and stimulate EGR-1 biosynthesis, which pro-mote cell proliferation (Kaufmann et al. 2001; Kaufmann and Thiel 2002; Gashler and Sukhatme 1995; Biesiada et al. 1996). Overexpression of EGR-1 has been observed in human prostate cancers (Eid et al. 1998) and modulates the androgen receptor mediated signaling pathway (Yang and Abdulkadir 2003), which directly correlates with the degree of prostate cancer malignancy in patients (Salah et al. 2007) and in an animal model (Abdulkadir et al. 2001). In kidney, colon, and blad-der cancers, upregulated EGR-1 expression has been observed and is consistent with aggressive phenotypes (Hong et al. 2007; Nutt et al. 2007; Scharnhorst et al. 2000). In human colorectal cancer with a high expression of EGFR, suppression of EGFR expression inhibited cancer growth through the reduction of the transac-tivating activity of EGR-1 (Chen et al. 2006). In addition, the roles of EGR-1 in the metastasis have been shown to increase heparanase, an enzyme that mediates degradation of the ECM in prostate and bladder cancers (Ogishima et al. 2005a; Ogishima et al. 2005b). Several growth factors, including IGF-II and TGF-β1 have been identified as target genes of EGR-1 (Khachigian et al. 1996; Khachigian et al. 1995; Svaren et al. 2000). Studies by our group and others indicate that EGR-1 regulates a spectrum of genes implicated in enhancing tumor progression and metastasis.

Pam 212 Syngeneic Model of Progressive and Metastatic Squamous Cell Carcinoma

Establishment of the Pam 212 Multistage Progression and Metastatic Model

As discussed above, invasion and metastatic tumor progression of HNSCC involve multiple genetic alterations resulting in downstream phenotypic changes that confer a selective advantage for neoplastic cells to escape from regulatory mechanisms. Development of a syngeneic experimental animal model of SCC tumor progression and metastasis provides many advantages over studies using in vitro model systems or those with human tumor specimens, which has helped us to identify some of the genetic and phenotypic changes necessary for escape from both cellular and host control mechanisms on a defined genetic background. To identify some of the molecular alterations associated with SCC progression and metastasis, we developed a multistage murine model for comparison of cells transformed in vitro and of variants of the same lineage selected following primary tumor formation and metastasis in the host environment in vivo. The murine cell line Pam 212 was previously derived by the spontaneous transformation of a primary culture of neonatal BALB/c keratinocytes by the Yuspa laboratory in the absence of host selective factors (Fig. 10.3) (Yuspa et al. 1980). The Pam 212 cell line was found to produce an invasive SCC which rarely gives rise to metastases when inoculated in syngeneic BALB/c mice (Fig. 10.3) (Chen et al. 1993; Chen et al. 1995). To establish more aggressive cell lines with metastatic potential, we re-isolated and adapted cell lines from the rarely occurring metastases that arose from Pam 212 tumors in vivo (Fig. 10.3) (Chen et al. 1997).

We compared the characteristics of the re-isolated and Pam 212 parental cell lines and found that they shared features of epithelial morphology, cell surface expression of the β4 integrin, and expression of K6 and K14 cytokeratin markers. All of the re-isolated tumor lines tested were tumorigenic and formed primary (100%) and metastatic tumors (60%) with increased incidence in BALB/c recipients. An overall decrease of 30–60% in survival time was observed in recipients inoculated with the Pam metastatic re-isolates when compared with the recipients of the parental Pam 212 line. Interestingly, however, when growth of the parental and re-isolated cell lines was compared in MTT assay in vitro, no significant growth advantage of the re-isolated Pam cell lines was observed, suggesting that the growth advantage of the variants observed in vivo occurs as a result of tumor changes that enhance tumor–host interaction. The host selection presumably favors the outgrowth of variant subpopulations with a more aggressive phenotype that is better adapted for the growth and formation of primary and metastatic tumors in vivo (Chen et al. 1997).

Metastatic Pam 212 Re-isolated Cell Lines Expressed Elevated Proinflammatory and Proangiogenic Cytokines

Based on the observation that the increased growth and metastatic potential of the metastatic Pam re-isolates were due to a tumor-host cell interaction, we studied the tumor-host interaction in depth, and found that the Pam 212 re-isolates induce a strong granulocyte response at the tumor site and in the spleen of the host. We observed that the strong granulocyte response at the tumor site was due to the elevated expression of the proinflammatory cytokines, IL-1α, IL-6, Gro-1, and GM-CSF, which were found to be produced by the re-isolated but not the paretnal PAM 212 cell lines (Smith et al. 1998). These proinflammatory cytokines have been detected at elevated levels in tissue homogenates, serum, or supernatants of cell lines derived from patients with HNSCC (Chen et al. 1998; Chen et al. 1999; Young et al. 1997; Young 2000). Individual members of the proinflammatory cytokine family such as IL-1, IL-6, IL-8, and GRO-1(also called KC or Gro-α) have been shown to directly promote growth of SCC tumors (Wolf et al. 2001; Lee et al. 2006; Loukinova et al. 2000; Hong et al. 2000; Squarize et al. 2006). Expression of IL-1, IL-6, IL-8, and GM-CSF has also been associated with increased metastasis in different experimental tumor models (Young 2000; Chen et al. 1997; Smith et al. 1998; Yoon et al. 2007). When gene expression profiles of the parental and metastatic variant cell lines are compared by mRNA differential display, the metastatic variants are found to have increased levels of the mRNA encoding murine Gro-1, the ortholog of human GRO-1, and IL-8 (Loukinova et al. 2000). The observation that Gro-1 expression is increased in association with tumor progression in vivo suggested the hypothesis that increased expression of this and possibly other proinflammatory cytokines by SCC may be promoted by interactions in the tumor-host environment. To test this, PAM-Gro-1 transfectants were generated and displayed an increased rate of growth and metastasis in BALB/c mice, similar to the highly malignant phenotype observed in spontaneously occurring metastatic variants. Furthermore, the PAM-Gro-1 tumors showed an increase in infiltration of host leukocytes and CD31+ blood vessels, consistent with increased CXC chemokine activity. The increased growth of PAM-Gro-1 cells was attenuated in CXCR-2-deficient mice, indicating that the increased growth was dependent in part upon host cells responsive to the CXC chemokine. Together, these results show that a

CXC chemokine such as Gro-1 can promote malignant growth of murine SCC by a host CXCR-2-dependent pathway (Loukinova et al. 2000).

Multiple Genes Upregulated with Murine SCC Tumor Progression and Metastasis are Related to the NF-κB Signal Pathway

To investigate the molecular mechanisms of SCC tumor progression from the Pam 212 to the Pam LY metastatic variants, molecular profiling was performed using a first generation 4,000 element murine cDNA microarray (Dong et al. 2001b). Through this analysis, we identified several groups of genes upregulated during tumor progression, that are involved in (1) immunologic, inflammatory, and angiogenesis responses, including Gro-1 (KC), complement component 3, IL-12B, CSF-1, and osteopontin (OPN); (2) signal transduction and regulation of gene expression and DNA replication, including c-Met, Yap1, neurotrophic receptor tyrosine kinase, HMG-1(Y), and replication protein A (14 kDa subunit); and (3) modulation of cell cycle and apoptosis, including cdc25, cyclin D1, PCNA, cIAP-1, Fas ligand (FasL), PEA-15, Nedd8, and ubiquitin-activating enzyme E1. Bioinformatic analysis revealed that many of the genes are targets of or involved in the regulation of the NF-κB signal transduction pathway (Dong et al. 2001b). Activation of the NF-κB target genes, including cytokines, has been implicated in the promotion of transformation and survival of tumor cells. We found that metastatic cell lines selected in the host environment exhibit an increase in constitutive and TNF-α-inducible expression of proinflammatory cytokines when compared with parental Pam 212 cells. The increased cytokine expression was associated with an increase in constitutive and TNF-inducible activation of NF-κB. Constitutive nuclear localization of NF-κB p65 was observed in LY-2 and LY-8 cells in culture and in vivo (Dong, et al. 1999). To inhibit activation of NF-κB, cells can be transfected to express a mutant form of IκB, which lacks the serine 32 and 36 position phosphorylation sites required for signal activation, ubiquitylation, and proteasome degradation, thus binding up NF-κB in inactive form in the cytoplasm. Overexpression of IκBαM in Pam 212 cells inhibited TNF-α-induced activation of NF-κB and cytokine expression (Dong et al. 1999), and the proteasome inhibitor bortezomib suppressed NF-κB activation and Gro-1 production in vitro and tumor growth in vivo (Chen et al. 2008; Sunwoo et al. 2001). These data indicate that activation of NF-κB is an important molecular controlling mechanism for proinflammatory cytokine expression during metastatic tumor progression of SCC.

We further examined the diversity of genes differentially expressed among the various stages of tumor progression and determined the effect of conditionally inhibiting NF-κB in Pam LY-2 cells by expressing IκBαM in a subsequent study using a second-generation 15,000 element cDNA microarray (Loercher et al. 2004). Cluster analysis identified 308 genes that exhibited more than two-fold difference in expression between keratinocytes, transformed Pam 212, metastatic Pam LY-2 cells, and Pam LY-2 cells expressing IκBαM induced by doxycycline treatment. Three dominant patterns were detected that clustered according to the step-wise differences in phenotype between keratinocytes, Pam 212, Pam LY-2 cells. Expression of IκBαM in Pam LY-2 results in restoration of the expression patterns observed in keratinocytes. The full list of upregulated and downregulated genes associated with malignant progression, shown through inhibition of NF-κB following induction of IκBαM expression, is available at http://www.nidcd.nih.gov/research/scientists/vanwaesc.asp. The genes were also classified according to putative function and published associations with NF-κB as determined by search of bioinformatic databases (National Center for Biotechnology Information, NCBI). Many genes detected as upregulated in Pam LY2 metastatic cells have previously been associated with NF-κB. These genes and additional ones identified in this study contain NF-κB binding sites at their promoter regions; many genes are downmodulated when NF-κB is inhibited (Loercher et al. 2004).

HGF/c-Met Signaling in Pam 212 Tumor Progression and Metastasis

As a result of the molecular profiling studies comparing the multistage Pam 212 progression and metastasis murine model , we were able to identify an interesting candidate from a pool of cDNA fragments overexpressed in the metastatic pheno-type (Dong et al. 2004). We confirmed that the candidate cDNA is derived from the untranslated region of the gene encoding murine c-Met, the homolog of human c-MET. As previously discussed, c-MET, together with its ligand, HGF, contributes to cell survival, migration, and endothelial proliferation (Birchmeier et al. 2003). We examined the role of HGF/c-Met pathway on expression of angiogenesis factors and on promotion of tumorigenesis and metastasis in our syngeneic murine Pam 212 SCC model, and we found that the mRNA and protein expression of c-Met were significantly elevated in the SCC cells derived from lymph node and lung metastases when compared with parental or transformed keratinocytes. Constitutive and HGF-induced c-Met phosphorylation was more profound in Pam 212 meta-static re-isolates. Significantly increased immunostaining intensities of HGF and c-Met receptor were observed in the tumor specimens isolated from the Pam 212 metastatic Pam-LY cell lines. In addition, HGF induced significantly higher levels of Gro-1 and VEGF production in the metastatic re-isolates than in the parental cell lines and induced the scattering effect only in the metastatic re-isolates. When engineered to overexpress HGF in the tumor microenvironment, Pam LY SCC cells exhibited increased tumorigenic and metastatic potential in vivo. Our data indicate that metastatic SCC cells that overexpress c-Met exhibit angiogenesis factor expression and enhanced scattering in response to HGF in vitro and tumorigenesis and metastasis in response to HGF in the tumor microenvironment in vivo. The contribution of HGF/c-Met activation to coexpression of angiogenesis factors, tumorigenesis, and metastasis makes it an important therapeutic target for SCC. Our data from the Pam 212 multistep tumor progression and metastatic model are consistent with the conclusions derived from investigations of human HNSCC specimens, supporting the notion that the findings in the Pam 212 tumor model are relevant for HNSCC progression and metastasis.

Summary and Future Directions

To date, studies of the signal transcription factor pathways altered in HNSCC have revealed that these cancers usually undergo functional loss or alteration of components of the p53 tumor suppressor pathway (p53, p14ARF, p16INK4a) and enhanced autocrine or paracrine activation of growth factor and cytokine pathways, which activate a network of signaling pathways that regulate expression of target genes and proteins that mediate the phenotypic features of the malignant phenotype (Figs. 10.1 and 10.2). This includes autocrine activation by IL-1R, TNFR, and EGFR, which contribute to activation of the MAPK-AP-1, PI3K-NF-κB, and AKT-mTOR pathways; EGFR and IL-6R, which contribute to STAT3 activation; and HGF/c-MET, which contributes to activation of the MAPK, PI3K, RAS, PKC, and EGR1 pathways (Figs. 10.1 and 10.2). Groups of genes predominantly regulated by one or a combination of the factors AP-1 and NF-κB (CyclinD, MMPs, IL-8, GRO-1), NF-κB and STAT3 (BCL-XL), AP-1, EGR1, and mTOR (VEGF) are key molecular mediators of cell proliferation, survival, invasion, and angiogenesis (Figs. 10.1 and 10.2).

The identification of these pathways and the recent appreciation that their inactivation or coactivation together forms a network that coregulates a diverse repertoire of genes (Yan et al. 2007, 2008) provide an explanation for the relatively low response rates observed with investigational monotherapy targeted to restore p53 or inhibit EGFR, MAPKs, NF-κB, or STAT3. The molecular pathogenesis of most HNSCCs appears to be highly complex and involves multiple pathways and transcription factors, as compared with some hematologic malignancies, in which fewer events may lead to malignancy. Therefore, the likelihood that targeting a single pathway will be a successful therapeutic strategy is low. In addition, these findings provide a rationale for future studies to more fully dissect the types and relative frequency of upstream events that lead to such global alterations, and how they regulate gene subprograms that determine pathogenesis and prognosis, which may serve as diagnostic and prognostic markers (Yan et al. 2007, 2008; Lee et al. 2007; Nottingham et al. 2008). Further, these studies provide a foundation for investigation of agents that target such key events or a combination of agents that target these pathways at key regulatory points. For example, recent preclinical studies provide evidence for the fact that restoring p53 while inhibiting NF-κB or STAT3 has greater gene modulating and cytotoxic effects than targeting the individual pathways alone (Lee et al. 2008). Consistent with this, agents such as the antimalarial and anti-inflammatory drug quinacrine that reactivate p53 while inhibiting NF-κB can have potent cytotoxic effects alone and together with standard chemotherapeutic agents such as cisplatin used for HNSCC (Friedman et al. 2007).

As drugs can target EGFR, IL-1, IL-6 or MAPKs, NF-κB, and STAT3 are identified, and it will be possible to explore the clinical activity of inhibiting the pathways that are coactivated in HNSCC.

Acknowledgments This work is supported by NIDCD Intramural project Z01-DC-000016, Z01-DC-000073 and Howard Hughes Medical Institute-NIH research scholarship (Reza Ehsanian). We would like to express our appreciation to Dr. Bin Yan for his effort in reference management.

References

Abdulkadir SA, Qu Z, Garabedian E, Song SK, Peters TJ, Svaren J, Carbone JM, Naughton CK, Catalona WJ, Ackerman JJ, Gordon JI, Humphrey PA, Milbrandt J (2001) Impaired prostate tumorigenesis in Egr1-deficient mice. Nat Med 7:101–107

Allen C, Duffy S, Teknos T, Islam M, Chen Z, Albert PS, Wolf G, Van Waes C (2007a) Nuclear factor-kappaB-related serum factors as longitudinal biomarkers of response and survival in advanced oropharyngeal carcinoma. Clin Cancer Res 13:3182–3190

Allen CT, Ricker JL, Chen Z, Van Waes C (2007b) Role of activated nuclear factor-kappaB in the pathogenesis and therapy of squamous cell carcinoma of the head and neck. Head Neck 29(10):959–971

Allen C, Saigal K, Nottingham L, Chen Z, Van Waes C (2008) Bortezomib-induced apoptosis with limited clinical response is accompanied by inhibition of canonical but not alternative NF-kappaB subunits or other prosurvival signal pathways activated in head and neck cancer. Clin Cancer Res 14(13):4175–4785

Amornphimoltham P, Patel V, Sodhi A, Nikitakis NG, Sauk JJ, Sausville EA, Molinolo AA, Gutkind JS (2005) Mammalian target of rapamycin, a molecular target in squamous cell carcinomas of the head and neck. Cancer Res 65(21):9953–9961

Bancroft CC, Chen Z, Yeh J, Sunwoo JB, Yeh NT, Jackson S, Jackson C, Van Waes C (2002) Effects of pharmacologic antagonists of epidermal growth factor receptor, PI3K and MEK signal kinases on NF-kappaB and AP-1 activation and IL-8 and VEGF expression in human head and neck squamous cell carcinoma lines. Int J Cancer 99(4):538–548

Beviglia L, Kramer RH (1999) HGF induces FAK activation and integrin-mediated adhesion in MTLn3 breast carcinoma cells. Int J Cancer 83(5):640–649

Biesiada E, Razandi M, Levin ER (1996) Egr-1 activates basic fibroblast growth factor transcription. Mechanistic implications for astrocyte proliferation. J Biol Chem 271(31):18576–18581

Birchmeier C, Gherardi E (1998) Developmental roles of HGF/SF and its receptor, the c-Met tyrosine kinase. Trends Cell Biol 8(10):404–410

Birchmeier C, Birchmeier W, Gherardi E, Vande Woude GF (2003) Met, metastasis, motility and more. Nat Rev Mol Cell Biol 4(12):915–925

Boccaccio C, Ando M, Tamagnone L, Bardelli A, Michieli P, Battistini C, Comoglio PM (1998) Induction of epithelial tubules by growth factor HGF depends on the STAT pathway. Nature 391(6664):285–288

Bonner JA, Raisch KP, Trummell HQ, Robert F, Meredith RF, Spencer SA, Buchsbaum DJ, Saleh MN, Stackhouse MA, LoBuglio AF, Peters GE, Carroll WR, Waksal HW (2000) Enhanced apoptosis with combination C225/radiation treatment serves as the impetus for clinical investigation in head and neck cancers. J Clin Oncol 18(Suppl 21):47S–53S

Bottaro DP, Rubin JS, Faletto DL, Chan AM, Kmiecik TE, Vande Woude GF, Aaronson SA (1991) Identification of the hepatocyte growth factor receptor as the c-met proto-oncogene product. Science 251(4995):802–804

Califano J, van der Riet P, Westra W, Nawroz H, Clayman G, Piantadosi S, Corio R, Lee D, Greenberg B, Koch W, Sidransky D (1996) Genetic progression model for head and neck cancer: Implications for field cancerization. Cancer Res 56(11):2488–2492

Camps JL, Chang SM, Hsu TC, Freeman MR, Hong SJ, Zhau HE, von Eschenbach AC, Chung LW (1990) Fibroblast-mediated acceleration of human epithelial tumor growth in vivo. Proc Natl Acad Sci USA 87(1):75–79

Cao XM, Guy GR, Sukhatme VP, Tan YH (1992) Regulation of the Egr-1 gene by tumor necrosis factor and interferons in primary human fibroblasts. J Biol Chem 267(2):1345–1349

Carroll DK, Carroll JS, Leong CO, Cheng F, Brown M, Mills AA, Brugge JS, Ellisen LW (2006) p63 Regulates an adhesion programme and cell survival in epithelial cells. Nat Cell Biol 8(6):551–561

Chang AA, Van Waes C (2005) Nuclear factor-KappaB as a common target and activator of onco-genes in head and neck squamous cell carcinoma. Adv Otorhinolaryngol 62:92–102

Chen Z, Rosten SI, Lord EM, Gaspari AA (1993) Murine Pam 212 cutaneous squamous cell carcinoma is nonimmunogenic in normal syngeneic hosts and resistant to immune effector mechanisms. Reg Immunol 5(5):285–292

Chen Z, Knepper JE, Gaspari AA (1995) Minor histocompatibility antigen-dependent rejection of Pam 212 epidermoid carcinoma by DBA/2 mice. Cell Immunol 164(1):90–99

Chen Z, Smith CW, Kiel D, Van Waes C (1997) Metastatic variants derived following in vivo tumor progression of an in vitro transformed squamous cell carcinoma line acquire a differen-tial growth advantage requiring tumor-host interaction. Clin Exp Metastasis 15(5):527–537

Chen Z, Colon I, Ortiz N, Callister M, Dong G, Pegram MY, Arosarena O, Strome S, Nicholson JC, Van Waes C (1998) Effects of interleukin-1alpha, interleukin-1 receptor antagonist, and neu-tralizing antibody on proinflammatory cytokine expression by human squamous cell carci-noma lines. Cancer Res 58(16):3668–3676

Chen Z, Malhotra PS, Thomas GR, Ondrey FG, Duffey DC, Smith CW, Enamorado I, Yeh NT, Kroog GS, Rudy S, McCullagh L, Mousa S, Quezado M, Herscher LL, Van Waes C (1999) Expression of proinflammatory and proangiogenic cytokines in patients with head and neck cancer. Clin Cancer Res 5(6):1369–1379

Chen A, Xu J, Johnson AC (2006) Curcumin inhibits human colon cancer cell growth by suppress-ing gene expression of epidermal growth factor receptor through reducing the activity of the transcription factor Egr-1. Oncogene 25(2):278–287

Chen Z, Ricker J, Malhotra PS, Nottingham L, Bagain L, Lee TL, Yeh NT, Van Waes C (2008) Differential bortezomib sensitivity in head and neck cancer lines corresponds to proteasome, nuclear factor-kappaB and activator protein-1 related mechanisms. Mol Cancer Therap 7(7):1949–1960

Chung CH, Parker JS, Ely K, Carter J, Yi Y, Murphy BA, Ang KK, El-Naggar AK, Zanation AM, Cmelak AJ, Levy S, Slebos RJ, Yarbrough WG (2006) Gene expression profiles identify epithelial-to-mesenchymal transition and activation of nuclear factor-{kappa}B signaling as characteristics of a high-risk head and neck squamous cell carcinoma. Cancer Res 66(16): 8210–8218

Coussens LM, Tinkle CL, Hanahan D, Werb Z (2000) MMP-9 supplied by bone marrow-derived cells contributes to skin carcinogenesis. Cell 103(3):481–490

Danilkovitch-Miagkova A, Zbar B (2002) Dysregulation of Met receptor tyrosine kinase activity in invasive tumors. J Clin Invest 109(7):863–867

Davies G, Mason MD, Martin TA, Parr C, Watkins G, Lane J, Matsumoto K, Nakamura T, Jiang WG (2003) The HGF/SF antagonist NK4 reverses fibroblast- and HGF-induced prostate tumor growth and angiogenesis in vivo. Int J Cancer 106(3):348–354

Di Renzo MF, Narsimhan RP, Olivero M, Bretti S, Giordano S, Medico E, Gaglia P, Zara P, Comoglio PM (1991) Expression of the Met/HGF receptor in normal and neoplastic human tissues. Oncogene 6(11):1997–2003

Dong G, Chen Z, Kato T, Van Waes C (1999) The host environment promotes the constitutive activation of nuclear factor-kappaB and proinflammatory cytokine expression during metastatic tumor progression of murine squamous cell carcinoma. Cancer Res 59(14):3495–3504

Dong G, Chen Z, Li ZY, Yeh NT, Bancroft CC, Van Waes C (2001a) Hepatocyte growth factor/ scatter factor-induced activation of MEK and PI3K signal pathways contributes to expression of proangiogenic cytokines interleukin-8 and vascular endothelial growth factor in head and neck squamous cell carcinoma. Cancer Res 61(15):5911–5918

Dong G, Loukinova E, Chen Z, Gangi L, Chanturita TI, Liu ET, Van Waes C (2001b) Molecular profiling of transformed and metastatic murine squamous carcinoma cells by differential display and cDNA microarray reveals altered expression of multiple genes related to growth, apoptosis, angiogenesis, and the NF-kappaB signal pathway. Cancer Res 61(12):4797–4808

Dong G, Lee TL, Yeh NT, Geoghegan J, Van Waes C, Chen Z (2004) Metastatic squamous cell carcinoma cells that overexpress c-Met exhibit enhanced angiogenesis factor expression, scattering and metastasis in response to hepatocyte growth factor. Oncogene 23(37):6199–6208

Druzgal CH, Chen Z, Yeh NT, Thomas GR, Ondrey FG, Duffey DC, Vilela RJ, Ende K, McCullagh L, Rudy SF, Muir C, Herscher LL, Morris JC, Albert PS, Van Waes C (2005) A pilot study of longitudinal serum cytokine and angiogenesis factor levels as markers of therapeutic response and survival in patients with head and neck squamous cell carcinoma. Head Neck 27(9):771–784

Duan J, Friedman J, Nottingham L, Chen Z, Ara G, Van Waes C (2007) Nuclear factor-kappaB p65 small interfering RNA or proteasome inhibitor bortezomib sensitizes head and neck squamous cell carcinomas to classic histone deacetylase inhibitors and novel histone deacetylase inhibitor PXD101. Mol Cancer Ther 6(1):37–50

Duffey DC, Chen Z, Dong G, Ondrey FG, Wolf JS, Brown K, Siebenlist U, Van Waes C (1999) Expression of a dominant-negative mutant inhibitor-kappaBalpha of nuclear factor-kappaB in human head and neck squamous cell carcinoma inhibits survival, proinflammatory cytokine expression, and tumor growth in vivo. Cancer Res 59(14):3468–3474

Duffey DC, Crowl-Bancroft CV, Chen Z, Ondrey FG, Nejad-Sattari M, Dong G, Van Waes C (2000) Inhibition of transcription factor nuclear factor-kappaB by a mutant inhibitor-kappaBalpha attenuates resistance of human head and neck squamous cell carcinoma to TNF-alpha caspase-mediated cell death. Br J Cancer 83(10):1367–1374

Eid MA, Kumar MV, Iczkowski KA, Bostwick DG, Tindall DJ (1998) Expression of early growth response genes in human prostate cancer. Cancer Res 58(11):2461–2468

Fan S, Ma YX, Gao M, Yuan RQ, Meng Q, Goldberg ID, Rosen EM (2001) The multisubstrate adapter Gab1 regulates hepatocyte growth factor (scatter factor)-c-Met signaling for cell survival and DNA repair. Mol Cell Biol 21(15):4968–4984

Folkman J (1996) Fighting cancer by attacking its blood supply. Sci Am 275(3):150–154

Friedman J, Nottingham L, Duggal P, Pernas FG, Yan B, Yang XP, Chen Z, Van Waes C (2007) Deficient TP53 expression, function, and cisplatin sensitivity are restored by quinacrine in head and neck cancer. Clin Cancer Res 13(22):6568–6578

Fu M, Wang C, Li Z, Sakamaki T, Pestell RG (2004) Minireview: Cyclin D1: normal and abnormal functions. Endocrinology 145(12):5439–5447

Furge KA, Kiewlich D, Le P, Vo MN, Faure M, Howlett AR, Lipson KE, Woude GF, Webb CP (2001) Suppression of Ras-mediated tumorigenicity and metastasis through inhibition of the Met receptor tyrosine kinase. Proc Natl Acad Sci USA 98(19):10722–10727

Gashler A, Sukhatme VP (1995) Early growth response protein 1 (Egr-1): Prototype of a zinc-finger family of transcription factors. Prog Nucleic Acid Res Mol Biol 50:191–224

Gillison ML, Koch WM, Capone RB, Spafford M, Westra WH, Wu L, Zahurak ML, Daniel RW, Viglione M, Symer DE, Shah KV, Sidransky D (2000) Evidence for a causal association between human papillomavirus and a subset of head and neck cancers. J Natl Cancer Inst 92(9):709–720

Gohda E, Matsunaga T, Kataoka H, Takebe T, Yamamoto I (1994) Induction of hepatocyte growth factor in human skin fibroblasts by epidermal growth factor, platelet-derived growth factor and fibroblast growth factor. Cytokine 6(6):633–640

Gong R, Rifai A, Tolbert EM, Centracchio JN, Dworkin LD (2003) Hepatocyte growth factor modulates matrix metalloproteinases and plasminogen activator/plasmin proteolytic pathways in progressive renal interstitial fibrosis. J Am Soc Nephrol 14(12):3047–3060

Gorgoulis V, Rassidakis G, Karameris A, Giatromanolaki A, Barbatis C, Kittas C (1994) Expression of p53 protein in laryngeal squamous cell carcinoma and dysplasia: Possible correlation with human papillomavirus infection and clinicopathological findings. Virchows Arch 425(5):481–489

Grandis JR, Chakraborty A, Zeng Q, Melhem MF, Tweardy DJ (1998a) Downmodulation of TGF-alpha protein expression with antisense oligonucleotides inhibits proliferation of head and neck squamous carcinoma but not normal mucosal epithelial cells. J Cell Biochem 69(1):55–62

Grandis JR, Melhem MF, Gooding WE, Day R, Holst VA, Wagener MM, Drenning SD, Tweardy DJ (1998b) Levels of TGF-alpha and EGFR protein in head and neck squamous cell carcinoma and patient survival. J Natl Cancer Inst 90(11):824–832

Grandis JR, Drenning SD, Zeng Q, Watkins SC, Melhem MF, Endo S, Johnson DE, Huang L, He Y, Kim JD (2000) Constitutive activation of Stat3 signaling abrogates apoptosis in squamous cell carcinogenesis in vivo. Proc Natl Acad Sci USA 97(8):4227–4232

Grant DS, Kleinman HK, Goldberg ID, Bhargava MM, Nickoloff BJ, Kinsella JL, Polverini P, Rosen EM (1993) Scatter factor induces blood vessel formation in vivo. Proc Natl Acad Sci USA 90(5):1937–1941

Gu H, Neel BG (2003) The "Gab" in signal transduction. Trends Cell Biol 13(3):122–130

Hanzawa M, Shindoh M, Higashino F, Yasuda M, Inoue N, Hida K, Ono M, Kohgo T, Nakamura M, Notani K, Fukuda H, Totsuka Y, Yoshida K, Fujinaga K (2000) Hepatocyte growth factor upregulates E1AF that induces oral squamous cell carcinoma cell invasion by activating matrix metalloproteinase genes. Carcinogenesis 21(6):1079–1085

He Y, Zeng Q, Drenning SD, Melhem MF, Tweardy DJ, Huang L, Grandis JR (1998) Inhibition of human squamous cell carcinoma growth in vivo by epidermal growth factor receptor antisense RNA transcribed from the U6 promoter. J Natl Cancer Inst 90(14):1080–1087

Hibi K, Trink B, Patturajan M, Westra WH, Caballero OL, Hill DE, Ratovitski EA, Jen J, Sidransky D (2000) AIS is an oncogene amplified in squamous cell carcinoma. Proc Natl Acad Sci USA 97(10):5462–5467

Hiscox S, Jiang WG (1997) Regulation of endothelial CD44 expression and endothelium-tumour cell interactions by hepatocyte growth factor/scatter factor. Biochem Biophys Res Commun 233(1):1–5

Hong SH, Ondrey FG, Avis IM, Chen Z, Loukinova E, Cavanaugh PF Jr, Van Waes C, Mulshine JL (2000) Cyclooxygenase regulates human oropharyngeal carcinomas via the proinflammatory cytokine IL-6: A general role for inflammation? FASEB J 14(11):1499–1507

Hong Y, Ho KS, Eu KW, Cheah PY (2007) A susceptibility gene set for early onset colorectal cancer that integrates diverse signaling pathways: Implication for tumorigenesis. Clin Cancer Res 13(4):1107–1114

Itoh T, Tanioka M, Matsuda H, Nishimoto H, Yoshioka T, Suzuki R, Uehira M (1999) Experimental metastasis is suppressed in MMP-9-deficient mice. Clin Exp Metastasis 17(2):177–181

Ivan M, Bond JA, Prat M, Comoglio PM, Wynford-Thomas D (1997) Activated ras and ret onco-genes induce over-expression of c-met (hepatocyte growth factor receptor) in human thyroid epithelial cells. Oncogene 14(20):2417–2423

Jackson-Bernitsas DG, Ichikawa H, Takada Y, Myers JN, Lin XL, Darnay BG, Chaturvedi MM, Aggarwal BB (2007) Evidence that TNF-TNFR1-TRADD-TRAF2-RIP-TAK1-IKK pathway mediates constitutive NF-kappaB activation and proliferation in human head and neck squamous cell carcinoma. Oncogene 26(10):1385–1397

Jiang W, Hiscox S, Matsumoto K, Nakamura T (1999) Hepatocyte growth factor/scatter factor, its molecular, cellular and clinical implications in cancer. Crit Rev Oncol Hematol 29(3): 209–248

Jiang WG, Martin TA, Parr C, Davies G, Matsumoto K, Nakamura T (2005) Hepatocyte growth factor, its receptor, and their potential value in cancer therapies. Crit Rev Oncol Hematol 53(1):35–69

Kaufmann K, Thiel G (2002) Epidermal growth factor and thrombin induced proliferation of immortalized human keratinocytes is coupled to the synthesis of Egr-1, a zinc finger transcriptional regulator. J Cell Biochem 85(2):381–391

Kaufmann K, Bach K, Thiel G (2001) The extracellular signal-regulated protein kinases Erk1/Erk2 stimulate expression and biological activity of the transcriptional regulator Egr-1. Biol Chem 382(7):1077–1081

Khachigian LM, Williams AJ, Collins T (1995) Interplay of Sp1 and Egr-1 in the proximal platelet-derived growth factor A-chain promoter in cultured vascular endothelial cells. J Biol Chem 270(46):27679–27686

Khachigian LM, Lindner V, Williams AJ, Collins T (1996) Egr-1-induced endothelial gene expression: A common theme in vascular injury. Science 271(5254):1427–1431

Kitadai Y, Takahashi Y, Haruma K, Naka K, Sumii K, Yokozaki H, Yasui W, Mukaida N, Ohmoto Y, Kajiyama G, Fidler IJ, Tahara E (1999) Transfection of interleukin-8 increases angiogenesis and tumorigenesis of human gastric carcinoma cells in nude mice. Br J Cancer 81(4):647–653

Kolatsi-Joannou M, Moore R, Winyard PJ, Woolf AS (1997) Expression of hepatocyte growth factor/scatter factor and its receptor, MET, suggests roles in human embryonic organogenesis. Pediatr Res 41(5):657–665

Lai JF, Kao SC, Jiang ST, Tang MJ, Chan PC, Chen HC (2000) Involvement of focal adhesion kinase in hepatocyte growth factor-induced scatter of Madin-Darby canine kidney cells. J Biol Chem 275(11):7474–7480

Lamorte L, Kamikura DM, Park M (2000) A switch from p130Cas/Crk to Gab1/Crk signaling correlates with anchorage independent growth and JNK activation in cells transformed by the Met receptor oncoprotein. Oncogene 19(52):5973–5981

Lee TL, Yeh J, Van Waes C, Chen Z (2006) Epigenetic modification of SOCS-1 differentially regulates STAT3 activation in response to interleukin-6 receptor and epidermal growth factor receptor signaling through JAK and/or MEK in head and neck squamous cell carcinomas. Mol Cancer Ther 5(1):8–19

Lee TL, Yang XP, Yan B, Friedman J, Duggal P, Bagain L, Dong G, Yeh NT, Wang J, Zhou J, Elkahloun A, Van Waes C, Chen Z (2007) A novel nuclear factor-kappaB gene signature is differentially expressed in head and neck squamous cell carcinomas in association with TP53 status. Clin Cancer Res 13(19):5680–5691

Lee TL, Yeh J, Friedman J, Yan B, Yang X, Yeh NT, Van Waes C, Chen Z (2008) A signal network involving co-activated NF-kappaB and STAT3 and altered p53 modulates BAX/BCL-XL expression and promotes cell survival of head and neck squamous cell carcinomas. Int J Cancer 122(9):1987–1998

Leong CO, Vidnovic N, DeYoung MP, Sgroi D, Ellisen LW (2007) The p63/p73 network mediates chemosensitivity to cisplatin in a biologically defined subset of primary breast cancers. J Clin Invest 117(5):1370–1380

Liang TJ, Reid AE, Xavier R, Cardiff RD, Wang TC (1996) Transgenic expression of tpr-met oncogene leads to development of mammary hyperplasia and tumors. J Clin Invest 97(12):2872–2877

Liggett WH Jr, Sewell DA, Rocco J, Ahrendt SA, Koch W, Sidransky D (1996) p16 and p16 beta are potent growth suppressors of head and neck squamous carcinoma cells in vitro. Cancer Res 56(18):4119–4123

Liu ZX, Yu CF, Nickel C, Thomas S, Cantley LG (2002) Hepatocyte growth factor induces ERK-dependent paxillin phosphorylation and regulates paxillin-focal adhesion kinase association. J Biol Chem 277(12):10452–10458

Loercher A, Lee TL, Ricker JL, Howard A, Geoghegen J, Chen Z, Sunwoo JB, Sitcheran R, Chuang EY, Mitchell JB, Baldwin AS Jr, Van Waes C (2004) Nuclear factor-kappaB is an important modulator of the altered gene expression profile and malignant phenotype in squamous cell carcinoma. Cancer Res 64(18):6511–6523

Loukinova E, Dong G, Enamorado-Ayalya I, Thomas GR, Chen Z, Schreiber H, Van Waes C (2000) Growth regulated oncogene-alpha expression by murine squamous cell carcinoma promotes tumor growth, metastasis, leukocyte infiltration and angiogenesis by a host CXC receptor-2 dependent mechanism. Oncogene 19(31):3477–3486

Madrid LV, Mayo MW, Reuther JY, Baldwin AS Jr (2001) Akt stimulates the transactivation potential of the RelA/p65 Subunit of NF-kappa B through utilization of the Ikappa B kinase and activation of the mitogen-activated protein kinase p38. J Biol Chem 276(22):18934–18940

Mages HW, Stamminger T, Rilke O, Bravo R, Kroczek RA (1993) Expression of PILOT, a putative transcription factor, requires two signals and is cyclosporin A sensitive in T cells. Int Immunol 5(1):63–70

Maroun CR, Holgado-Madruga M, Royal I, Naujokas MA, Fournier TM, Wong AJ, Park M
    (1999) The Gab1 PH domain is required for localization of Gab1 at sites of cell-cell contact
    and epithelial morphogenesis downstream from the met receptor tyrosine kinase. Mol Cell
    Biol 19(3):1784–1799
Matsumoto K, Nakamura T (1997) Hepatocyte growth factor (HGF) as a tissue organizer for
    organogenesis and regeneration. Biochem Biophys Res Commun 239(3):639–644
Matsumoto K, Nakamura T (2006) Hepatocyte growth factor and the Met system as a mediator of
    tumor-stromal interactions. Int J Cancer 119(3):477–483
Matsumoto K, Horikoshi M, Rikimaru K, Enomoto S (1989) A study of an in vitro model for
    invasion of oral squamous cell carcinoma. J Oral Pathol Med 18(9):498–501
Matsumoto K, Date K, Ohmichi H, Nakamura T (1996) Hepatocyte growth factor in lung mor-
    phogenesis and tumor invasion: Role as a mediator in epithelium-mesenchyme and tumor-
    stroma interactions. Cancer Chemother Pharmacol Suppl 38:S42–S47
Matteucci E, Ridolfi E, Desiderio MA (2006) Hepatocyte growth factor differently influences
    Met-E-cadherin phosphorylation and downstream signaling pathway in two models of breast
    cells. Cell Mol Life Sci 63(17):2016–2026
Milas L, Mason K, Hunter N, Petersen S, Yamakawa M, Ang K, Mendelsohn J, Fan Z (2000) In
    vivo enhancement of tumor radioresponse by C225 antiepidermal growth factor receptor anti-
    body. Clin Cancer Res 6(2):701–708
Mine S, Fujisaki T, Kawahara C, Tabata T, Iida T, Yasuda M, Yoneda T, Tanaka Y (2003)
    Hepatocyte growth factor enhances adhesion of breast cancer cells to endothelial cells in vitro
    through up-regulation of CD44. Exp Cell Res 288(1):189–197
Muller M, Morotti A, Ponzetto C (2002) Activation of NF-kappaB is essential for hepatocyte
    growth factor-mediated proliferation and tubulogenesis. Mol Cell Biol 22(4):1060–1072
Nakamura T, Matsumoto K, Kiritoshi A, Tano Y, Nakamura T (1997) Induction of hepatocyte
    growth factor in fibroblasts by tumor-derived factors affects invasive growth of tumor cells: In
    vitro analysis of tumor-stromal interactions. Cancer Res 57(15):3305–3313
Nathan CO, Franklin S, Abreo FW, Nassar R, de Benedetti A, Williams J, Stucker FJ (1999)
    Expression of eIF4E during head and neck tumorigenesis: Possible role in angiogenesis.
    Laryngoscope 109(8):1253–1258
Nathan CO, Amirghahari N, Abreo F, Rong X, Caldito G, Jones ML, Zhou H, Smith M, Kimberly D,
    Glass J (2004) Overexpressed eIF4E is functionally active in surgical margins of head and
    neck cancer patients via activation of the Akt/mammalian target of rapamycin pathway. Clin
    Cancer Res 10(17):5820–5827
Ni WF, Tsai CH, Yang SF, Chang YC (2007) Elevated expression of NF-kappaB in oral submu-
    cous fibrosis–evidence for NF-kappaB induction by safrole in human buccal mucosal fibro-
    blasts. Oral Oncol 43(6):557–562
Nishimura K, Matsumiya K, Miura H, Tsujimura A, Nonomura N, Matsumoto K, Nakamura T,
    Okuyama A (2003) Effects of hepatocyte growth factor on urokinase-type plasminogen activa-
    tor (uPA) and uPA receptor in DU145 prostate cancer cells. Int J Androl 26(3):175–179
Nottingham L, Chen Z, Brown K, Van Waes C (2008) Canonical and Non-canonical IKK/NF-κB
    activation promote proliferation and aberrant motility in head and neck squamous cell carci-
    nomas. In: *Keystone symposia*, NF-kappaB, Banff, Canada
Nutt JE, Foster PA, Mellon JK, Lunec J (2007) hEGR1 is induced by EGF, inhibited by gefitinib
    in bladder cell lines and related to EGF receptor levels in bladder tumours. Br J Cancer
    96(5):762–768
O-charoenrat P, Modjtahedi H, Rhys-Evans P, Court WJ, Box GM, Eccles SA (2000) Epidermal
    growth factor-like ligands differentially up-regulate matrix metalloproteinase 9 in head and
    neck squamous carcinoma cells. Cancer Res 60(4):1121–1128
Ogishima T, Shiina H, Breault JE, Tabatabai L, Bassett WW, Enokida H, Li LC, Kawakami T,
    Urakami S, Ribeiro-Filho LA, Terashima M, Fujime M, Igawa M, Dahiya R (2005a)
    Increased heparanase expression is caused by promoter hypomethylation and up-regulation
    of transcriptional factor early growth response-1 in human prostate cancer. Clin Cancer Res
    11(3):1028–1036

Ogishima T, Shiina H, Breault JE, Terashima M, Honda S, Enokida H, Urakami S, Tokizane T, Kawakami T, Ribeiro-Filho LA, Fujime M, Kane CJ, Carroll PR, Igawa M, Dahiya R (2005b) Promoter CpG hypomethylation and transcription factor EGR1 hyperactivate heparanase expression in bladder cancer. Oncogene 24(45):6765–6772

Okami K, Wu L, Riggins G, Cairns P, Goggins M, Evron E, Halachmi N, Ahrendt SA, Reed AL, Hilgers W, Kern SE, Koch WM, Sidransky D, Jen J (1998) Analysis of PTEN/MMAC1 alterations in aerodigestive tract tumors. Cancer Res 58(3):509–511

Ondrey FG, Dong G, Sunwoo J, Chen Z, Wolf JS, Crowl-Bancroft CV, Mukaida N, Van Waes C (1999) Constitutive activation of transcription factors NF-(kappa)B, AP-1, and NF-IL6 in human head and neck squamous cell carcinoma cell lines that express pro-inflammatory and pro-angiogenic cytokines. Mol Carcinog 26(2):119–129

Pai SI, Wu GS, Ozoren N, Wu L, Jen J, Sidransky D, El-Deiry WS (1998) Rare loss-of-function mutation of a death receptor gene in head and neck cancer. Cancer Res 58(16):3513–3518

Patane S, Avnet S, Coltella N, Costa B, Sponza S, Olivero M, Vigna E, Naldini L, Baldini N, Ferracini R, Corso S, Giordano S, Comoglio PM, Di Renzo MF (2006) MET overexpression turns human primary osteoblasts into osteosarcomas. Cancer Res 66(9):4750–4757

Pekarek LA, Starr BA, Toledano AY, Schreiber H (1995) Inhibition of tumor growth by elimination of granulocytes. J Exp Med 181(1):435–440

Pernas FG, Allen CT, Winters ME, Dabir B, Bagain L, Saigal K, Yan B, Morris JC, Calvo KR, Van Waes C, Chen Z (2008) Proteomic signatures of epidermal growth factor receptor and survival signal pathways correspond to Gefitinib sensitivity in head and neck cancer. Clin Cancer Res 15(7):2361-2372

Potempa S, Ridley AJ (1998) Activation of both MAP kinase and phosphatidylinositide 3-kinase by Ras is required for hepatocyte growth factor/scatter factor-induced adherens junction disassembly. Mol Biol Cell 9(8):2185–2200

Rabinovitz I, Mercurio AM (1996) The integrin alpha 6 beta 4 and the biology of carcinoma. Biochem Cell Biol 74(6):811–821

Reed AL, Califano J, Cairns P, Westra WH, Jones RM, Koch W, Ahrendt S, Eby Y, Sewell D, Nawroz H, Bartek J, Sidransky D (1996) High frequency of p16 (CDKN2/MTS-1/INK4A) inactivation in head and neck squamous cell carcinoma. Cancer Res 56(16):3630–3633

Ridley AJ, Comoglio PM, Hall A (1995) Regulation of scatter factor/hepatocyte growth factor responses by Ras, Rac, and Rho in MDCK cells. Mol Cell Biol 15(2):1110–1122

Rocco JW, Leong CO, Kuperwasser N, DeYoung MP, Ellisen LW (2006) p63 Mediates survival in squamous cell carcinoma by suppression of p73-dependent apoptosis. Cancer Cell 9(1):45–56

Rocha S, Garrett MD, Campbell KJ, Schumm K, Perkins ND (2005) Regulation of NF-kappaB and p53 through activation of ATR and Chk1 by the ARF tumour suppressor. EMBO J 24(6):1157–1169

Rosario M, Birchmeier W (2003) How to make tubes: Signaling by the Met receptor tyrosine kinase. Trends Cell Biol 13(6):328–335

Rosenthal EL, Johnson TM, Allen ED, Apel IJ, Punturieri A, Weiss SJ (1998) Role of the plasminogen activator and matrix metalloproteinase systems in epidermal growth factor- and scatter factor-stimulated invasion of carcinoma cells. Cancer Res 58(22):5221–5230

Royal I, Lamarche-Vane N, Lamorte L, Kaibuchi K, Park M (2000) Activation of cdc42, rac, PAK, and rho-kinase in response to hepatocyte growth factor differentially regulates epithelial cell colony spreading and dissociation. Mol Biol Cell 11(5):1709–1725

Sachs M, Brohmann H, Zechner D, Muller T, Hulsken J, Walther I, Schaeper U, Birchmeier C, Birchmeier W (2000) Essential role of Gab1 for signaling by the c-Met receptor in vivo. J Cell Biol 150(6):1375–1384

Sakkab D, Lewitzky M, Posern G, Schaeper U, Sachs M, Birchmeier W, Feller SM (2000) Signaling of hepatocyte growth factor/scatter factor (HGF) to the small GTPase Rap1 via the large docking protein Gab1 and the adapter protein CRKL. J Biol Chem 275(15):10772–10778

Salah Z, Maoz M, Pizov G, Bar-Shavit R (2007) Transcriptional regulation of human protease-activated receptor 1: A role for the early growth response-1 protein in prostate cancer. Cancer Res 67(20):9835–9843

Scarpino S, D'Alena FC, Di Napoli A, Ballarini F, Prat M, Ruco LP (2003) Papillary carcinoma of the thyroid: Evidence for a role for hepatocyte growth factor (HGF) in promoting tumour angiogenesis. J Pathol 199(2):243–250

Schaper F, Siewert E, Gomez-Lechon MJ, Gatsios P, Sachs M, Birchmeier W, Heinrich PC, Castell J (1997) Hepatocyte growth factor/scatter factor (HGF/SF) signals via the STAT3/APRF transcription factor in human hepatoma cells and hepatocytes. FEBS Lett 405(1):99–103

Scharnhorst V, Menke AL, Attema J, Haneveld JK, Riteco N, van Steenbrugge GJ, van der Eb AJ, Jochemsen AG (2000) EGR-1 enhances tumor growth and modulates the effect of the Wilms' tumor 1 gene products on tumorigenicity. Oncogene 19(6):791–800

Scholnick SB, Richter TM (2003) The role of CSMD1 in head and neck carcinogenesis. Genes Chromosomes Cancer 38(3):281–283

Scholnick SB, Haughey BH, Sunwoo JB, el-Mofty SK, Baty JD, Piccirillo JF, Zequeira MR (1996) Chromosome 8 allelic loss and the outcome of patients with squamous cell carcinoma of the supraglottic larynx. J Natl Cancer Inst 88(22):1676–1682

Sengupta S, Gherardi E, Sellers LA, Wood JM, Sasisekharan R, Fan TP (2003) Hepatocyte growth factor/scatter factor can induce angiogenesis independently of vascular endothelial growth factor. Arterioscler Thromb Vasc Biol 23(1):69–75

Seslar S, Nakamura T, Byers S (1995) Tumor-stroma interactions and stromal cell density regulate hepatocyte growth factor protein levels: A role for transforming growth factor-beta activation. Endocrinology 136(5):1945–1953

Sidransky D, Hollstein M (1996) Clinical implications of the p53 gene. Annu Rev Med 47:285–301

Smith CW, Chen Z, Dong G, Loukinova E, Pegram MY, Nicholas-Figueroa L, Van Waes C (1998) The host environment promotes the development of primary and metastatic squamous cell carcinomas that constitutively express proinflammatory cytokines IL-1alpha, IL-6, GM-CSF, and KC. Clin Exp Metastasis 16(7):655–664

Squarize CH, Castilho RM, Sriuranpong V, Pinto DS Jr, Gutkind JS (2006) Molecular cross-talk between the NFkappaB and STAT3 signaling pathways in head and neck squamous cell carcinoma. Neoplasia 8(9):733–746

Stabile LP, Lyker JS, Land SR, Dacic S, Zamboni BA, Siegfried JM (2006) Transgenic mice overexpressing hepatocyte growth factor in the airways show increased susceptibility to lung cancer. Carcinogenesis 27(8):1547–1555

Sukhatme VP, Cao XM, Chang LC, Tsai-Morris CH, Stamenkovich D, Ferreira PC, Cohen DR, Edwards SA, Shows TB, Curran T et al (1988) A zinc finger-encoding gene coregulated with c-fos during growth and differentiation, and after cellular depolarization. Cell 53(1):37–43

Sunwoo JB, Chen Z, Dong G, Yeh N, Crowl Bancroft C, Sausville E, Adams J, Elliott P, Van Waes C (2001) Novel proteasome inhibitor PS-341 inhibits activation of nuclear factor-kappa B, cell survival, tumor growth, and angiogenesis in squamous cell carcinoma. Clin Cancer Res 7(5):1419–1428

Svaren J, Ehrig T, Abdulkadir SA, Ehrengruber MU, Watson MA, Milbrandt J (2000) EGR1 target genes in prostate carcinoma cells identified by microarray analysis. J Biol Chem 275(49):38524–38531

Takayama H, LaRochelle WJ, Sharp R, Otsuka T, Kriebel P, Anver M, Aaronson SA, Merlino G (1997) Diverse tumorigenesis associated with aberrant development in mice overexpressing hepatocyte growth factor/scatter factor. Proc Natl Acad Sci USA 94(2):701–706

Tamura M, Arakaki N, Tsubouchi H, Takada H, Daikuhara Y (1993) Enhancement of human hepatocyte growth factor production by interleukin-1 alpha and -1 beta and tumor necrosis factor-alpha by fibroblasts in culture. J Biol Chem 268(11):8140–8145

Truelson JM, Fisher SG, Beals TE, McClatchey KD, Wolf GT (1992) DNA content and histologic growth pattern correlate with prognosis in patients with advanced squamous cell carcinoma of the larynx. The Department of Veterans Affairs Cooperative Laryngeal Cancer Study Group. Cancer 70(1):56–62

Tsurutani J, Castillo SS, Brognard J, Granville CA, Zhang C, Gills JJ, Sayyah J, Dennis PA (2005) Tobacco components stimulate Akt-dependent proliferation and NFkappaB-dependent survival in lung cancer cells. Carcinogenesis 26(7):1182–1195

Van Waes C (2007) Nuclear factor-kappaB in development, prevention, and therapy of cancer. Clin Cancer Res 13(4):1076–1082

Van Waes C, Kozarsky KF, Warren AB, Kidd L, Paugh D, Liebert M, Carey TE (1991) The A9 antigen associated with aggressive human squamous carcinoma is structurally and functionally similar to the newly defined integrin alpha 6 beta 4. Cancer Res 51(9):2395–2402

Van Waes C, Surh DM, Chen Z, Kirby M, Rhim JS, Brager R, Sessions RB, Poore J, Wolf GT, Carey TE (1995) Increase in suprabasilar integrin adhesion molecule expression in human epidermal neoplasms accompanies increased proliferation occurring with immortalization and tumor progression. Cancer Res 55(22):5434–5444

Van Waes C, Enamorado-Ayala I, Hecht D, Sulica L, Chen Z, Batt DG, Mousa S (2000) Effects of the novel alphav integrin antagonist SM256 and cis-platinum on growth of murine squamous cell carcinoma PAM LY8. Int J Oncol 16(6):1189–1195

Webster GA, Perkins ND (1999) Transcriptional cross talk between NF-kappaB and p53. Mol Cell Biol 19(5):3485–3495

Weidner KM, Behrens J, Vandekerckhove J, Birchmeier W (1990) Scatter factor: Molecular characteristics and effect on the invasiveness of epithelial cells. J Cell Biol 111(5 Pt 1):2097–2108

Wolf GT, Carey TE, Schmaltz SP, McClatchey KD, Poore J, Glaser L, Hayashida DJ, Hsu S (1990) Altered antigen expression predicts outcome in squamous cell carcinoma of the head and neck. J Natl Cancer Inst 82(19):1566–1572

Wolf JS, Chen Z, Dong G, Sunwoo JB, Bancroft CC, Capo DE, Yeh NT, Mukaida N, Van Waes C (2001) IL (interleukin)-1alpha promotes nuclear factor-kappaB and AP-1-induced IL-8 expression, cell survival, and proliferation in head and neck squamous cell carcinomas. Clin Cancer Res 7(6):1812–1820

Worden B, Yang XP, Lee TL, Bagain L, Yeh NT, Cohen JG, Van Waes C, Chen Z (2005) Hepatocyte growth factor/scatter factor differentially regulates expression of proangiogenic factors through Egr-1 in head and neck squamous cell carcinoma. Cancer Res 65(16):7071–7080

Wright JJ, Gunter KC, Mitsuya H, Irving SG, Kelly K, Siebenlist U (1990) Expression of a zinc finger gene in HTLV-I- and HTLV-II-transformed cells. Science 248(4955):588–591

Xiao GH, Jeffers M, Bellacosa A, Mitsuuchi Y, Vande Woude GF, Testa JR (2001) Anti-apoptotic signaling by hepatocyte growth factor/Met via the phosphatidylinositol 3-kinase/Akt and mitogen-activated protein kinase pathways. Proc Natl Acad Sci USA 98(1):247–252

Yan B, Yang X, Lee TL, Friedman J, Tang J, Van Waes C, Chen Z (2007) Genome-wide identification of novel expression signatures reveal distinct patterns and prevalence of binding motifs for p53, nuclear factor-kappaB and other signal transcription factors in head and neck squamous cell carcinoma. Genome Biol 8(5):R78

Yan B, Chen G, Saigal K, Yang X, Jensen ST, Van Waes C, Stoeckert CJ, Chen Z (2008) Systems biology-defined NF-kappaB regulons, interacting signal pathways and networks are implicated in the malignant phenotype of head and neck cancer. In: International conference on systems biology, Long Beach, CA

Yang SZ, Abdulkadir SA (2003) Early growth response gene 1 modulates androgen receptor signaling in prostate carcinoma cells. J Biol Chem 278(41):39906–39911

Yang X, Lu H, Yan B, Duggal P, Chuang R, Friedman J, Ehsanian R,Van Waes C, Chen Z (2009) ΔNp63 modulates survival and inflammatory gene programs overlapping with the NF-κB transcriptome in head and neck cancer. In 100th Annual meeting of American association for cancer research, Denver, CO

Yoon Y, Liang Z, Zhang X, Choe M, Zhu A, Cho HT, Shin DM, Goodman MM, Chen ZG, Shim H (2007) CXC chemokine receptor-4 antagonist blocks both growth of primary tumor and metastasis of head and neck cancer in xenograft mouse models. Cancer Res 67(15):7518–7524

Young MR (2000) Chemokines and cancer. Arch Pathol Lab Med 124(4):642

Young MR, Wright MA, Lozano Y, Prechel MM, Benefield J, Leonetti JP, Collins SL, Petruzzelli GJ (1997) Increased recurrence and metastasis in patients whose primary head and neck squamous cell carcinomas secreted granulocyte-macrophage colony-stimulating factor and contained CD34+ natural suppressor cells. Int J Cancer 74(1):69–74

Yu M, Yeh J, Van Waes C (2006) Protein kinase casein kinase 2 mediates inhibitor-kappaB kinase and aberrant nuclear factor-kappaB activation by serum factor(s) in head and neck squamous carcinoma cells. Cancer Res 66(13):6722–6731

Yuspa SH, Hawley-Nelson P, Koehler B, Stanley JR (1980) A survey of transformation markers in differentiating epidermal cell lines in culture. Cancer Res 40(12):4694–4703

Zhang YW, Wang LM, Jove R, Vande Woude GF (2002) Requirement of Stat3 signaling for HGF/SF-Met mediated tumorigenesis. Oncogene 21(2):217–226

Zhang YW, Su Y, Volpert OV, Vande Woude GF (2003) Hepatocyte growth factor/scatter factor mediates angiogenesis through positive VEGF and negative thrombospondin 1 regulation. Proc Natl Acad Sci USA 100(22):12718–12723

Zhang PL, Pellitteri PK, Law A, Gilroy PA, Wood GC, Kennedy TL, Blasick TM, Lun M, Schuerch C III, Brown RE (2005) Overexpression of phosphorylated nuclear factor-kappa B in tonsillar squamous cell carcinoma and high-grade dysplasia is associated with poor prognosis. Mod Pathol 18(7):924–932

Chapter 11
Wnt/β-Catenin Signaling and Oral Cancer Metastasis

Ge Zhou

Abstract The Wnt/β-catenin signaling pathway participates in many physiologic events in embryogenesis and adult homeostasis, including cell fate specification, maintenance, and activation of stem cells. Dysregulation of Wnt/β-catenin signaling promotes uncontrolled cell growth, survival, and consequently results in epithelial-to-mesenchymal transition (EMT) and the development of familial and/or sporadic epithelial cancers in a range of tissues such as colon, skin, liver, and ovary cancers. In squamous cell carcinoma of the oral cavity, SCCOC, its roles, however, are largely undefined. Although it is evident that constitutive activation of the Wnt/β-catenin is frequently observed in oral cancer progression, only infrequent mutations have been found in genes encoding various components of this pathway that commonly mutated in other cancers. This suggests that Wnt/β-catenin signaling is probably activated by multiple mechanisms, including genetic and epigenetic alterations of the components in this signaling, and the alterations in other autocrine and/or paracrine factors that are involved in the regulation of this pathway. More importantly, the interaction between epithelial tumor cells and the different components of the surrounding microenvironment can locally affect the intracellular levels of Wnt/β-catenin signaling components and differentially trigger tumor cell stemness, cell proliferation, EMT, invasive behavior, and metastasis. The exact mechanisms by which this occurs still remain unclear. Therefore, further investigation is required for understanding the role of Wnt/β-catenin signaling in the tumorigenesis, tumor progression, and metastasis of SCCOC.

Ge Zhou (✉)
Department of Head and Neck Surgery, The University of Texas, M. D. Anderson Cancer Center, 1515 Holcombe Blvd., Unit 0123, Houston, TX, 77030-4009, USA
e-mail: gzhou@mdanderson.org

J. Myers (ed.), *Oral Cancer Metastasis*,
DOI 10.1007/978-1-4419-0775-2_11, © Springer Science+Business Media, LLC 2010

Introduction

The Wnt family of secreted proteins is one of the most important families of intercellular signaling factors in animal development. These secreted cysteine-rich glycoproteins function as short-range ligands to activate receptor-mediated Wnt signaling pathways. It has been shown that activation of Wnt signaling functions as a "master switch" for proliferation versus differentiation (van de Wetering et al. 2002), and regulates proper tissue development in embryos and tissue homeostasis in adults. This is achieved by directing a specific set of genes that strictly regulate cell growth, survival, apoptosis, and cell motility. The signaling cascades initiating these processes include the widely studied canonical Wnt/β-catenin pathway, as well as a variety of noncanonical pathways. In normal epithelium, the Wnt/β-catenin signaling pathways have been shown to control the cell fate specification, maintenance, and activation of stem cells, and dysregulation of the Wnt/β-catenin pathway promotes uncontrolled cell growth, survival, and consequently results in epithelial-to-mesenchymal transition (EMT) and the development of familial and/or sporadic epithelial cancers in a range of tissues including colon, skin, liver, and ovarian cancers (Morin and Weeraratna 2003; Moon et al. 2004; Nelson and Nusse 2004; Taketo 2004; Huber et al. 2005; Reya and Clevers 2005; Clevers 2006; Blanpain et al. 2007; Polakis 2007).

So far, the Wnt signaling pathway has been well studied in a number of cancers, most notably colorectal carcinoma (Giles et al. 2003). In the majority of colorectal cancers, the mutational inactivation of adenomatous polyposis coli (APC), an important component of β-catenin destruction complex in the Wnt pathway, is an early event (Vogelstein et al. 1988). This leads to the stabilization of the cytoplasmic pool of β-catenin, and subsequent accumulation and translocation to the nucleus where it associates with T-cell factor/lymphoid enchancer factor-1 (TCF/LEF1) and stimulates the transcription of Wnt/β-catenin signaling target genes. In addition, some colorectal cancers exhibit activating β-catenin gene mutations, which result in constitutive activation β-catenin /TCF transcriptional activities (Sparks et al. 1998). Thus, both an inactivating APC mutation and activating β-catenin mutation eventually lead to initiation of constitutive Wnt/β-catenin signaling activation and colon cancer progression (Segditsas and Tomlinson 2006; Polakis 2007).

In contrast to colorectal cancers, the tumorigenesis and tumor progression of oral cancer is a complicated process that involves multiple steps characterized with different epigenetic and genetic alterations. While it is evident that constitutive activation of the Wnt/β-catenin is frequently observed in oral cancer, only infrequent mutations have been found in genes encoding various components of this pathway that commonly mutated in other cancers, such as those encoding APC and β-catenin in colorectal cancer. Therefore, Wnt/β-catenin signaling is probably activated by changes in the expression of genes encoding proteins directly involved in the signaling pathway or associated with the positive/negative regulation of this pathway. However, detailed molecular mechanisms involved are far from being understood. So, dissection of the Wnt/β-catenin pathway in oral cancer should provide great insights into the molecular and cellular mechanisms involved in the initiation, progression, and metastasis of oral cancers. In this chapter, we present a brief overview of the pathway's components and the process of Wnt/β-catenin signaling transduction. The current literature regarding the Wnt/β-catenin signaling pathway in tumorigenesis, tumor progression, and metastasis of different cancers including oral cancer are reviewed and discussed.

Components of Canonical Wnt/β-Catenin Signaling

Wnt proteins, once bound to their receptors, can activate at least one of the three different pathways: (1) the canonical Wnt/β-catenin signaling pathway, (2) the Wnt/planar cell polarity pathway, and (3) the Wnt/calcium pathway (Veeman et al. 2003). The type of Wnt proteins secreted determines which of these three signaling cascades is activated. Thus, the Wnt ligands and their receptors usually can be loosely classified in accordance with the pathway(s) that they activate. However, this is not a strict classification because there is a degree of promiscuity in the Wnt-receptor interactions. In canonical Wnt/β-catenin signaling, the Wnts activating this pathway trigger a signaling cascade of events within the cell, which leads to stabilization and increased levels of the free cytoplasmic pool of β-catenin, and the subsequent nuclear translocation of this protein to regulate gene transcription. Since this pathway is the most widely studied and understood, we focus here on the canonical Wnt/β-catenin signaling (Fig. 11.1), its regulation as well as its physiological functions.

Extracellular and Cell Membrane Components

Wnts are a large family of secreted glycoprotein ligands characterized by a high number of conserved cysteine residues that are expressed in species ranging from Drosophila to man (Giles et al. 2003). All Wnt signaling pathways are initiated following Wnt ligand binding to a membrane of the Frizzled (Fzd) family of seven-spanning transmembrane receptors. So far, at least 19 Wnt ligands and 10 Fzd receptors have been identified in the human genome (http://www.stanford. edu/~rnusse/wntwindow.html). The pathway also requires an additional single spanning transmembrane protein, the low-density lipoprotein receptor-related protein (LRP). In the presence of Wnt binding, Fzd and LRP are associated with each other, forming a trimeric complex that activates a cascade of intercellular signaling (Giles et al. 2003). In addition, at least two types of proteins that are unrelated to Wnt factors can activate the Fzd/LRP receptors. One of these factors is Norrin, which binds to Fzd 4 and activates the canonical signaling pathway in an LRP5/6-dependent manner (Xu et al. 2004). Other factors are R-spondins that interact with LRP6 and Fzd8 and activate the Wnt reporter genes (Nam et al. 2006). Finally, Wnt signaling is blocked by two groups of extracellular Wnt antagonists depending

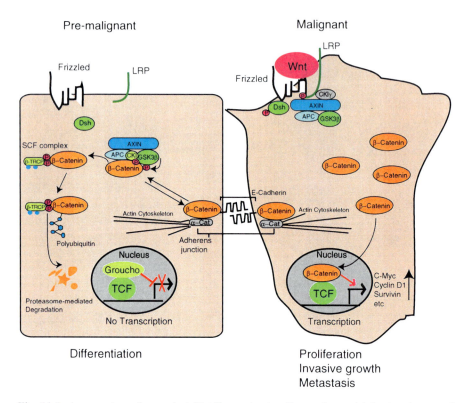

Fig. 11.1 An overview of canonical Wnt/β-catenin signaling pathway. (**a**) In the absence of soluble Wnt ligand, β-catenin is captured by APC and axin within the β-catenin destruction complex, facilitating its phosphorylation by the kinases CK1α and GSK3β. CK1α and GSK3β then sequentially phosphorylate a conserved set of serine and threonine residues at the N-terminus of β-catenin. The phosphorylation of β-catenin facilitates binding of the β-TRCP, which subsequently mediates the ubiquitinylation and efficient proteasome-mediated degradation of β-catenin. The decreased level of β-catenin ensures that the nuclear TCF transcription factor family actively represses target genes by recruiting transcriptional repressor Groucho/TLE to their promoter and/or enhancer. In addition, α-catenins also constitutively bind to E-cadherin through β-catenin to form adherens junction. The interactions at the junction are dynamic and involve many other proteins. (**b**) In response to Wnt ligand binding to its specific receptor complex containing a Frizzled family member and LRP triggers the formation of Dsh-Frizzled complexes and phosphorylation of LRP by CK1γ, facilitating relocation of Axin to the membrane and the inactivation of destruction complex and. This enables β-catenin to accumulate and translocate to the nucleus, where β-catenin interacts with members of TCF family and converts them into potent transcriptional activator by displacing Groucho/TLE protein and recruiting an array of coactivators including CBP, BRG-1, Legless and Pygopus, etc. This ensures efficient activation of TCF target genes such as *c-Myc*, which promote the cell to actively proliferate and remain in an undifferentiated state (Barker and Clevers 2006). *APC* adenomatous polyposis coli; *β-Trcp* β-transducin repeat containing protein; *GSK3β* glycogen synthase kinase 3β; *CK* casein kinase; *SCF* Skp1-Cullen-F-box; *P* phosphorylation

on their modes of action. One group, including soluble frizzled-related protein (SFRP), Wnt inhibitory factor (WIF) and Cerberus, inhibits Wnt signaling by directly binding to Wnt molecules, thereby preventing the binding of Wnt to Frz and the activation of the Wnt signaling (Piccolo et al. 1999; Kawano and Kypta 2003; Clevers 2006). Another group includes the secreted Dickkopf (DDK) and Wise, which binds LRP5 or LRP6 and competes with Wnt ligands for Frz-LRP-receptor interactions and thus inhibits Wnt signaling (Clevers 2006).

Cytoplasmic Components

The central player in the canonical Wnt/β-catenin signaling is β-catenin, a transcriptional cofactor that localizes at the cell membrane and in the cytoplasm and plays a pivotal role in balancing both cell adhesion and Wnt signaling within the cell. In the absence of a Wnt signal, cytoplasmic β-catenin is actively degraded by a large multiprotein "destruction complex," which keeps the levels of free β-catenin below the threshold beyond which aberrant transcriptional activity will occur. Within this complex, the tumor suppressor protein Axin forms a central scaffold as it directly interacts with all other components: β-catenin, the tumor suppressor APC, glycogen synthase kinase 3β (GSK3β), casein kinase Iα-(CKIα), protein phosphatase 2A (PP2A) (Fig. 11.1) (Giles et al. 2003; Barker and Clevers 2006; Clevers 2006), and the Wilms tumor suppressor (WTX) (Major et al. 2007). APC can also bind β-catenin and PP2A, but GSK3β, in contrast to other members of this complex, only has binding sites for Axin and thus cannot directly associate with either APC or β-catenin. Once the complex is formed, it is stabilized by the GSK3β-mediated phosphorylation of Axin and APC, and by the activity of PP2 (Sakanaka et al. 1998; Seeling et al. 1999). Another important cytoplasmic component upstream of AXIN-APC-GSK3β complex is Dishevelled (Dsh), which is a phosphoprotein that sits at the signaling crossroads of the canonical and noncanonical Wnt pathway. CK1 can bind to and phosphorylate Dsh, promoting its function in the canonical pathway (Giles et al. 2003).

In addition to cytoplsmic pool of β-catenin, β-catenin also binds tightly to the cytoplasmic domain of E-cadherin and plays an essential role in the structural organization and function of adherens junctions (AJ) by linking E-cadherin through α-catenin to the actin cytoskeleton (Fig. 11.1). Binding of β-catenin to E-cadhein at adherins junctions, AJs sequesters β-catenin to the cell membrane, making it unavailable for translocation to nucleus and thereby inhibits Wnt signaling. In contrast, signals which cause breakdown of AJs lead to an increase in the level of free cytoplasmic β-catenin, and consequent transcriptional activity (Nelson and Nusse 2004). Therefore, it has been suggested that there is a dynamic interaction between the cytoplasmic pool and cell membrane pool of β-catenin, and that Wnt-related β-catenin is subjected to the regulation by AJ-mediated cell–cell adhesion.

Nuclear Components

In the absence of Wnt, β-catenin should not translocate to the nucleus, and thus its target genes are not activated. However, once activated and translocated into the nucleus, β-catenin partners with members of the TCF/LEF family of transcription factors to activate the transcription of Wnt target genes (Behrens et al. 1996; Brunner et al. 1997; van de Wetering et al. 1997). The TCF/LEF family of transcription factors consists of four proteins (TCF1, LEF1, TCF3, and TCF4), which bind to DNA with the consensus binding motif (A/T)(A/T)CAA(A/T)G (Brantjes et al. 2002). β-catenin binds to these proteins and is an essential cofactor for the TCF/LEF family of transcription factors, but does not bind DNA directly. In the absence of nuclear β-catenin, the TCF/LEF proteins are found in complex with the transcriptional repressor Groucho and histone deacetylases (HDAC) to form a repressive complex that blocks the transcription of the Wnt target genes (Cavallo et al. 1998; Chen et al. 1999; Gordon and Nusse 2006). When β-catenin enters the nucleus, it directly replaces Groucho from its binding of TCF/LEF and converts the complex to a transcriptional activating complex, thereby stimulating the transcription of Wnt target genes. Other members of this activating complex are the histone acetylase CBP/p300 and the SWI/SNF chromatin-remodeling complex member Brg-1, and both of them facilitate chromatin remodeling as a prerequistite for transcriptional activation (Hecht and Kemler 2000; Takemaru and Moon 2000; Barker et al. 2001; Li et al. 2007). In addition, nuclear β-catenin/TCF activity is regulated by Legless (Lgs) and its binding partner Pygopus (Pygo) (Kramps et al. 2002; Thompson et al. 2002). Lgs binds directly to the *N*-terminus of β-catenin and serves as an adaptor to recruit Pygo to the β-catenin transactivation complex (Parker et al. 2002). It has also been reported that Pygo has a role in transporting β-catenin from the cytoplasm to nucleus (Townsley et al. 2004a) and functions as a critical link in the TCF/LEF complex by recruiting the transcriptional coactivating complexes to the DNA-bound TCF factors (Townsley et al. 2004b).

Canonical Wnt Signaling Transduction (Fig. 11.1)

In the absence of Wnt signaling, GSK3β phosphorylates the *N*-terminus of β-catenin within the stabilized "destruction complex" in cytoplasm. There is a GSK3β recognition motif between amino acids 33 and 45 of β-catenin wherein lie four serine/threonine residues targeted for phosphorylation. In order for GSK3β-mediated phosphorylation to proceed, the motif must be primed by phosphorylation of the serine 45 by Casein kinase Iα (CKIα). Thereafter, the remaining target residues (Thr-41, Ser-37, and Ser-33) are sequentially phosphorylated by GSK3β (Liu et al. 2002). Once phosporylated, β-catenin is recognized by the F-box/WD protein β-transducin repeat containing protein (β-TrCP), which, together with Skp1, Cullen and Rbx-1, constitutes the enzyme ubiquitin ligase (E3) (Hart et al. 1999; Latres et al. 1999). This, together with the ubiquitin conjugating enzyme (E2) and ubiquitin activation enzyme (E1), causes ubiquitination of β-catenin and its subsequent destruction by the proteasome-mediated degradation (Aberle et al. 1997). All four serine and threonine residues in the GSK3β-recognition motif of β-catenin must be phosphorylated in order to be recognized by β-TrCP to be targeted for subsequent degradation.

In the presence of Wnt signaling, extracellular Wnt ligands initiate the pathways. However, the canonical Wnt signaling pathway will only be activated by interaction of Wnt ligands with Fzd receptor in the presence of the LRP5 or LRP6 (Pinson et al. 2000; Mao et al. 2001). The formation of the trimolecular complex (Wnt-Frizzled-LRP5/6) leads to recruitment of Dsh to the cell surface (through an unknown mechanism) and its phosphorylation by Kinases PAR-1 and CKII. The phosphorylated Dsh can form a complex with GSK3β, which serves to inhibit the activity of GSK3β (Kishida et al. 2001; Chen et al. 2003b; Wong et al. 2003). The Wnt-Fzd-LRP5/6 interaction also facilitates the recruitment of Axin to the cytoplasmic tail of LRP, which is mediated by phosphorylation of LRP on key residues by the kinase CK1γ and GSK3 (Mao et al. 2001; Davidson et al. 2005; Zeng et al. 2005). As a result, Axin dissociates from the Axin-APC-GSK3β complex, thereby compromising the ability of the destruction complex to phosphorylate β-catenin (Brennan et al. 2004). Nonphosphorylated β-catenin cannot be recognized by β-TrCP, which leads to increased levels of the cytoplasmic pool and subsequent nuclear translocalization of β-catenin.

The mechanism by which β-catenin translocates into the nucleus is not completely clear, since it does not contain a nuclear localization signal and thus may be transported by other proteins. The APC protein has been shown to have a nuclear export function for β-catenin (Neufeld et al. 2000; Rosin-Arbesfeld et al. 2000). In addition, the Pygo protein can function as nuclear anchor to transport β-catenin to nucleus (Townsley et al. 2004a). When β-catenin enters the nucleus, it directly replaces Groucho/tranducin-like enhancer (TLE) proteins from its binding of TCF/LEF, Lgs recruits Pygo to β-catenin and TCF/LEF is converted from a transcriptional repressor into an activator to induce the expression of downstream target genes (Fig. 11.1). Additionally, the activity of TCF/LEF itself may be modulated by signaling from the mitogen-activated protein kinase cascade composed of TAK1 and NLK/Nemo (Ishitani et al. 2003a, b), β-catenin can also interact with other DNA-binding protein such as Pix2 and Prop1 to activate transcription in a TCF/LEF independent manner (Kioussi et al. 2002; Olson et al. 2006). More importantly, it is also shown that β-catenin can interact with Prop1, or NF-κB, and act as a repressor to suppress transcription (Kim et al. 2005; Olson et al. 2006). These diverse pathways demonstrate the emerging complexity involved in the regulation of β-catenin nuclear activation.

It is believed that different cell types respond to Wnt signaling by transcribing different (although often overlapping) sets of target genes. To date, many Wnt/β-catenin target genes that contain TCF/LEF binding-site in their promoters have been identified. Moreover, some target genes are involved in Wnt/β-catenin signaling (e.g., Axin 2, LEF1, etc.), suggesting a feedback mechanism implicated in regulation Wnt/β-catenin signaling. For the up-to-date list of Wnt/β-catenin target genes, the reader is referred to the Wnt signaling homepage (http://www.stanford.edu/~rnusse/

wntwindow.html). In addition, studies using DNA microarrays have identified a large number of genes that undergo altered expression after disruption of Wnt signaling (Chen et al. 2003a; Paoni et al. 2003; Sansom et al. 2004). Since many of Wnt/β-catenin target genes are transcription factors (e.g., c-Myc, c-Jun, and Sox9, etc.) (He et al. 1998; Mann et al. 1999; Blache et al. 2004) that will in turn regulate their own genes. Some of the altered genes identified by microarrays may not be the true Wnt/β-catenin targets, and they may represent secondary effects of genes regulated downstream of Wnt signaling. Nevertheless, it has been shown that genes that are deregulated, whether as primary or secondary consequences of aberrant Wnt signaling, are implicated in a variety of different biological functions within cells. All these highlight the important role of Wnt/β-catenin signaling in cell growth, proliferation, animal development, and tumorigenesis and progression of many types of cancers.

Wnt/β-Catenin Signaling and Epithelial Stem Cells

The canonical Wnt/β-catenin signaling program has emerged as a critical regulator of stem cells, and studies have shown that this signaling virtually regulates all of the defined human adult stem cells systems, including skin, blood, intestine, and brain (Radtke and Clevers 2005; Reya and Clevers 2005). In many tissues, aberrant activation of Wnt/β-catenin signaling is associated with cancer, raising the possibility that the tightly regulated self-renewal mediated by Wnt/β-catenin signaling in stem and progenitor cells may be dysregulated in cancer cells to allow malignant proliferation. Thus, knowledge gained from understanding how the Wnt signaling is implicated in both stem cell and cancer cell biology is of great importance in understanding the dual nature of self-renewal signals of this signaling pathway.

Wnt/β-catenin signaling pathways often have multiple roles in stem cell linage determination within most if not all epithelial tissues. For example, in the intestine and mammary glands, nuclear β-catenin (the hallmarks of Wnt/β-catenin signaling) and TCF4 are prominently observed in the stem cell compartment (Barker et al. 1999; Batlle et al. 2002). In mice deficient for Tcf4, the intestinal villus epithelial compartment appears normal but the crypt progenitor compartment is lost, implying that physiological Wnt signaling is required for the maintenance of the intestinal crypt progenitor phenotype. Mice deficient for Lef1 do not develop hair follicles, mammary glands, or teeth (van Genderen et al. 1994). When β-catenin is conditionally targeted, it results in an absence of follicle morphogenesis and the follicular stem cell niche (Huelsken et al. 2001; Lowry et al. 2005). Similarly, over-expression of the Wnt ligand inhibitor DDK-1 results in the loss of intestinal crypts and a failure to develop hair follicles and mammary glands (Andl et al. 2002; Chu et al. 2004). Together, all these studies suggest a specific role for Wnt/β-catenin in development and/or maintenance of epithelial stem cells (Blanpain et al. 2007).

In healthy epithelial stem cells, it appears that there is an existence of a constant Wnt-active proliferative state and that β-catenin/TCF-4 complex constitutes the master switch that controls proliferation versus differentiation (van de Wetering et al. 2002), indicating that Wnt/β-catenin signaling is required for stem cell renewal. By contrast, some stem cells such as hair bulge stem cells appear to reside in a Wnt-restricted environment, while β-catenin signaling is only activated in bulge stem cells during the transition from quiescent to growing phases of the hair cycle (DasGupta and Fuchs 1999; Merrill et al. 2001; Lowry et al. 2005), suggesting a role of Wnt/β-catenin signaling in stem cell activation. Consistent with this, mice expressing a constitutively stabilized form of β-catenin in the epidermis develop excess hair follicles (Gat et al. 1998; Van Mater et al. 2003; Lo Celso et al. 2004; Lowry et al. 2005). Therefore, Wnt/β-catenin signaling is required for both stem cell renewal and activation in skin.

Some Tcfs may also function in stem cells even when the levels of cytoplasmic/ nuclear β-catenin are low or absent. For example, it was found that Tcf3 is expressed in adult hair follicle stem cells at all stages of the hair cycle as well as in multipotent embryonic skin progenitors. Moreover, when Tcf3 expression is maintained postnatally, it represses all three skin differentiation lineages (epidermal, sebaceous gland, and hair follicle differentiation) (Nguyen et al. 2006). These data suggest that in the absence of Wnt signals, Tcf3 may function in skin stem cells to maintain an undifferentiated state and, when β-catenin is stabilized (Wnt/β-catenin signaling is activated), Tcf3 repression is relieved, and stem cells become activated to proliferate and embark upon hair-follicle linage differentiation (Blanpain et al. 2007).

While Wnt/β-catenin signaling is important in stem cell activation and proliferation, it is also used by stem cells to specify certain cell lineage. In skin, β-catenin/ TCF signaling promotes hair-shaft differentiation, and at excessive levels, tumors of this cell lineage arise (Gat et al. 1998; DasGupta and Fuchs 1999; Van Mater et al. 2003; Lo Celso et al. 2004). Similarly, increased Wnt signaling (1) leads neural crest stem cells to adopt a sensory neuronal fate (Lee et al. 2004); (2) instructs skeletal progenitors toward osteoblast rather than chrondrocyte differentiation (Day et al. 2005); (3) promotes Paneth cell differentiation in the intestine (van Es et al. 2005); and (4) stimulates lobulo-alveolar differentiation in the mammary epithelium (Tsukamoto et al. 1988; Teuliere et al. 2005). Therefore, Wnt/β-catenin is implicated in both stem cell proliferation and differentiation.

More importantly, whether stem cells proliferate or differentiate in response to Wnt signaling is likely to depend upon factors that influence the levels and activation of TCF/β-catenin complexes and their associated cofactors in a dosage- and context-dependent fashion. In the past years, studies have been focused on the identification of Wnt/β-catenin downstream target genes signaling in epithelial stem cells (Batlle et al. 2002; van de Wetering et al. 2002; Lowry et al. 2005; Silva-Vargas et al. 2005; Nguyen et al. 2006). For example, in the hair follicle, the stabilization of β-catenin stimulates resting bulge stem cells to proliferate and regenerate hair follicles. Through transcriptional profiling of purified bulge stem cells during resting and active phases of the hair cycle using DNA microarray, it was discovered that during stem cell activation a number of genes associated with cell cycle progression are upregulated (Lowry et al. 2005). Similarly, when the levels of β-catenin are transgenically elevated in quiescent stem cells, the transcription of some of these genes is elevated, providing insights into how Wnt signaling may promote stem cell activation.

More importantly, Wnt signaling in bulge stem cells did not upregulate the hair keratin genes that are induced at later stages of hair-follicle differentiation (Lowry et al. 2005). Thus, as stem cells are activated and progress along a particular differentiation lineage, they appear to respond to different environmental cues and activate different sets of Wnt target genes. The multiplicity of transcriptional partners for β-catenin, together with the complex network of regulatory factors, is likely to contribute to the effect and potency of β-catenin/Lef1/Tcf activity in cells. These regulatory mechanisms of Wnt signaling are likely to impact on whether and when the stem cells will self-renew, become activated to proliferate, or embark upon a terminal differentiation program (Niemann 2006; Blanpain et al. 2007).

Given the importance of Wnt/β-catenin in epithelial stem cell renewal, activation, and differentiation, it is perhaps not surprising to find its pivotal role in cancer stem cells. Cancer stem cells have been defined as cells within a cancer that have the extensive ability to self-renew and to differentiate into the heterogeneous lineages of cancers that comprise a tumor (Clarke et al. 2006). To date, the relationship between normal stem and cancer stem cells is still unclear. However, evidence to the fact that genetic alterations that disturb key stem cell features and affect cell cycle are linked to the induction of neoplastic transformation and that neoplastic cells with these alterations are clearly distinct from normal stem cells is gradually emerging. In addition to Wnt/β-catenin signaling, it is generally believed that the Notch, hedgehog, transforming growth factor (TGF)β/bone morphogenic protein (BMP), and fibroblast growth factor (FGF) signaling networks are also implicated in the maintenance of tissue homeostasis by regulating self-renewal of normal stem cells as well as proliferation and differentiation of progenitor cells (Reya et al. 2001; Taipale and Beachy 2001; Chamorro et al. 2005; Duncan et al. 2005; Katoh and Katoh 2006; McDonald et al. 2006; Radtke et al. 2006; Shackleton et al. 2006). Dysregulation of the "stem cell signaling" network in normal stem cells can lead to the transformation to cancer stem cells. Alternatively, acquisition of self-renewal potential in progenitor cells due to epigenetic change or genetic alteration of stem cell signaling-related genes gives rise to cancer stem cells. For example, constitutively stabilizing mutations in β-catenin are associated with a variety of human epithelial cancers, including adenocarcinomas of the colon (Reya and Clevers 2005) and mammary gland (Teuliere et al. 2005). More importantly, epithelial tumors generated by excessive Wnt signaling often display an increased frequency of cells with stem and progenitor cell properties, in contrast to tumors from mice expressing other oncogenes. In this regard, the Wnt signaling appears to be special if not unique in its ability to target stem cell and/or progenitor cells for neoplastic transformation (Blanpain et al. 2007).

Wnt/β-Catenin Signaling and Cancers

Wnt/β-catenin signaling pathways participate in many physiologic events in embryogenesis and adult cell homeostasis, including cell fate specification, control of proliferation, and migration. Dysregulation of Wnt/β-catenin signaling is implicated in cancers.

Genetic and Epigenetic Alternations of Wnt/β-Catenin Signaling in Cancers

The *APC* gene was amongst the first tumor suppressors to be cloned. Mutations in the gene encoding the APC protein was first identified as the cause of one form of inherited colorectal cancer, familial adenomatous polyposis coli (FAP) (Groden et al. 1991; Kinzler et al. 1991), and subsequently was found in sporadic colorectal, lung, ovarian, and breast cancers (Munemitsu et al. 1995; Wallis et al. 1999; Furuuchi et al. 2000; Wu et al. 2001; Ohgaki et al. 2004). Most of the *APC* mutations lead to a truncated protein, whereas loss of both *APC* alleles and deletions of the whole gene or exon(s) were also reported (Kinzler and Vogelstein 1996; Sieber et al. 2003). Mutational inactivation of *APC* leads to the inappropriate stabilization and activation of β-catenin (Rubinfeld et al. 1996). In addition to gene mutation, tanscriptional silencing of *APC* by epigenetic promoter methylation has been suggested as an alternative to the suppression of *APC* by somatic mutation (Esteller et al. 2000).

Although the *APC* gene is mutated in the majority of sporadic colorectal cancers, it is infrequently mutated in other cancers originating outside of the gastrointestinal tract (Munemitsu et al. 1995; Wallis et al. 1999; Furuuchi et al. 2000; Wu et al. 2001; Ohgaki et al. 2004). Instead, mutations in *β-catenin* that abrogate its regulation by APC represent an alternative to Wnt activation and do occur more commonly in sporadic cancers outside of the gut. The best characterized alternatives to *APC* mutations are activating mutations of *β-catenin* (Ilyas et al. 1997; Morin et al. 1997). These either delete the whole of exon 3 or target individual serine and threonine residues encoded by this exon. These serines/threonines (codon 45, 41, 33, and 37) are phosphorylated by the CK1α and GSK3β in destruction complex that contains *APC*, and hence their mutation causes GSK3β to escape from proteasomal degradation. These mutations were first identified in sporadic colorectal cancers (Ilyas et al. 1997; Korinek et al. 1997; Morin et al. 1997) and in melanoma (Rubinfeld et al. 1997), but subsequent studies indicated that they occur quite infrequently (<5%) in these cancers (Demunter et al. 2002; Johnson et al. 2005; Luchtenborg et al. 2005; Thorstensen et al. 2005). This demonstrated that *β-catenin* mutations are not found together with *APC* mutations in colorectal cancers, indicating that changes in the two genes are alternatives in some way, although their functional effects are unlikely to be identical (Segditsas and Tomlinson 2006).

Unlike in colorectal cancers, mutations in *β-catenin* are particularly common in endometrioid ovarian cancer, although their prevalence ranges widely (16–54%) in the various studies (Bell 2005). Interestingly, it has been shown that *β-catenin* mutations in this cancer are more frequent in low-grade, highly differentiated early lesions (Oliva et al. 2006) and are strongly associated with primary independent tumors and are not found in any metastatic tumors (Irving et al. 2005). This suggests that endometrioid ovarian cancers with *β-catenin* mutations are associated with a favorable prognosis and might have reduced the capacity to metastasize. Finally, tumors such as pilomatrixoma, heptoblastoma, and Wilms kidney tumors also frequently contain mutations in *β-catenin* (Giles et al. 2003).

Axin is another important part of the destruction complex for β-catenin. It is believed that it functions as a scaffold protein in the complex and loss of its expression leads to increased Wnt/β-catenin signaling. Accordingly, loss-of-function mutations in *Axin* have been found in a variety of human cancers, including colorectal cancers, ovarian cancers, medulloblastoma, and hepatocellular carcinomas (Giles et al. 2003; Salahshor and Woodgett 2005). For example, one of the mutations in *Axin1*, L396M, leads to *Axin* inactivation by preventing binding of GSK3β (Webster et al. 2000). Additional missense mutations in the *Axin1* gene have been detected in germline of patients with multiple adenomatous polyps. Some of these mutations have also been found in unaffected individuals, but their increased frequency in cancer patients suggests that they contribute to a multifactorial inherited susceptibility to colorectal cancers (Fearnhead et al. 2004). In addition, at least some of the colorectal cancers with *Axin1* mutations also have *APC* mutation, suggesting that *Axin1* changes cannot be the sole cause of Wnt/β-catenin activation in these tumors. Recently, a new component, WTX, has been identified in the β-catenin destruction complex, which was shown to promote β-catenin ubiquitination and degradation (Major et al. 2007). This gene was discovered to be mutated in approximately 30% of Wilms tumors (Rivera et al. 2007). Studies showed that constitutive activation of Wnt/β-catenin signaling is common in Wilms tumors: approximately 10% of tumors harbor activating mutations in β-catenin (Koesters et al. 1999), and nuclear β-catenin is observed in approximately 50% of tumors lacking detectable *β-catenin* mutations (Koesters et al. 2003). *WTX* and *β-catenin* mutations were found to be mutually exclusive in the tumor samples examined suggesting that mutated WTX activates Wnt/β-catenin signaling by stabilizing β-catenin, providing a possible mechanistic explanation for the tumor suppressor activity of WTX (Rivera et al. 2007).

T-cell factor 4 (TCF4), one of the β-catenin binding transcriptional factors, is mutated in nearly half of colorectal cancers with high-frequency microsatellite instability (Duval et al. 1999; Fukushima et al. 2001), and these mutations eliminate the coding of TCF4 isoforms capable of binding the transcriptional repressor carboxy-terminal binding protein (CtBP) (Cuilliere-Dartigues et al. 2006). Additional but rare cases of genetic activation in the Wnt/β-catenin pathway include inactivating mutations in the SFRP1, which inhibits receptor activation by competitively binding to Wnt/β-catenin proteins (Caldwell et al. 2004). Finally, frequent promoter hypermethylation and gene silencing of the genes encoding soluble frizzled-related proteins (SFRPs) have been found in the early stages of colorectal cancer, suggesting that the epigenetic loss of SFRP function may provide constitutive Wnt signaling that is required for tumor development and progression of cancers (Suzuki et al. 2004).

In addition to the Wnt/β-catenin pathway genes discussed above, other components in this pathway may activate the Wnt signaling if mutated. However, recent studies with high-throughput sequencing suggest that it is unlikely that highly prevalent mutations, such as those in *APC* in colorectal tumors, remain undiscovered (Sjoblom et al. 2006). Therefore, the spectrum of mutations in human cancers is more complex and heterogeneous than once appreciated, and temporal order and different combinations also appear to be relevant to tumor progression (Polakis 2007). Finally, in addition to genetic and epigenetic alterations as discussed here, there are many other ways to activate Wnt/β-catenin signaling in tumors, in which many intrinsic (cell autonomous, autocrine) as well as extrinsic (cell non-autonomous, paracrine) Wnt/β-catenin signaling–promoting factors have been shown to regulate this signaling pathway that ultimately controls the malignant behavior of cancer cells.

Regulation in Wnt/β-Catenin Signaling in Cancer Malignant Behavior

As shown in Fig. 11.1, nuclear localization of β-catenin is the hallmark of activation of Wnt/β-catenin signaling. Theoretically, each cancer cell within the tumor initiated by mutations in *APC*, *β-catenin*, or *Axin* should exhibit intracellular and/or nuclear β-catenin accumulation. However, immunohistochemical analysis of colorectal cancers reveals a very heterogeneous intracellular distribution of β-catenin: whereas well-differentiated parenchymal cells located in the tumor center exhibit membranous expression of β-catenin comparable to normal colon epithelium, nuclear β-catenin expression is predominately observed in tumor cells localized at the invasion front and scattered in the adjacent stromal component (Brabletz et al. 1998). Notably, tumor cells with nuclear β-catenin accumulation appear to undergo EMTs, as shown by the progressive loss of E-cadherin expression and acquisition of mesenchymal markers such as fibronectin (Kirchner and Brabletz 2000; Brabletz et al. 2001). These alleged "migrating cancer stem cells" (MCSCs) may retain the capacity to self-renew and differentiate, allowing them to transiently trans-differentiate and to invade adjacent tissues more efficiently by EMT, and eventually to form metastases in distant organs through mesenchymal-to-epithelial transitions (METs) once the cells have settled in the metastatic site (Brabletz et al. 2005; Fodde and Brabletz 2007). The nonrandom distribution of tumor cells with intracellular β-catenin accumulation within primary tumors and distant metastases suggests that the initiating *APC* or *β-catenin* mutation is necessary but insufficient for full-scale Wnt activation and thus only tumor cells located at the invasive front are exposed to growth factors and cytokines are able to further enhance β-catenin nuclear translocation. In addition, somatic mutations in other tumor suppressors and oncogenes may act synergistically in promoting Wnt signaling. Therefore, both intrinsic (autocrine, tumor cell-autonomous) and extrinsic (paracrine, secreted by the tumor microenvironment) factors are likely to play important rate-limiting roles in cancer stemness, local invasion, and metastasis by differentially modulating Wnt/β-catenin in different cancers (Fodde and Brabletz 2007).

Cell Autonomous Wnt/β-Catenin Signaling-Promoting Factors

Studies using breast and ovarian cancer cell lines have identified that Wnt ligand expression is associated with increased levels of the transcriptionally active form of unphosphorylated, uncomplexed β-catenin in the absence of mutations in the commonly implicated downstream signaling components, *APC* or *β-catenin*. This concept is further supported by the finding that increases in the levels of the extracellular Wnt antagonists SFRP1 and DKK1 is accompanied by dramatic downregulation of the uncomplexed transcriptionally active form of β-catenin in these tumor cells and increased expression of epithelial differentiation markers (Bafico et al. 2004). In addition, colorectal carcinoma cells with deletion of the mutant *β-catenin* allele also retain upregulated *β-catenin* levels, which can be inhibited by the Wnt antagonists as well. All these results, taken together, strongly suggest there is an autocrine mechanism that constitutively activates Wnt/β-catenin pathway in human cancer cells (Bafico et al. 2004).

Another example of intrinsic Wnt/β-catenin promoting factors came of studies from tumors with *KRAS* mutations. It has been shown that loss of *APC* function is usually followed by oncogenic activation of the *KRAS* oncogene through mutations that occur during colorectal tumor progression from adenoma to carcinoma (Zhang et al. 2003). It is believed that both *APC* and *KRAS* mutations are synergistic in promoting β-catenin nuclear translocation at the invasive front of tumors, thus enhancing canonical Wnt/β-catenin signal transduction (Janssen et al. 2006). It is believed that activated KRAS trigger tyrosine phosphorylation of β-catenin, leading to its release from E-cadherin-mediated cell adhesion and increased transit of β-catenin to nucleus (Kinch et al. 1995). Similarly, mutations in the other genes the RAS pathway, such as *BRAF* (Rajagopalan et al. 2002), or in members of tyrosine kinome and phosphatome (Bardelli et al. 2003; Wang et al. 2004) that frequently occur in sporadic colorectal cancers are likely to enhance Wnt-signaling through β-catenin tyrosine phosphorylation (Fodde and Brabletz 2007). Finally, overexpression of the tyrosine kinases Src, Fer, and activation of transmembrane tyrosine kinases EGFR and c-Met downregulate E-cadherin-mediated adhesion and increase tyrosine phosphorylation of β-catenin (Lilien and Balsamo 2005), leading to nuclear translocation of β-catenin and activation of Wnt/β-catenin signaling. These are the kinases now known to target specific residues in β-catenin that are critical for its interaction with cadherin or α-catenin. Moreover, aberrant growth of tumor cells and ultimately metastasis are always correlated with constitutive activation and/or overexpression of these kinases (Birchmeier et al. 2003).

Cellular Wnt/β-Catenin Signaling-Promoting Factors

In addition to the cell-autonomous mechanisms, the nuclear β-catenin and activation of the Wnt/β-catenin signaling at the invasive front of colorectal cancers is likely to be at least partly explained by interactions with the tumor microenvironment. The invasive front of epithelial tumors represents an environment in which stromal myofibroblasts interact with tumor cells by producing extracellular matrix (ECM) components and by secreting Wnt ligands, cytokines, and growth factors that locally promote cell proliferation and invasion (De Wever et al. 2004; Gregorieff et al. 2005). It has been shown that all these factors presumably can enhance Wnt/β-catenin signaling to the nucleus. For example, hepatocyte growth factor (HGF) can induce Wnt-independent translocation of β-catenin to the nucleus in hepatocytes (Piedra et al. 2001). Binding of HGF to its tyrosine kinase receptor c-Met induces phosphorylation of β-catenin at tyrosine 142, releasing it from the plasma membrane and resulting in translocation to the nucleus, which occurs concomitantly with the conversion of MDCK cells to a mesenchymal phenotype (Brembeck et al. 2004). In colorectal cancer, HGF is found in the tumor microenvironment (Wielenga et al. 2000), whereas c-Met and β-catenin physically interact in a complex in cancer cells (Rasola et al. 2007). Upon HGF stimulation of colorectal cancer cells, β-catenin is tyrosine phosphorylated and dissociated from c-Met followed by nuclear translocation and activation of downstream target gene expression. Moreover, HGF also upregulates β-catenin expression via the phosphatidylinositol 3-kinase (PI3K) pathway in conditions that mimic those found by the invading and metastasizing cells. In addition, HGF and β-catenin can cooperate in promoting entry into the cell cycle, in stimulating cell scattering and motility, and in protecting cells from apoptosis. Therefore, HGF and β-catenin pathways are mutually activated in colorectal cancer, the cross-talk between HGF secreted from the tumor microenvironment and Wnt/β-catenin signaling in cancer cells may generate a self-amplifying positive feedback loop, leading to the upregulation of the invasive growth properties of cancer cells (Rasola et al. 2007).

Platelet-derived growth factor (PDGF) has been shown to be expressed by several mesenchymal and epithelial cells (Heldin and Westermark 1999) and to activate EMT and tumor invasion in epithelial cells by enhancing Wnt/β-catenin signaling (Yang et al. 2006b). Unlike HGF that results in the phosphorylation of β-catenin, stimulation by PDGF was shown to promote tyrosine phosphorylation of p68, a RNA helicase, by c-Abl kinase in colorectal cancer HT-29 cells. The tyrosine-phosphorylated p68 then binds to β-catenin, inhibiting its Ser/Thr phosphorylation by GSK3β and displacing Axin from β-catenin. This leads to stabilization and nuclear accumulation of β-catenin, mediating PDGF-induced EMT (Yang et al. 2006b). Given that other growth factors such as epidermal growth factor (EGF) and TGF-β can also lead to p68 phosphorylation through their receptor tyrosine kinases, the p68-driven upregulation of Wnt/β-catenin signaling may represent a common intracellular response of paracrine stimulation of EMT in epithelial tumor cells (He 2006; Yang et al. 2006b).

In addition to growth factors, Wnt ligands secreted by mesenchymal cells in the tumor microenvironment are likely to be able to activate Wnt/β-catenin signaling. For example, expression of canonical and noncanonical Wnt ligands has been shown to be expressed in both mesenchymal and epithelial compartments of the small intestine and colon (Gregorieff et al. 2005). Targeting Foxf1 and Foxf2, mesenchymal forkhead transcription factors, was shown to have pleiotropic effects on intestinal paracrine signaling in mice, causing a range of defects, including megacolon, colorectal muscle hypoplasia and agangliosis (Ormestad et al. 2006). Further analysis indicated that in Foxf mutants, mesenchymal expression of Wnt5a expression is increased. In these mice, activation of the canonical Wnt pathway, with nuclear localization of β-catenin in epithelial cells, is associated with over-proliferation and resistance to apoptosis, which suggests that Foxf proteins are mesenchymal factors that control epithelial proliferation and survival, and regulate Wnt signaling (Ormestad et al. 2006). Another example of mesenchymal/epithelial cross talk is the winged helix transcription factor Foxl1 that is expressed in the mesenchyme of the gastrointestinal tract. Foxl1 null mice display severe structural defects in the epithelia of the stomach, duodenum, and jejunum, which result from an increase in the number of proliferating cells and not from a change in the rate of cell migration (Perreault et al. 2001). Further analysis indicates that Foxl1 activates the Wnt/β-catenin pathway by increasing extracellular proteoglycans, which act as coreceptors for Wnt (Perreault et al. 2001). Likewise, loss of this mesenchymal transcription factor Foxl1 leads to a marked increases in tumor numbers in the colon of APC(min) mice, which strongly demonstrates the importance of mesenchymal/epithelial interactions in the tumor genesis of colorectal cancers (Perreault et al. 2005).

Finally, inflammation has been known to play an important role in promoting tumorigenesis and tumor progression. Progressive up-regulation of Wnt2 and Wnt5a expression has been observed in macrophages during the progression from colorectal adenoma to carcinoma (Smith et al. 1999). This observation indicates the existence of another mechanism of paracrine Wnt activation by macrophages, and possibly other inflammatory cells (Fodde and Brabletz 2007). Indeed, it has been shown that cyclooxygenase 2 (Cox-2) and its proinflammatory metabolite prostaglandin E2 (PGE2) enhance colon cancer progression, whereas anti-inflammatory drugs against Cox-2 effectively inhibit formation of intestinal polyps in patients carrying germline *APC* mutations and in *APC*-mutant mice (Brown and DuBois 2005). Further study showed that PGE2 stimulates colon cancer cell growth through its guanine nucleotide-binding protein (G protein)-coupled receptor, EP2, by a signaling route that involves the activation of PI3K and the protein kinase Akt by free G protein βγ subunits and the direct association of the G protein α subunit with the regulator of G protein signaling domain of Axin. This leads to the inactivation and release of GSK3β from its complex with Axin, thereby relieving the inhibitory phosphorylation of β-catenin and activating its signaling pathway (Castellone et al. 2005). Therefore, together with the increased expression of Wnt ligands by tumor-infiltrating macrophages (Smith et al. 1999), these findings reveal a molecular mechanism for the activation of paracrine Wnt/β-catenin signaling by tumor inflammatory cells.

In summary, in addition to being regulated by genetic and epigenetic alterations in components implicated in the signaling pathway, the activity of Wnt/β-catenin signaling is subjected to both autocrine and paracrine factors acting locally within the tumor microenvironment. As observed in several adult stem cell niches, such as the intestinal crypt, the hair follicle and the mammary gland, Wnt/β-catenin signaling regulates self-renewal, activation of proliferation, and differentiation in a dosage- and context-dependent manner (Niemann 2006; Blanpain et al. 2007). More importantly, the interaction between epithelial tumor cells and the different components of the surrounding microenvironment, including tumor-infiltrating inflammatory cells, myofibroblasts and other stromal cells, can locally affect the intracellular levels of canonical Wnt/β-catenin signaling and differentially trigger stemness, cell proliferation, EMT, and invasive behavior. Likewise, similar local effects are achieved by mutations and/or dysregulation of other genes such as *KRAS*, *BRAF*, and kinases (Sjoblom et al. 2006). Therefore, a combination of autocrine and paracrine factors differentially modulates Wnt signaling activation and locally promotes migration and invasion in tumor cells (Fodde and Brabletz 2007).

Wnt/β-Catenin Signaling and Oral Cancer Metastasis

Although Wnt/β-catenin signaling has been shown to play an important role in many different cancers such as colorectal, breast, ovarian, gastric, pancreatic, and hepatocellular cancers, its role in oral cancer is not as well understood and remains controversial. Here we briefly review the evidence in support of Wnt/β-catenin signaling's role in tumor development and progression of oral cancer.

APC, Axin, and Oral Cancer

Loss of heterozygosity (LOH) of *APC* gene has been found in human SCCOC at a frequency ranging from 13% to 73% in several different studies (Largey et al. 1994; Uzawa et al. 1994; Huang et al. 1997; Chang et al. 2000; Gao et al. 2005). In both early and advanced stages of SCCOC, LOH of *APC* occurs (Huang et al. 1997), indicating that the alteration of APC may be an early event and may play a role in the pathogenesis of human SCCOC. *APC* mutations, which result in amino-acid substitutions or truncation of the APC protein, were also infrequently identified in 12.5% of human SCCOC (Uzawa et al. 1994; Kok et al. 2002). Interestingly, in one study, all patients with *APC* mutations were both areca quid chewers and tobacco smokers (Kok et al. 2002). Additionally, epigenetic alterations appear to regulate the *APC* expression as well. Uesugi et al. (2005) reported significant down regulation of APC in 15 (30.0%) of 50 SCCOC tumor samples and in five (62.5%) of eight cell lines. Hypermethylation of the *APC* promoter CpG island was detected in two of eight (25%) SCCOC-derived cell lines, whereas *APC* gene mRNA was restored in all five SCCOC-derived cell lines with low *APC* expression after treatment with 5-aza-2′-deoxycytidine, a DNA demethylating agent. Similarly, in another study, hypermethylation of the *APC* promoter was found in five (14.7%) of 34 SCCOC tumor samples (Gao et al. 2005). These results indicate that hypermethylation of the gene promoter CpG island may represent a significant mechanism of inactivation of the *APC* gene in oral carcinogenesis. Interestingly, in one study using laser microdissection method from 23 human SCCOC samples, no *APC* mutations were identified, and well-differentiated SCCOC showed significantly high APC expression level when compared with normal squamous epithelium, but APC expression level was decreased in moderately and poorly differentiated SCCOC. Notably, there was tendency that APC was observed in nucleus of SCCOC when compared with that in normal squamous epithelium, suggesting that the changes in the expression level and intracellular localization of APC were related to the tumorigeneis of SCCOC (Tsuchiya et al. 2004). Finally, in addition to *APC*, *Axin1*, another component of β-catenin destruction complex, has also been reported to be mutated in four (9.1%) of 44 (Zhou and Gao 2007) or three (12.5%) of 24 (Iwai et al. 2005) SCCOC samples, whereas Axin1 expression level was significantly reduced in 35 (79.5%) of 44 tumor specimen of SCCOC, especially in poorly differentiated tumors with metastasis (Zhou and Gao 2007). These results suggest that mutational inactivation and reduced expression of *Axin1* gene may play a role in SCCOC tumorigenesis and metastasis.

β-*Catenin and Oral Cancer*

As discussed previously, β-catenin plays a pivotal role in both E-cadherin-mediated cell adhesion (at the cell membrane) and Wnt signaling (in the cytoplasm and nucleus). Although no β-catenin mutations have been identified in human SCCOC (Lo Muzio et al. 2005; Odajima et al. 2005), immunohistological studies of subcellular localization of β-catenin in SCCOC have provided us a complex picture regarding the possible role of β-catenin and Wnt signaling in the development and progression of SCCOC.

It appears that the loss of membranous expression β-catenin and E-cadherin is a common feature of SCCOC (Williams et al. 1998; Chow et al. 2001; Bankfalvi et al. 2002a; Bankfalvi et al. 2002b; Tanaka et al. 2003; Fillies et al. 2005; Odajima et al. 2005; Yu et al. 2005; Wang et al. 2007). As an example, in one study of 159 SCCOC tumor samples, a significantly greater reduction in expression levels of β-catenin, E-cadherin, and α-catenin was found in the metastasis group ($n=64$) compared with the nonmetastatic group ($n=95$) (Tanaka et al. 2003).

Similar observations have been made in several other studies (Williams et al. 1998; Chow et al. 2001; Bankfalvi et al. 2002a; Bankfalvi et al. 2002b; Fillies et al. 2005; Wang et al. 2007). Notably, loss of membranous β-catenin often occurs at the invasive front of poorly differentiated SCCOC (Williams et al. 1998; Lo Muzio et al. 1999; Kudo et al. 2004; Mahomed et al. 2007), which could constitute a hallmark of aggressive biological behavior of tumor cells. Moreover, invasion and metastasis of SCCOC cells have been shown to require methylation of E-cadherin and/or degradation of membranous β-catenin (Kudo et al. 2004). Odajims et al. reported that 75 (68.2%) of 110 SCCOC cases have reduced membranous expression of β-catenin, and the remaining 35 (31.8%) have a membranous pattern of expression similar to that in normal oral epithelium, and that the reduced membranous expression of β-catenin was significantly associated with an invasive growth pattern, EGFR expression, an increased Ki-67 labeling index (proliferation index) (Odajima et al. 2005). Furthermore, it has been suggested that SCCOC patients with loss of membranous β-catenin should be considered at high-risk for lymph-node metastasis and worse disease-free survival (Bankfalvi et al. 2002b; Fillies et al. 2005;

Yu et al. 2005; Ueda et al. 2006). Similarly, patients whose tumors have low levels of β-catenin protein expression have decreased survival rates and reduced response to therapy when compared with patients whose tumors have high levels of β-catenin (Rodriguez-Pinilla et al. 2005). Based upon the finding that β-catenin mutations are rare and the loss of membranous β-catenin is associated with SCCOC development, it has been suggested that β-catenin functions mainly as an adhesion molecule in SCCOC and that loss of adhesion rather than (Yu et al. 2005) increased Wnt signaling plays a greater role in the development of SCCOC (Yeh et al. 2003). However, closer examination of available evidence indicates that this conclusion may be an oversimplification.

Odajima et al. (2005) reported that while 75 (68.2%) of the 110 SCCOC tumors exhibited reduced membranous β-catenin expression, a cytoplasmic/nuclear pattern of β-catenin staining was observed in 21 (19.1%) of these tumors. Nuclear expression was accompanied by a reduction of membranous expression and significantly correlated with disease progression. Even at the invasive front of SCCOC where membranous β-catenin is frequently lost, cytoplasmic accumulation of β-catenin, with frequent paranuclear accentuation, was observed in more than 50% of tumor cells in 11 (37%) of 30 SCCOC tumors, which were either moderately or poorly differentiated tumors (Mahomed et al. 2007). Gao et al. (2005) found that cytoplasmic rather than membrane staining of β-catenin is a prominent aberrant tumor-related alteration that is associated with moderately and poorly differentiated tumors, and more importantly, with LOH and hypermethylation of the APC promoter, suggesting that LOH at the APC locus or hypermethylation of the APC promoter may lead to free β-catenin accumulation in the cytoplasm of SCCOC cells and thereby to oral malignant progression (Gao et al. 2005). Similarly, in another study, Uraguchi et al.(2004) showed that nuclear localization of β-catenin is predominant in carcinoma cells at the invasive front of SCCOC, suggesting that it is associated with local invasiveness of the tumor.

Gasparoni et al. (2002) compared the subcellular localization of β-catenin in cultures of human oral normal and malignant keratinocytes and found that β-catenin was mostly located in the perinuclear and nuclear areas of malignant SCC25 cells. Consistent with this, in the growth assay, SCC25 cells proliferated faster than in normal and SCC15 cells, where β-catenin is localized at the plasma membrane (Gasparoni et al. 2002).

We have also investigated the subcellular localization of β-catenin in different human SCCOC cell lines (e.g., Tu167, DM14, and OSC19) that have different levels of differentiation and malignancy. Tu167 is a more differentiated SCCOC cell line with the indolent local growth and rarely metastasizes when injected into the mouse tongue. DM14 is a less differentiated SCCOC cell line with aggressive local growth and metastasis to cervical lymph nodes when injected into the mouse tongue. OSC19 is the most malignant SCCOC cell line among these three, with the most aggressive local growth and frequent metastasis to cervical lymph nodes. As shown in Fig. 11.2a, β-catenin is predominately localized at the cell membrane in Tu167 cells, whereas cytoplasmic and nuclear staining of β-catenin increase from DM14 to OSC19 cells. This pattern of localization is also shown in orthotopic

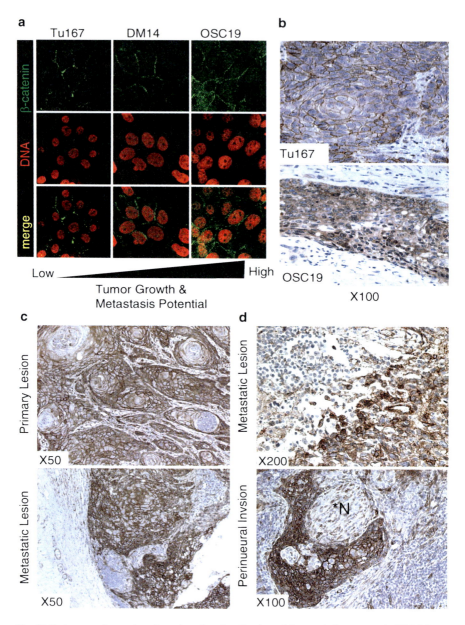

Fig. 11.2 Increased cytoplasmic and nuclear localization of β-catenin in metastatic SCCOC. (a) Immunofluorescent staining of β-catenin in SCCOC cells with different aggressiveness and metastatic potential as indicated. DNA was stained by TO-PRO-3 iodide and is presented by red pseudo color. (b) Immunohistochemical (IHC) staining of β-catenin in mouse orthotopic tongue tumors generated from human Tu167 and OSC19 SCCOC cell lines. (c) IHC staining of β-catenin in a primary human SCCOC tumor lesion and its matched-paired metastatic lesion from a human SCCOC patient. (d) IHC staining of β-catenin in a human metastatic lesion (*upper*) and a perineural invasion region (*bottom*) from two human SCCOC specimens. *N nerve

tongue tumors generated from these cell lines, where strong cytoplasm and nuclear β-catenin is observed in OSC19 tumors (Fig. 11.2b). These results demonstrate that nuclear localization of β-catenin is correlated with tumor invasion, metastatic potential, and tumor malignancy, implying that Wnt/β-catenin signaling plays a role in tumor progression of SCCOC. In support of this, we also observed that strong cytoplasmic and nuclear staining of β-catenin in human SCCOC tumor samples, especially at invasive fronts in both primary and metastatic lesions (Fig 11.2c,d).

Other investigators have found that β-catenin can be found in the cytoplasm and nucleus in the early stages of SCCOC tumor development (Sato et al. 2002; Ishida et al. 2007). In a rat SCCOC model in which almost all of the dysplastic lesions transform to invasive cancers, accumulation of β-catenin in the cytoplasm and nucleus is evident in 10 of 16 dysplastic lesions (Sato et al. 2002), strongly suggesting that β-catenin accumulation may contribute to the early stage of carcinogenesis of SCCOC. More recently, Ishida et al. (2007) reported that nuclear localization of β-catenin can be found in precancerous changes in human oral leukoplakic lesions as well as SCCOC. In this study, the normal oral epithelium showed β-catenin expression only at the cell membrane, and not in the nuclei. In the oral leukoplakia lesions without dysplasia, seven of 17 samples (41%) showed β-catenin expression in the cell membrane, and five samples (29%) showed expression in the nuclei. In the oral leukoplakia with dysplasia, nuclear expression of β-catenin was shown in 11 of 12 samples (92%). The incidence of nuclear β-catenin expression was significantly different between dysplasia and normal oral epithelium, and also between oral leukoplakia with dysplasia and those without dysplasia. In addition, nuclear expression of β-catenin was also observed in 10 of 15 samples of SOOC (Ishida et al. 2007). Therefore, these results suggest that nuclear β-catenin is potentially involved in the progression of normal to dysplastic areas within oral leukoplakia.

In addition to the change in subcellular localization, phosphorylation of β-catenin may also be associated with SCCOC progression. In a rat model of tongue cancer induced with 4-nitroquinoline 1-oxide, in which treatment leads to the development of dysplasia and well-differentiated SCCOC in rat tongues, β-catenin is expressed only in the cell membranes of control tongue suprabasal epithelial cells, whereas dysplastic and cancer cells express β-catenin not only at cell membranes but also in the nuclear and cytoplasmic compartments. During carcinogenesis, however, the levels of expression as well as phosphotyrosine of β-catenin increase gradually, as does the expression of the tyrosine receptor kinase c-Met (Tamura et al. 2003). As discussed before, the tyrosine phosphorylation of β-catenin by c-Met is accompanied by the release of β-catenin from the cell membrane as well as nuclear translocation and activation of downstream target gene expression, resulting in the upregulation of the invasive growth properties of cancer cells (Rasola et al. 2007). Thus these experiments strongly suggested that cell–cell adhesion in epithelial cells can be reduced by phosphorylation of β-catenin associated with increased production of c-Met during SCCOC carcinogenesis, leading to cytoplasmic and nuclear translocation of β-catenin, and invasive growth of the tongue tumors.

Cytoplasmic/nuclear β-catenin expression has also been found to significantly correlate with EGFR expression in SCCOC (Odajima et al. 2005). It has been shown that tyrosine phosphorylation of β-catenin by the EGFR is associated with the perturbation of E-cadherin-mediated cell adhesion and the acquisition of a mesenchymal fibroblast-like morphology and leads to increased cell motility that are requisite for invasion and metastasis in human cancers (Hirohashi 1998; Thiery 2003). Since overexpression of the EGFR is one of most frequent events associated with tumor progression in SCCOC, abnormal cytoplasmic/nuclear β-catenin expression may be associated with tyrosine phosphorylation of β-catenin through the activated EGFR, resulting in decreased cell adhesion followed by increased cell invasion and metastasis. In addition, the EGFR downstream kinase, AKT, has been shown to inhibit GSK-3β (Cross et al. 1995) (which presumably stabilizes β-catenin and activates β-catenin signaling) and play a central role in tumor development (Testa and Bellacosa 2001). In SCCOC cell lines, AKT is highly activated (Nakayama et al. 2001), which induces EMT and enhances tumor cell invasive property (Grille et al. 2003). Therefore, the cytoplasmic/nuclear expression of β-catenin in tumor cells at the invasive front observed in SCCOC may possibly be associated with EMT followed by the acquisition of tumor invasion, which is important for SCCOC tumor metastasis and tumor progression.

Wnt, SFRP and Oral Cancer

A study using cDNA microarrays from laser capture microdissected head and neck squamous cell carcinoma (HNSCC) showed that most HNSCCs overexpress members of the Wnt and Notch growth and differentiation regulatory systems, suggesting that the Wnt and notch pathways may contribute to squamous cell carcinogenesis (Leethanakul et al. 2000). Rhee et al. (2002) investigated the expression and function of five Wnt (Wnt-1, 5a, 7a, 10b, 13) and two Fzd (Fz-2, 5) genes in 10 HNSCC cell lines, and found that compared with normal bronchial or oral epithelial cells, the levels of both proteins and mRNAs of Wnt-1, 10b, and Fz-2 were markedly increased in HNSCC. Moreover, treatment of one HNSCC cell line (SNU 1076) with antiWnt-1 antibodies reduced the Wnt/Fzd-dependent transcription activity of the LEF/TCF, diminished the expression of cyclin D1 and β-catenin proteins, and inhibited cell proliferation and induced apoptosis. These results support the concept that Wnt/β-catenin signaling can be constitutively active in this HNSCC cell line through an autocrine mechanism that is required for its growth and survival. More importantly, Wntβ-catenin signaling was shown to inhibit not only tumor necrosis factor (TNF)/c-Myc-mediated apoptosis, but also cell detachment-mediated apoptosis (anoikis) in HNSCC cell lines. In addition, Wnt/β-catenin signaling pathway induced HNSCC cell scattering and promoted cell invasion both in vitro and in vivo invasive growth of HNSCC cells (Yang et al. 2006a). In a study of oral leukoplakia, Wnt3 expression was detected at the epithelial cell membrane or in cytoplasm of oral leukoplakia where nuclear expression of β-catenin was evident, but not in epithelial cells without nuclear expression of β-catenin. In the samples with nuclear expression of β-catenin, Wnt3 expression was shown in 13 of 16 samples (81%), and there was significant positive correlation between the nuclear expression of β-catenin and Wnt staining (Ishida et al. 2007). Uraguchi et al. (2004) showed by reverse-transcriptase polymerase chain reaction (RT/PCR) that SCCOC carcinoma cells express 11 of 19 Wnt family members. They also found that Wnt-expressing carcinoma cells exhibit increased β-catenin levels in the cytoplasmic and nuclear pools. In addition, Wnt3 staining was observed predominantly at the invasive front in SCCOC cells in 28 of 42 carcinoma tissue specimens (57%). Interestingly, endothelial cells, fibroblast-like cells, and macrophage-like cells were all positively stained for Wnt3, whereas normal oral tissues did not stain with the antiWnt3 antibody (Uraguchi et al. 2004). In these same tissues, β-catenin primarily stained the cell–cell boundaries of the carcinoma cells and localized to the nucleus and diffusively in cytoplasm in tumor cells at the invasive front (Uraguchi et al. 2004). It has been shown that the invasive front is the place where cells evade cell–cell adhesion and gain the characteristics of EMTs (Brabletz et al. 2001), and that EMTs are particularly prominent at the invasive front and predispose carcinomas to a more advanced state of progression (Birchmeier et al. 1996). Because Wnt3 is a typical and powerful member of the family which activates Wnt/β-catenin-mediated signaling (Seidensticker and Behrens 2000), the colocalization of both Wnt3 and nuclear β-catenin at the invasive front suggested that Wnt signaling can trigger nuclear translocation of β-catenin and EMTs. Similar findings have been reported in colorectal carcinomas (Eger et al. 2000; Kirchner and Brabletz 2000; Brabletz et al. 2001). In addition, the fibroblast-type Wnts and β-catenin-mediated signaling are documented to initiate malignant transformation and enhance cellular proliferation, dedifferentiation, invasion and metastasis (Lo Muzio 2001). Therefore, the evidence described above when taken together suggests that both autocrine and paracrine signaling are implicated in modulating Wnt/β-catenin signaling to activate EMTs, tumor invasion, and tumor progression of SCCOC.

Finally, epigenetic modification has been shown to play an important role in the regulation of Wnt/β-catenin signaling. For example, In HNSCC epigenetic inactivation of the *SFRP* genes, encoding antagonists of the Wnt pathway, was found to be associated with drinking, smoking, and human papillomavirus (HPV) expression (Marsit et al. 2006). Methylation-specific PCR showed that the prevalence of methylation of SFRP1, SFRP2, SFRP4, and SFRP5 was 35%, 32%, 35%, and 29%, respectively, among 350 HNSCC cases. Promoter methylation of SFRP1 occurred more often in both heavy and light drinkers compared with nondrinkers. SFRP4 promoter methylation, on the other hand, occurred at a higher prevalence in non smokers and former smokers than in current smokers, and also was independently associated with the presence of HPV16 viral DNA. A joint effects model of SFRP4 promoter methylation demonstrated that it significantly interacted with smoking and HPV status in HNSCC. These results suggest that aberrant activation of the Wnt pathway through silencing of pathway antagonists, the *SFRP* genes, is highly prevalent in HNSCC, and that the clonal selection for these alterations is complex and may be related to the carcinogenic exposures that are known risk factors, such as HPV and alcohol, for this disease (Marsit et al. 2006).

Conclusion

Although aberrant Wnt/β-catenin signaling has been implicated in the tumorigenesis and tumor progression of many cancers, its role in SCCOC remains largely undefined. While there is evidence to suggest that this pathway plays a role in the development of this tumor type, some data support a limited role for Wnt/β-catenin signaling in SCCOC development and progression. Most of the supporting evidence has come from immunohistochemical evaluations that show that β-catenin staining at the cell membrane decreases during SCCOC tumor progression without apparent nuclear localization. It should be noted that such studies using immunostaining always depend on the quality of antibodies as well as on different staining protocols. In addition, specimen quality, the method of evaluation of immunostaining, and the definition of reduced or underexpression are quite variable and subjective in different studies. Sometimes a semiquantitative estimation of the immunostaining intensity was used with varying criteria, while the expression analysis was carried out in different areas of the tumor by different investigators. Thus all these factors related to methodology may account for the discrepancy in the results obtained from different studies. Nevertheless, the frequent observation of cytoplasmic and nuclear localization of β-catenin in premalignant oral leukoplakia as well as at the invasive front of tumors suggests that Wnt/β-catenin signaling may play a role in tumor initiation and progression, tumor invasive growth, as well as EMT of SCCOC. All these are required for the tumor metastasis. However, the molecular and cellular mechanisms involved are still unclear. In particular, infrequent mutations in the *APC*, *β-catenin*, *Axin* do not account for the activation of Wnt/β-catenin signaling in most of SCCOCs. It is likely that the Wnt/β-catenin pathway is implicated in SCCOC through multiple, diverse mechanisms including genetic and epigenetic alterations of the components in this signaling pathway, and alterations in other autocrine and/or paracrine factors that are involved in the regulation of this pathway in a Wnt-dependent or even Wnt-independent manner. More importantly, the interaction between epithelial tumor cells and the different components of the surrounding microenvironment can locally affect the intracellular levels of canonical Wnt/β-catenin signaling and differentially trigger tumor cell stemness, cell proliferation, EMT, invasive behavior, and metastasis. So far, little is known about the factors and mechanisms involved. Likewise, it is still unclear how the Wnt/β-catenin signaling pathway induces downstream genes that are implicated in invasive growth and metastasis of SCCOC. Therefore, further investigation is necessary for understanding the role of Wnt/β-catenin signaling in SCCOC. Gain-and loss-of-function studies with various components of Wnt/β-catenin signaling in cell culture and animal models will be of particular value for evaluating the contribution of each component to SCCOC. All these will provide us with greater insights into the molecular and cellular mechanisms involved in the initiation, progression, and metastasis of oral cancers.

References

Aberle H, Bauer A, Stappert J, Kispert A, Kemler R (1997) Beta-catenin is a target for the ubiquitin-proteasome pathway. EMBO J 16:3797–3804

Andl T, Reddy ST, Gaddapara T, Millar SE (2002) WNT signals are required for the initiation of hair follicle development. Dev Cell 2:643–653

Bafico A, Liu G, Goldin L, Harris V, Aaronson SA (2004) An autocrine mechanism for constitutive Wnt pathway activation in human cancer cells. Cancer Cell 6:497–506

Bankfalvi A, Krassort M, Buchwalow IB, Vegh A, Felszeghy E, Piffko J (2002a) Gains and losses of adhesion molecules (CD44, E-cadherin, and beta-catenin) during oral carcinogenesis and tumour progression. J Pathol 198:343–351

Bankfalvi A, Krassort M, Vegh A, Felszeghy E, Piffko J (2002b) Deranged expression of the E-cadherin/beta-catenin complex and the epidermal growth factor receptor in the clinical evolution and progression of oral squamous cell carcinomas. J Oral Pathol Med 31:450–457

Bardelli A, Parsons DW, Silliman N, Ptak J, Szabo S, Saha S, Markowitz S, Willson JK, Parmigiani G, Kinzler KW et al (2003) Mutational analysis of the tyrosine kinome in colorectal cancers. Science 300:949

Barker N, Clevers H (2006) Mining the Wnt pathway for cancer therapeutics. Nat Rev Drug Discov 5:997–1014

Barker N, Huls G, Korinek V, Clevers H (1999) Restricted high level expression of Tcf-4 protein in intestinal and mammary gland epithelium. Am J Pathol 154:29–35

Barker N, Hurlstone A, Musisi H, Miles A, Bienz M, Clevers H (2001) The chromatin remodelling factor Brg-1 interacts with beta-catenin to promote target gene activation. EMBO J 20:4935–4943

Batlle E, Henderson JT, Beghtel H, van den Born MM, Sancho E, Huls G, Meeldijk J, Robertson J, van de Wetering M, Pawson T, Clevers H (2002) Beta-catenin and TCF mediate cell positioning in the intestinal epithelium by controlling the expression of EphB/ephrinB. Cell 111:251–263

Behrens J, von Kries JP, Kuhl M, Bruhn L, Wedlich D, Grosschedl R, Birchmeier W (1996) Functional interaction of beta-catenin with the transcription factor LEF-1. Nature 382:638–642

Bell DA (2005) Origins and molecular pathology of ovarian cancer. Mod Pathol 18(Suppl 2):S19–S32

Birchmeier C, Birchmeier W, Brand-Saberi B (1996) Epithelial-mesenchymal transitions in cancer progression. Acta Anat (Basel) 156:217–226

Birchmeier C, Birchmeier W, Gherardi E, Vande Woude GF (2003) Met, metastasis, motility and more. Nat Rev Mol Cell Biol 4:915–925

Blache P, van de Wetering M, Duluc I, Domon C, Berta P, Freund JN, Clevers H, Jay P (2004) SOX9 is an intestine crypt transcription factor, is regulated by the Wnt pathway, and represses the CDX2 and MUC2 genes. J Cell Biol 166:37–47

Blanpain C, Horsley V, Fuchs E (2007) Epithelial stem cells: turning over new leaves. Cell 128:445–458

Brabletz T, Jung A, Hermann K, Gunther K, Hohenberger W, Kirchner T (1998) Nuclear overexpression of the oncoprotein beta-catenin in colorectal cancer is localized predominantly at the invasion front. Pathol Res Pract 194:701–704

Brabletz T, Jung A, Reu S, Porzner M, Hlubek F, Kunz-Schughart LA, Knuechel R, Kirchner T (2001) Variable beta-catenin expression in colorectal cancers indicates tumor progression driven by the tumor environment. Proc Natl Acad Sci U S A 98:10356–10361

Brabletz T, Jung A, Spaderna S, Hlubek F, Kirchner T (2005) Opinion: migrating cancer stem cells – an integrated concept of malignant tumour progression. Nat Rev Cancer 5:744–749

Brantjes H, Barker N, van Es J, Clevers H (2002) TCF: Lady Justice casting the final verdict on the outcome of Wnt signalling. Biol Chem 383:255–261

Brembeck FH, Schwarz-Romond T, Bakkers J, Wilhelm S, Hammerschmidt M, Birchmeier W (2004) Essential role of BCL9-2 in the switch between beta-catenin's adhesive and transcriptional functions. Genes Dev 18:2225–2230

Brennan K, Gonzalez-Sancho JM, Castelo-Soccio LA, Howe LR, Brown AM (2004) Truncated mutants of the putative Wnt receptor LRP6/Arrow can stabilize beta-catenin independently of Frizzled proteins. Oncogene 23:4873–4884

Brown JR, DuBois RN (2005) COX-2: a molecular target for colorectal cancer prevention. J Clin Oncol 23:2840–2855

Brunner E, Peter O, Schweizer L, Basler K (1997) pangolin encodes a Lef-1 homologue that acts downstream of Armadillo to transduce the Wingless signal in Drosophila. Nature 385:829–833

Caldwell GM, Jones C, Gensberg K, Jan S, Hardy RG, Byrd P, Chughtai S, Wallis Y, Matthews GM, Morton DG (2004) The Wnt antagonist sFRP1 in colorectal tumorigenesis. Cancer Res 64:883–888

Castellone MD, Teramoto H, Williams BO, Druey KM, Gutkind JS (2005) Prostaglandin E2 promotes colon cancer cell growth through a Gs-axin-beta-catenin signaling axis. Science 310:1504–1510

Cavallo RA, Cox RT, Moline MM, Roose J, Polevoy GA, Clevers H, Peifer M, Bejsovec A (1998) Drosophila Tcf and Groucho interact to repress Wingless signalling activity. Nature 395:604–608

Chamorro MN, Schwartz DR, Vonica A, Brivanlou AH, Cho KR, Varmus HE (2005) FGF-20 and DKK1 are transcriptional targets of beta-catenin and FGF-20 is implicated in cancer and development. EMBO J 24:73–84

Chang KW, Lin SC, Mangold KA, Jean MS, Yuan TC, Lin SN, Chang CS (2000) Alterations of adenomatous polyposis Coli (APC) gene in oral squamous cell carcinoma. Int J Oral Maxillofac Surg 29:223–226

Chen G, Fernandez J, Mische S, Courey AJ (1999) A functional interaction between the histone deacetylase Rpd3 and the corepressor groucho in Drosophila development. Genes Dev 13:2218–2230

Chen T, Yang I, Irby R, Shain KH, Wang HG, Quackenbush J, Coppola D, Cheng JQ, Yeatman TJ (2003a) Regulation of caspase expression and apoptosis by adenomatous polyposis coli. Cancer Res 63:4368–4374

Chen W, ten Berge D, Brown J, Ahn S, Hu LA, Miller WE, Caron MG, Barak LS, Nusse R, Lefkowitz RJ (2003b) Dishevelled 2 recruits beta-arrestin 2 to mediate Wnt5A-stimulated endocytosis of Frizzled 4. Science 301:1391–1394

Chow V, Yuen AP, Lam KY, Tsao GS, Ho WK, Wei WI (2001) A comparative study of the clinicopathological significance of E-cadherin and catenins (alpha, beta, gamma) expression in the surgical management of oral tongue carcinoma. J Cancer Res Clin Oncol 127:59–63

Chu EY, Hens J, Andl T, Kairo A, Yamaguchi TP, Brisken C, Glick A, Wysolmerski JJ, Millar SE (2004) Canonical WNT signaling promotes mammary placode development and is essential for initiation of mammary gland morphogenesis. Development 131:4819–4829

Clarke MF, Dick JE, Dirks PB, Eaves CJ, Jamieson CH, Jones DL, Visvader J, Weissman IL, Wahl GM (2006) Cancer stem cells – perspectives on current status and future directions: AACR Workshop on cancer stem cells. Cancer Res 66:9339–9344

Clevers H (2006) Wnt/beta-catenin signaling in development and disease. Cell 127:469–480

Cross DA, Alessi DR, Cohen P, Andjelkovich M, Hemmings BA (1995) Inhibition of glycogen synthase kinase-3 by insulin mediated by protein kinase B. Nature 378:785–789

Cuilliere-Dartigues P, El-Bchiri J, Krimi A, Buhard O, Fontanges P, Flejou JF, Hamelin R, Duval A (2006) TCF-4 isoforms absent in TCF-4 mutated MSI-H colorectal cancer cells colocalize with nuclear CtBP and repress TCF-4-mediated transcription. Oncogene 25:4441–4448

DasGupta R, Fuchs E (1999) Multiple roles for activated LEF/TCF transcription complexes during hair follicle development and differentiation. Development 126:4557–4568

Davidson G, Wu W, Shen J, Bilic J, Fenger U, Stannek P, Glinka A, Niehrs C (2005) Casein kinase 1 gamma couples Wnt receptor activation to cytoplasmic signal transduction. Nature 438:867–872

Day TF, Guo X, Garrett-Beal L, Yang Y (2005) Wnt/beta-catenin signaling in mesenchymal progenitors controls osteoblast and chondrocyte differentiation during vertebrate skeletogenesis. Dev Cell 8:739–750

De Wever O, Nguyen QD, Van Hoorde L, Bracke M, Bruyneel E, Gespach C, Mareel M (2004) Tenascin-C and SF/HGF produced by myofibroblasts in vitro provide convergent pro-invasive signals to human colon cancer cells through RhoA and Rac. FASEB J 18:1016–1018

Demunter A, Libbrecht L, Degreef H, De Wolf-Peeters C, van den Oord JJ (2002) Loss of membranous expression of beta-catenin is associated with tumor progression in cutaneous melanoma and rarely caused by exon 3 mutations. Mod Pathol 15:454–461

Duncan AW, Rattis FM, DiMascio LN, Congdon KL, Pazianos G, Zhao C, Yoon K, Cook JM, Willert K, Gaiano N, Reya T (2005) Integration of Notch and Wnt signaling in hematopoietic stem cell maintenance. Nat Immunol 6:314–322

Duval A, Gayet J, Zhou XP, Iacopetta B, Thomas G, Hamelin R (1999) Frequent frameshift mutations of the TCF-4 gene in colorectal cancers with microsatellite instability. Cancer Res 59:4213–4215

Eger A, Stockinger A, Schaffhauser B, Beug H, Foisner R (2000) Epithelial mesenchymal transition by c-Fos estrogen receptor activation involves nuclear translocation of beta-catenin and upregulation of beta-catenin/lymphoid enhancer binding factor-1 transcriptional activity. J Cell Biol 148:173–188

Esteller M, Sparks A, Toyota M, Sanchez-Cespedes M, Capella G, Peinado MA, Gonzalez S, Tarafa G, Sidransky D, Meltzer SJ et al (2000) Analysis of adenomatous polyposis coli promoter hypermethylation in human cancer. Cancer Res 60:4366–4371

Fearnhead NS, Wilding JL, Winney B, Tonks S, Bartlett S, Bicknell DC, Tomlinson IP, Mortensen NJ, Bodmer WF (2004) Multiple rare variants in different genes account for multifactorial inherited susceptibility to colorectal adenomas. Proc Natl Acad Sci U S A 101:15992–15997

Fillies T, Buerger H, Gaertner C, August C, Brandt B, Joos U, Werkmeister R (2005) Catenin expression in T1/2 carcinomas of the floor of the mouth. Int J Oral Maxillofac Surg 34:907–911

Fodde R, Brabletz T (2007) Wnt/beta-catenin signaling in cancer stemness and malignant behavior. Curr Opin Cell Biol 19:150–158

Fukushima H, Yamamoto H, Itoh F, Horiuchi S, Min Y, Iku S, Imai K (2001) Frequent alterations of the beta-catenin and TCF-4 genes, but not of the APC gene, in colon cancers with high-frequency microsatellite instability. J Exp Clin Cancer Res 20:553–559

Furuuchi K, Tada M, Yamada H, Kataoka A, Furuuchi N, Hamada J, Takahashi M, Todo S, Moriuchi T (2000) Somatic mutations of the APC gene in primary breast cancers. Am J Pathol 156:1997–2005

Gao S, Eiberg H, Krogdahl A, Liu CJ, Sorensen JA (2005) Cytoplasmic expression of E-cadherin and beta-Catenin correlated with LOH and hypermethylation of the APC gene in oral squamous cell carcinomas. J Oral Pathol Med 34:116–119

Gasparoni A, Chaves A, Fonzi L, Johnson GK, Schneider GB, Squier CA (2002) Subcellular localization of beta-catenin in malignant cell lines and squamous cell carcinomas of the oral cavity. J Oral Pathol Med 31:385–394

Gat U, DasGupta R, Degenstein L, Fuchs E (1998) De Novo hair follicle morphogenesis and hair tumors in mice expressing a truncated beta-catenin in skin. Cell 95:605–614

Giles RH, van Es JH, Clevers H (2003) Caught up in a Wnt storm: Wnt signaling in cancer. Biochim Biophys Acta 1653:1–24

Gordon MD, Nusse R (2006) Wnt signaling: multiple pathways, multiple receptors, and multiple transcription factors. J Biol Chem 281:22429–22433

Gregorieff A, Pinto D, Begthel H, Destree O, Kielman M, Clevers H (2005) Expression pattern of Wnt signaling components in the adult intestine. Gastroenterology 129:626–638

Grille SJ, Bellacosa A, Upson J, Klein-Szanto AJ, van Roy F, Lee-Kwon W, Donowitz M, Tsichlis PN, Larue L (2003) The protein kinase Akt induces epithelial mesenchymal transition and promotes enhanced motility and invasiveness of squamous cell carcinoma lines. Cancer Res 63:2172–2178

Groden J, Thliveris A, Samowitz W, Carlson M, Gelbert L, Albertsen H, Joslyn G, Stevens J, Spirio L, Robertson M et al (1991) Identification and characterization of the familial adenomatous polyposis coli gene. Cell 66:589–600

Hart M, Concordet JP, Lassot I, Albert I, del los Santos R, Durand H, Perret C, Rubinfeld B, Margottin F, Benarous R, Polakis P (1999) The F-box protein beta-TrCP associates with phosphorylated beta-catenin and regulates its activity in the cell. Curr Biol 9:207–210

He TC, Sparks AB, Rago C, Hermeking H, Zawel L, da Costa LT, Morin PJ, Vogelstein B, Kinzler KW (1998) Identification of c-MYC as a target of the APC pathway. Science 281:1509–1512

He X (2006) Unwinding a path to nuclear beta-catenin. Cell 127:40–42

Hecht A, Kemler R (2000) Curbing the nuclear activities of beta-catenin. Control over Wnt target gene expression. EMBO Rep 1:24–28

Heldin CH, Westermark B (1999) Mechanism of action and in vivo role of platelet-derived growth factor. Physiol Rev 79:1283–1316

Hirohashi S (1998) Inactivation of the E-cadherin-mediated cell adhesion system in human cancers. Am J Pathol 153:333–339

Huang JS, Chiang CP, Kok SH, Kuo YS, Kuo MY (1997) Loss of heterozygosity of APC and MCC genes in oral squamous cell carcinomas in Taiwan. J Oral Pathol Med 26:322–326

Huber MA, Kraut N, Beug H (2005) Molecular requirements for epithelial-mesenchymal transition during tumor progression. Curr Opin Cell Biol 17:548–558

Huelsken J, Vogel R, Erdmann B, Cotsarelis G, Birchmeier W (2001) beta-Catenin controls hair follicle morphogenesis and stem cell differentiation in the skin. Cell 105:533–545

Ilyas M, Tomlinson IP, Rowan A, Pignatelli M, Bodmer WF (1997) Beta-catenin mutations in cell lines established from human colorectal cancers. Proc Natl Acad Sci U S A 94:10330–10334

Irving JA, Catasus L, Gallardo A, Bussaglia E, Romero M, Matias-Guiu X, Prat J (2005) Synchronous endometrioid carcinomas of the uterine corpus and ovary: alterations in the beta-catenin (CTNNB1) pathway are associated with independent primary tumors and favorable prognosis. Hum Pathol 36:605–619

Ishida K, Ito S, Wada N, Deguchi H, Hata T, Hosoda M, Nohno T (2007) Nuclear localization of beta-catenin involved in precancerous change in oral leukoplakia. Mol Cancer 6:62

Ishitani T, Kishida S, Hyodo-Miura J, Ueno N, Yasuda J, Waterman M, Shibuya H, Moon RT, Ninomiya-Tsuji J, Matsumoto K (2003a) The TAK1-NLK mitogen-activated protein kinase cascade functions in the Wnt-5a/Ca(2+) pathway to antagonize Wnt/beta-catenin signaling. Mol Cell Biol 23:131–139

Ishitani T, Ninomiya-Tsuji J, Matsumoto K (2003b) Regulation of lymphoid enhancer factor 1/T-cell factor by mitogen-activated protein kinase-related Nemo-like kinase-dependent phosphorylation in Wnt/beta-catenin signaling. Mol Cell Biol 23:1379–1389

Iwai S, Katagiri W, Kong C, Amekawa S, Nakazawa M, Yura Y (2005) Mutations of the APC, beta-catenin, and axin 1 genes and cytoplasmic accumulation of beta-catenin in oral squamous cell carcinoma. J Cancer Res Clin Oncol 131:773–782

Janssen KP, Alberici P, Fsihi H, Gaspar C, Breukel C, Franken P, Rosty C, Abal M, El Marjou F, Smits R et al (2006) APC and oncogenic KRAS are synergistic in enhancing Wnt signaling in intestinal tumor formation and progression. Gastroenterology 131:1096–1109

Johnson V, Volikos E, Halford SE, Eftekhar Sadat ET, Popat S, Talbot I, Truninger K, Martin J, Jass J, Houlston R et al (2005) Exon 3 beta-catenin mutations are specifically associated with colorectal carcinomas in hereditary non-polyposis colorectal cancer syndrome. Gut 54:264–267

Katoh M, Katoh M (2006) Notch ligand, JAG1, is evolutionarily conserved target of canonical WNT signaling pathway in progenitor cells. Int J Mol Med 17:681–685

Kawano Y, Kypta R (2003) Secreted antagonists of the Wnt signalling pathway. J Cell Sci 116:2627–2634

Kim JH, Kim B, Cai L, Choi HJ, Ohgi KA, Tran C, Chen C, Chung CH, Huber O, Rose DW et al (2005) Transcriptional regulation of a metastasis suppressor gene by Tip60 and beta-catenin complexes. Nature 434:921–926

Kinch MS, Clark GJ, Der CJ, Burridge K (1995) Tyrosine phosphorylation regulates the adhesions of ras-transformed breast epithelia. J Cell Biol 130:461–471

Kinzler KW, Nilbert MC, Su LK, Vogelstein B, Bryan TM, Levy DB, Smith KJ, Preisinger AC, Hedge P, McKechnie D et al (1991) Identification of FAP locus genes from chromosome 5q21. Science 253:661–665

Kinzler KW, Vogelstein B (1996) Lessons from hereditary colorectal cancer. Cell 87:159–170

Kioussi C, Briata P, Baek SH, Rose DW, Hamblet NS, Herman T, Ohgi KA, Lin C, Gleiberman A, Wang J et al (2002) Identification of a Wnt/Dvl/beta-Catenin → Pitx2 pathway mediating cell-type-specific proliferation during development. Cell 111:673–685

Kirchner T, Brabletz T (2000) Patterning and nuclear beta-catenin expression in the colonic adenoma-carcinoma sequence. Analogies with embryonic gastrulation. Am J Pathol 157: 1113–1121

Kishida M, Hino S, Michiue T, Yamamoto H, Kishida S, Fukui A, Asashima M, Kikuchi A (2001) Synergistic activation of the Wnt signaling pathway by Dvl and casein kinase Iepsilon. J Biol Chem 276:33147–33155

Koesters R, Niggli F, von Knebel Doeberitz M, Stallmach T (2003) Nuclear accumulation of beta-catenin protein in Wilms' tumours. J Pathol 199:68–76

Koesters R, Ridder R, Kopp-Schneider A, Betts D, Adams V, Niggli F, Briner J, von Knebel Doeberitz M (1999) Mutational activation of the beta-catenin proto-oncogene is a common event in the development of Wilms' tumors. Cancer Res 59:3880–3882

Kok SH, Lee JJ, Hsu HC, Chiang CP, Kuo YS, Kuo MY (2002) Mutations of the adenomatous polyposis coli gene in areca quid and tobacco-associated oral squamous cell carcinomas in Taiwan. J Oral Pathol Med 31:395–401

Korinek V, Barker N, Morin PJ, van Wichen D, de Weger R, Kinzler KW, Vogelstein B, Clevers H (1997) Constitutive transcriptional activation by a beta-catenin-Tcf complex in APC–/– colon carcinoma. Science 275:1784–1787

Kramps T, Peter O, Brunner E, Nellen D, Froesch B, Chatterjee S, Murone M, Zullig S, Basler K (2002) Wnt/wingless signaling requires BCL9/legless-mediated recruitment of pygopus to the nuclear beta-catenin-TCF complex. Cell 109:47–60

Kudo Y, Kitajima S, Ogawa I, Hiraoka M, Sargolzaei S, Keikhaee MR, Sato S, Miyauchi M, Takata T (2004) Invasion and metastasis of oral cancer cells require methylation of E-cadherin and/or degradation of membranous beta-catenin. Clin Cancer Res 10:5455–5463

Largey JS, Meltzer SJ, Sauk JJ, Hebert CA, Archibald DW (1994) Loss of heterozygosity involving the APC gene in oral squamous cell carcinomas. Oral Surg Oral Med Oral Pathol 77:260–263

Latres E, Chiaur DS, Pagano M (1999) The human F box protein beta-Trcp associates with the Cul1/Skp1 complex and regulates the stability of beta-catenin. Oncogene 18:849–854

Lee HY, Kleber M, Hari L, Brault V, Suter U, Taketo MM, Kemler R, Sommer L (2004) Instructive role of Wnt/beta-catenin in sensory fate specification in neural crest stem cells. Science 303:1020–1023

Leethanakul C, Patel V, Gillespie J, Pallente M, Ensley JF, Koontongkaew S, Liotta LA, Emmert-Buck M, Gutkind JS (2000) Distinct pattern of expression of differentiation and growth-related genes in squamous cell carcinomas of the head and neck revealed by the use of laser capture microdissection and cDNA arrays. Oncogene 19:3220–3224

Li J, Sutter C, Parker DS, Blauwkamp T, Fang M, Cadigan KM (2007) CBP/p300 are bimodal regulators of Wnt signaling. Embo J 26:2284–2294

Lilien J, Balsamo J (2005) The regulation of cadherin-mediated adhesion by tyrosine phosphorylation/dephosphorylation of beta-catenin. Curr Opin Cell Biol 17:459–465

Liu C, Li Y, Semenov M, Han C, Baeg GH, Tan Y, Zhang Z, Lin X, He X (2002) Control of beta-catenin phosphorylation/degradation by a dual-kinase mechanism. Cell 108:837–847

Lo Celso C, Prowse DM, Watt FM (2004) Transient activation of beta-catenin signalling in adult mouse epidermis is sufficient to induce new hair follicles but continuous activation is required to maintain hair follicle tumours. Development 131:1787–1799

Lo Muzio L (2001) A possible role for the WNT-1 pathway in oral carcinogenesis. Crit Rev Oral Biol Med 12:152–165

Lo Muzio L, Goteri G, Capretti R, Rubini C, Vinella A, Fumarolo R, Bianchi F, Mastrangelo F, Porfiri E, Mariggio MA (2005) Beta-catenin gene analysis in oral squamous cell carcinoma. Int J Immunopathol Pharmacol 18:33–38

Lo Muzio L, Staibano S, Pannone G, Grieco M, Mignogna MD, Cerrato A, Testa NF, De Rosa G (1999) Beta- and gamma-catenin expression in oral squamous cell carcinomas. Anticancer Res 19:3817–3826

Lowry WE, Blanpain C, Nowak JA, Guasch G, Lewis L, Fuchs E (2005) Defining the impact of beta-catenin/Tcf transactivation on epithelial stem cells. Genes Dev 19:1596–1611

Luchtenborg M, Weijenberg MP, Wark PA, Saritas AM, Roemen GM, van Muijen GN, de Bruine AP, van den Brandt PA, de Goeij AF (2005) Mutations in APC, CTNNB1 and K-ras genes and expression of hMLH1 in sporadic colorectal carcinomas from the Netherlands Cohort Study. BMC Cancer 5:160

Mahomed F, Altini M, Meer S (2007) Altered E-cadherin/beta-catenin expression in oral squamous carcinoma with and without nodal metastasis. Oral Dis 13:386–392

Major MB, Camp ND, Berndt JD, Yi X, Goldenberg SJ, Hubbert C, Biechele TL, Gingras AC, Zheng N, Maccoss MJ et al (2007) Wilms tumor suppressor WTX negatively regulates WNT/beta-catenin signaling. Science 316:1043–1046

Mann B, Gelos M, Siedow A, Hanski ML, Gratchev A, Ilyas M, Bodmer WF, Moyer MP, Riecken EO, Buhr HJ, Hanski C (1999) Target genes of beta-catenin-T cell-factor/lymphoid-enhancer-factor signaling in human colorectal carcinomas. Proc Natl Acad Sci U S A 96:1603–1608

Mao J, Wang J, Liu B, Pan W, Farr GH III, Flynn C, Yuan H, Takada S, Kimelman D, Li L, Wu D (2001) Low-density lipoprotein receptor-related protein-5 binds to Axin and regulates the canonical Wnt signaling pathway. Mol Cell 7:801–809

Marsit CJ, McClean MD, Furniss CS, Kelsey KT (2006) Epigenetic inactivation of the SFRP genes is associated with drinking, smoking and HPV in head and neck squamous cell carcinoma. Int J Cancer 119:1761–1766

McDonald SA, Preston SL, Lovell MJ, Wright NA, Jankowski JA (2006) Mechanisms of disease: from stem cells to colorectal cancer. Nat Clin Pract Gastroenterol Hepatol 3:267–274

Merrill BJ, Gat U, DasGupta R, Fuchs E (2001) Tcf3 and Lef1 regulate lineage differentiation of multipotent stem cells in skin. Genes Dev 15:1688–1705

Moon RT, Kohn AD, De Ferrari GV, Kaykas A (2004) WNT and beta-catenin signalling: diseases and therapies. Nat Rev Genet 5:691–701

Morin PJ, Sparks AB, Korinek V, Barker N, Clevers H, Vogelstein B, Kinzler KW (1997) Activation of beta-catenin-Tcf signaling in colon cancer by mutations in beta-catenin or APC. Science 275:1787–1790

Morin PJ, Weeraratna AT (2003) Wnt signaling in human cancer. Cancer Treat Res 115:169–187

Munemitsu S, Albert I, Souza B, Rubinfeld B, Polakis P (1995) Regulation of intracellular beta-catenin levels by the adenomatous polyposis coli (APC) tumor-suppressor protein. Proc Natl Acad Sci U S A 92:3046–3050

Nakayama H, Ikebe T, Beppu M, Shirasuna K (2001) High expression levels of nuclear factor kappaB, IkappaB kinase alpha and Akt kinase in squamous cell carcinoma of the oral cavity. Cancer 92:3037–3044

Nam JS, Turcotte TJ, Smith PF, Choi S, Yoon JK (2006) Mouse cristin/R-spondin family proteins are novel ligands for the Frizzled 8 and LRP6 receptors and activate beta-catenin-dependent gene expression. J Biol Chem 281:13247–13257

Nelson WJ, Nusse R (2004) Convergence of Wnt, beta-catenin, and cadherin pathways. Science 303:1483–1487

Neufeld KL, Zhang F, Cullen BR, White RL (2000) APC-mediated downregulation of beta-catenin activity involves nuclear sequestration and nuclear export. EMBO Rep 1:519–523

Nguyen H, Rendl M, Fuchs E (2006) Tcf3 governs stem cell features and represses cell fate determination in skin. Cell 127:171–183

Niemann C (2006) Controlling the stem cell niche: right time, right place, right strength. Bioessays 28:1–5

Odajima T, Sasaki Y, Tanaka N, Kato-Mori Y, Asanuma H, Ikeda T, Satoh M, Hiratsuka H, Tokino T, Sawada N (2005) Abnormal beta-catenin expression in oral cancer with no gene mutation: correlation with expression of cyclin D1 and epidermal growth factor receptor, Ki-67 labeling index, and clinicopathological features. Hum Pathol 36:234–241

Ohgaki H, Kros JM, Okamoto Y, Gaspert A, Huang H, Kurrer MO (2004) APC mutations are infrequent but present in human lung cancer. Cancer Lett 207:197–203

Oliva E, Sarrio D, Brachtel EF, Sanchez-Estevez C, Soslow RA, Moreno-Bueno G, Palacios J (2006) High frequency of beta-catenin mutations in borderline endometrioid tumours of the ovary. J Pathol 208:708–713

Olson LE, Tollkuhn J, Scafoglio C, Krones A, Zhang J, Ohgi KA, Wu W, Taketo MM, Kemler R, Grosschedl R et al (2006) Homeodomain-mediated beta-catenin-dependent switching events dictate cell-lineage determination. Cell 125:593–605

Ormestad M, Astorga J, Landgren H, Wang T, Johansson BR, Miura N, Carlsson P (2006) Foxf1 and Foxf2 control murine gut development by limiting mesenchymal Wnt signaling and promoting extracellular matrix production. Development 133:833–843

Paoni NF, Feldman MW, Gutierrez LS, Ploplis VA, Castellino FJ (2003) Transcriptional profiling of the transition from normal intestinal epithelia to adenomas and carcinomas in the APCMin/+ mouse. Physiol Genomics 15:228–235

Parker DS, Jemison J, Cadigan KM (2002) Pygopus, a nuclear PHD-finger protein required for Wingless signaling in Drosophila. Development 129:2565–2576

Perreault N, Katz JP, Sackett SD, Kaestner KH (2001) Foxl1 controls the Wnt/beta-catenin pathway by modulating the expression of proteoglycans in the gut. J Biol Chem 276:43328–43333

Perreault N, Sackett SD, Katz JP, Furth EE, Kaestner KH (2005) Foxl1 is a mesenchymal Modifier of Min in carcinogenesis of stomach and colon. Genes Dev 19:311–315

Piccolo S, Agius E, Leyns L, Bhattacharyya S, Grunz H, Bouwmeester T, De Robertis EM (1999) The head inducer Cerberus is a multifunctional antagonist of Nodal, BMP and Wnt signals. Nature 397:707–710

Piedra J, Martinez D, Castano J, Miravet S, Dunach M, de Herreros AG (2001) Regulation of beta-catenin structure and activity by tyrosine phosphorylation. J Biol Chem 276:20436–20443

Pinson KI, Brennan J, Monkley S, Avery BJ, Skarnes WC (2000) An LDL-receptor-related protein mediates Wnt signalling in mice. Nature 407:535–538

Polakis P (2007) The many ways of Wnt in cancer. Curr Opin Genet Dev 17:45–51

Radtke F, Clevers H (2005) Self-renewal and cancer of the gut: two sides of a coin. Science 307:1904–1909

Radtke F, Clevers H, Riccio O (2006) From gut homeostasis to cancer. Curr Mol Med 6:275–289

Rajagopalan H, Bardelli A, Lengauer C, Kinzler KW, Vogelstein B, Velculescu VE (2002) Tumorigenesis: RAF/RAS oncogenes and mismatch-repair status. Nature 418:934

Rasola A, Fassetta M, De Bacco F, D'Alessandro L, Gramaglia D, Di Renzo MF, Comoglio PM (2007) A positive feedback loop between hepatocyte growth factor receptor and beta-catenin sustains colorectal cancer cell invasive growth. Oncogene 26:1078–1087

Reya T, Clevers H (2005) Wnt signalling in stem cells and cancer. Nature 434:843–850

Reya T, Morrison SJ, Clarke MF, Weissman IL (2001) Stem cells, cancer, and cancer stem cells. Nature 414:105–111

Rhee CS, Sen M, Lu D, Wu C, Leoni L, Rubin J, Corr M, Carson DA (2002) Wnt and frizzled receptors as potential targets for immunotherapy in head and neck squamous cell carcinomas. Oncogene 21:6598–6605

Rivera MN, Kim WJ, Wells J, Driscoll DR, Brannigan BW, Han M, Kim JC, Feinberg AP, Gerald WL, Vargas SO et al (2007) An X chromosome gene, WTX, is commonly inactivated in Wilms tumor. Science 315:642–645

Rodriguez-Pinilla M, Rodriguez-Peralto JL, Hitt R, Sanchez JJ, Sanchez-Verde L, Alameda F, Ballestin C, Sanchez-Cespedes M (2005) beta-Catenin, Nf-kappaB and FAS protein expression are independent events in head and neck cancer: study of their association with clinical parameters. Cancer Lett 230:141–148

Rosin-Arbesfeld R, Townsley F, Bienz M (2000) The APC tumour suppressor has a nuclear export function. Nature 406:1009–1012

Rubinfeld B, Albert I, Porfiri E, Fiol C, Munemitsu S, Polakis P (1996) Binding of GSK3beta to the APC-beta-catenin complex and regulation of complex assembly. Science 272:1023–1026

Rubinfeld B, Robbins P, El-Gamil M, Albert I, Porfiri E, Polakis P (1997) Stabilization of beta-catenin by genetic defects in melanoma cell lines. Science 275:1790–1792

Sakanaka C, Weiss JB, Williams LT (1998) Bridging of beta-catenin and glycogen synthase kinase-3beta by axin and inhibition of beta-catenin-mediated transcription. Proc Natl Acad Sci U S A 95:3020–3023

Salahshor S, Woodgett JR (2005) The links between axin and carcinogenesis. J Clin Pathol 58:225–236

Sansom OJ, Reed KR, Hayes AJ, Ireland H, Brinkmann H, Newton IP, Batlle E, Simon-Assmann P, Clevers H, Nathke IS et al (2004) Loss of Apc in vivo immediately perturbs Wnt signaling, differentiation, and migration. Genes Dev 18:1385–1390

Sato K, Okazaki Y, Tonogi M, Tanaka Y, Yamane GY (2002) Expression of beta-catenin in rat oral epithelial dysplasia induced by 4-nitroquinoline 1-oxide. Oral Oncol 38:772–778

Seeling JM, Miller JR, Gil R, Moon RT, White R, Virshup DM (1999) Regulation of beta-catenin signaling by the B56 subunit of protein phosphatase 2A. Science 283:2089–2091

Segditsas S, Tomlinson I (2006) Colorectal cancer and genetic alterations in the Wnt pathway. Oncogene 25:7531–7537

Seidensticker MJ, Behrens J (2000) Biochemical interactions in the wnt pathway. Biochim Biophys Acta 1495:168–182

Shackleton M, Vaillant F, Simpson KJ, Stingl J, Smyth GK, Asselin-Labat ML, Wu L, Lindeman GJ, Visvader JE (2006) Generation of a functional mammary gland from a single stem cell. Nature 439:84–88

Sieber O, Lipton L, Heinimann K, Tomlinson I (2003) Colorectal tumourigenesis in carriers of the APC I1307K variant: lone gunman or conspiracy? J Pathol 199:137–139

Silva-Vargas V, Lo Celso C, Giangreco A, Ofstad T, Prowse DM, Braun KM, Watt FM (2005) Beta-catenin and Hedgehog signal strength can specify number and location of hair follicles in adult epidermis without recruitment of bulge stem cells. Dev Cell 9:121–131

Sjoblom T, Jones S, Wood LD, Parsons DW, Lin J, Barber TD, Mandelker D, Leary RJ, Ptak J, Silliman N et al (2006) The consensus coding sequences of human breast and colorectal cancers. Science 314:268–274

Smith K, Bui TD, Poulsom R, Kaklamanis L, Williams G, Harris AL (1999) Up-regulation of macrophage wnt gene expression in adenoma-carcinoma progression of human colorectal cancer. Br J Cancer 81:496–502

Sparks AB, Morin PJ, Vogelstein B, Kinzler KW (1998) Mutational analysis of the APC/beta-catenin/Tcf pathway in colorectal cancer. Cancer Res 58:1130–1134

Suzuki H, Watkins DN, Jair KW, Schuebel KE, Markowitz SD, Chen WD, Pretlow TP, Yang B, Akiyama Y, Van Engeland M et al (2004) Epigenetic inactivation of SFRP genes allows constitutive WNT signaling in colorectal cancer. Nat Genet 36:417–422

Taipale J, Beachy PA (2001) The Hedgehog and Wnt signalling pathways in cancer. Nature 411:349–354

Takemaru KI, Moon RT (2000) The transcriptional coactivator CBP interacts with beta-catenin to activate gene expression. J Cell Biol 149:249–254

Taketo MM (2004) Shutting down Wnt signal-activated cancer. Nat Genet 36:320–322

Tamura I, Sakaki T, Chaqour B, Howard PS, Ikeo T, Macarak EJ (2003) Correlation of P-cadherin and beta-catenin expression and phosphorylation with carcinogenesis in rat tongue cancer induced with 4-nitroquinoline 1-oxide. Oral Oncol 39:506–514

Tanaka N, Odajima T, Ogi K, Ikeda T, Satoh M (2003) Expression of E-cadherin, alpha-catenin, and beta-catenin in the process of lymph node metastasis in oral squamous cell carcinoma. Br J Cancer 89:557–563

Testa JR, Bellacosa A (2001) AKT plays a central role in tumorigenesis. Proc Natl Acad Sci U S A 98:10983–10985

Teuliere J, Faraldo MM, Deugnier MA, Shtutman M, Ben-Ze'ev A, Thiery JP, Glukhova MA (2005) Targeted activation of beta-catenin signaling in basal mammary epithelial cells affects mammary development and leads to hyperplasia. Development 132:267–277

Thiery JP (2003) Epithelial-mesenchymal transitions in development and pathologies. Curr Opin Cell Biol 15:740–746

Thompson B, Townsley F, Rosin-Arbesfeld R, Musisi H, Bienz M (2002) A new nuclear component of the Wnt signalling pathway. Nat Cell Biol 4:367–373

Thorstensen L, Lind GE, Lovig T, Diep CB, Meling GI, Rognum TO, Lothe RA (2005) Genetic and epigenetic changes of components affecting the WNT pathway in colorectal carcinomas stratified by microsatellite instability. Neoplasia 7:99–108

Townsley FM, Cliffe A, Bienz M (2004a) Pygopus and Legless target Armadillo/beta-catenin to the nucleus to enable its transcriptional co-activator function. Nat Cell Biol 6:626–633

Townsley FM, Thompson B, Bienz M (2004b) Pygopus residues required for its binding to Legless are critical for transcription and development. J Biol Chem 279:5177–5183

Tsuchiya R, Yamamoto G, Nagoshi Y, Aida T, Irie T, Tachikawa T (2004) Expression of adenomatous polyposis coli (APC) in tumorigenesis of human oral squamous cell carcinoma. Oral Oncol 40:932–940

Tsukamoto AS, Grosschedl R, Guzman RC, Parslow T, Varmus HE (1988) Expression of the int-1 gene in transgenic mice is associated with mammary gland hyperplasia and adenocarcinomas in male and female mice. Cell 55:619–625

Ueda G, Sunakawa H, Nakamori K, Shinya T, Tsuhako W, Tamura Y, Kosugi T, Sato N, Ogi K, Hiratsuka H (2006) Aberrant expression of beta- and gamma-catenin is an independent prognostic marker in oral squamous cell carcinoma. Int J Oral Maxillofac Surg 35:356–361

Uesugi H, Uzawa K, Kawasaki K, Shimada K, Moriya T, Tada A, Shiiba M, Tanzawa H (2005) Status of reduced expression and hypermethylation of the APC tumor suppressor gene in human oral squamous cell carcinoma. Int J Mol Med 15:597–602

Uraguchi M, Morikawa M, Shirakawa M, Sanada K, Imai K (2004) Activation of WNT family expression and signaling in squamous cell carcinomas of the oral cavity. J Dent Res 83:327–332

Uzawa K, Yoshida H, Suzuki H, Tanzawa H, Shimazaki J, Seino S, Sato K (1994) Abnormalities of the adenomatous polyposis coli gene in human oral squamous-cell carcinoma. Int J Cancer 58:814–817

van de Wetering M, Cavallo R, Dooijes D, van Beest M, van Es J, Loureiro J, Ypma A, Hursh D, Jones T, Bejsovec A et al (1997) Armadillo coactivates transcription driven by the product of the Drosophila segment polarity gene dTCF. Cell 88:789–799

van de Wetering M, Sancho E, Verweij C, de Lau W, Oving I, Hurlstone A, van der Horn K, Batlle E, Coudreuse D, Haramis AP et al (2002) The beta-catenin/TCF-4 complex imposes a crypt progenitor phenotype on colorectal cancer cells. Cell 111:241–250

van Es JH, Jay P, Gregorieff A, van Gijn ME, Jonkheer S, Hatzis P, Thiele A, van den Born M, Begthel H, Brabletz T et al (2005) Wnt signalling induces maturation of Paneth cells in intestinal crypts. Nat Cell Biol 7:381–386

van Genderen C, Okamura RM, Farinas I, Quo RG, Parslow TG, Bruhn L, Grosschedl R (1994) Development of several organs that require inductive epithelial-mesenchymal interactions is impaired in LEF-1-deficient mice. Genes Dev 8:2691–2703

Van Mater D, Kolligs FT, Dlugosz AA, Fearon ER (2003) Transient activation of beta -catenin signaling in cutaneous keratinocytes is sufficient to trigger the active growth phase of the hair cycle in mice. Genes Dev 17:1219–1224

Veeman MT, Axelrod JD, Moon RT (2003) A second canon. Functions and mechanisms of beta-catenin-independent Wnt signaling. Dev Cell 5:367–377

Vogelstein B, Fearon ER, Hamilton SR, Kern SE, Preisinger AC, Leppert M, Nakamura Y, White R, Smits AM, Bos JL (1988) Genetic alterations during colorectal-tumor development. N Engl J Med 319:525–532

Wallis YL, Morton DG, McKeown CM, Macdonald F (1999) Molecular analysis of the APC gene in 205 families: extended genotype-phenotype correlations in FAP and evidence for the role of APC amino acid changes in colorectal cancer predisposition. J Med Genet 36:14–20

Wang L, Liu T, Wang Y, Cao L, Nishioka M, Aguirre RL, Ishikawa A, Geng L, Okada N (2007) Altered expression of desmocollin 3, desmoglein 3, and beta-catenin in oral squamous cell carcinoma: correlation with lymph node metastasis and cell proliferation. Virchows Arch 451:959–966

Wang Z, Shen D, Parsons DW, Bardelli A, Sager J, Szabo S, Ptak J, Silliman N, Peters BA, van der Heijden MS et al (2004) Mutational analysis of the tyrosine phosphatome in colorectal cancers. Science 304:1164–1166

Webster MT, Rozycka M, Sara E, Davis E, Smalley M, Young N, Dale TC, Wooster R (2000) Sequence variants of the axin gene in breast, colon, and other cancers: an analysis of mutations that interfere with GSK3 binding. Genes Chromosomes Cancer 28:443–453

Wielenga VJ, van der Voort R, Taher TE, Smit L, Beuling EA, van Krimpen C, Spaargaren M, Pals ST (2000) Expression of c-Met and heparan-sulfate proteoglycan forms of CD44 in colorectal cancer. Am J Pathol 157:1563–1573

Williams HK, Sanders DS, Jankowski JA, Landini G, Brown AM (1998) Expression of cadherins and catenins in oral epithelial dysplasia and squamous cell carcinoma. J Oral Pathol Med 27:308–317

Wong HC, Bourdelas A, Krauss A, Lee HJ, Shao Y, Wu D, Mlodzik M, Shi DL, Zheng J (2003) Direct binding of the PDZ domain of Dishevelled to a conserved internal sequence in the C-terminal region of Frizzled. Mol Cell 12:1251–1260

Wu R, Zhai Y, Fearon ER, Cho KR (2001) Diverse mechanisms of beta-catenin deregulation in ovarian endometrioid adenocarcinomas. Cancer Res 61:8247–8255

Xu Q, Wang Y, Dabdoub A, Smallwood PM, Williams J, Woods C, Kelley MW, Jiang L, Tasman W, Zhang K, Nathans J (2004) Vascular development in the retina and inner ear: control by Norrin and Frizzled-4, a high-affinity ligand-receptor pair. Cell 116:883–895

Yang F, Zeng Q, Yu G, Li S, Wang CY (2006a) Wnt/beta-catenin signaling inhibits death receptor-mediated apoptosis and promotes invasive growth of HNSCC. Cell Signal 18:679–687

Yang L, Lin C, Liu ZR (2006b) P68 RNA helicase mediates PDGF-induced epithelial mesenchymal transition by displacing Axin from beta-catenin. Cell 127:139–155

Yeh KT, Chang JG, Lin TH, Wang YF, Chang JY, Shih MC, Lin CC (2003) Correlation between protein expression and epigenetic and mutation changes of Wnt pathway-related genes in oral cancer. Int J Oncol 23:1001–1007

Yu Z, Weinberger PM, Provost E, Haffty BG, Sasaki C, Joe J, Camp RL, Rimm DL, Psyrri A (2005) beta-Catenin functions mainly as an adhesion molecule in patients with squamous cell cancer of the head and neck. Clin Cancer Res 11:2471–2477

Zeng X, Tamai K, Doble B, Li S, Huang H, Habas R, Okamura H, Woodgett J, He X (2005) A dual-kinase mechanism for Wnt co-receptor phosphorylation and activation. Nature 438:873–877

Zhang B, Ougolkov A, Yamashita K, Takahashi Y, Mai M, Minamoto T (2003) beta-Catenin and ras oncogenes detect most human colorectal cancer. Clin Cancer Res 9:3073–3079

Zhou CX, Gao Y (2007) Frequent genetic alterations and reduced expression of the Axin1 gene in oral squamous cell carcinoma: involvement in tumor progression and metastasis. Oncol Rep 17:73–79

Chapter 12
Role of Tumor Stromal Interactions and Proteases in Oral Cancer Metastasis

J. Robert Newman and Eben L. Rosenthal

Abstract To metastasize, tumor cells must migrate through the surrounding stroma which is composed of extracellular matrix (ECM) components, fibroblasts, inflammatory cells, and endothelial cells. Tumor-associated matrix permeability to tumor cells is thought to result from complex interactions between the tumor cell and the cellular and acellular components of the stroma. These interactions result in tumor cell changes in substrate adhesion, cell migration, and focused proteolysis of ECM components. Although the process of ECM degradation has been associated with multiple types of proteases including cathepsins, and serine proteases (such as plasmin), it is the matrix metalloproteinases (MMPs) that are most commonly upregulated and associated with the invasive process. Although tumor cells were originally thought to be the primary source of MMPs within the tumor, it was recently recognized that MMPs are expressed primarily by stromal cells when stimulated by tumor cell derived factors. One mechanism that tumor cells employ to stimulate MMPs from tumor-associated stroma is the expression of ECM metalloproteinase inducer (EMMPRIN). EMMPRIN is a tumor cell expressed protein known to induce growth factors and proteases in the surrounding fibroblasts and endothelial cells. In addition to an analysis of EMMPRIN as a paradigm for tumor–stromal interactions, this chapter will characterize the presence of stromal tissue in head and neck cancer on the basis of histological analysis, the role of proteases in tumor–stromal interactions, and the specific role of membrane type-1 MMP (MT1-MMP) in tumor invasion and metastasis. Furthermore, the clinical trials associated with MMP inhibitors in cancer have been disappointing, and some possible explanations for their failure and future directions are suggested.

E.L. Rosenthal (✉)
Division of Otolaryngology, University of Alabama at Birmingham, BDB Suite 563,
1808 7th Avenue South, Birmingham, AL, 35294-0012, USA
e-mail: oto@uab.edu

J. Myers (ed.), *Oral Cancer Metastasis*,
DOI 10.1007/978-1-4419-0775-2_12, © Springer Science+Business Media, LLC 2010

Introduction

Many epithelial tumors, including head and neck squamous cell carcinoma (HNSCC), are composed of not only of carcinoma cells but also infiltrating dense stroma that contains ECM, fibroblasts, inflammatory cells, and endothelial cells. Under physiological conditions, the basement membrane and underlying stroma provide orientation for epithelial cells. As part of the neoplastic process, these organizational and barrier functions are disrupted. Unregulated cell growth in squamous cancer is necessary but not sufficient to cause the invasive behavior that characterizes this disease (Crowe et al. 2002; Elenbaas and Weinberg 2001). Changes in stromal signaling are thought to represent a process similar to instructive signals from stromal cells that facilitate organogenesis. Many authors hypothesize that the ability of HNSCC tumor cells to harness the remodeling capabilities of the stroma enables local tissue destruction and spread to distant sites.

The dense infiltration of fibroblasts which interdigitate with tumor islands in HNSCC is thought to promote a growth permissive tumor microenvironment (Almholt and Johnsen 2003; Coussens et al. 2000; McCawley and Matrisian 2001; Matrisian et al. 1994; Lynch and Matrisian 2002). Studies of carcinoma associated fibroblasts (CAFs) in squamous cell carcinoma (SCC) have demonstrated that paracrine fibroblast signaling can profoundly affect tumor formation (Matrisian et al. 1994; Skobe and Fusenig 1998; Ponec et al. 1991). Overexpression of platelet derived growth factor (PDGF) in non-tumorigenic immortalized human keratinocytes (HaCaT cell line) induces tumor formation through the PDGF-mediated paracrine activation of fibroblasts (Skobe and Fusenig 1998). The fibroblast-dependent acceleration of epithelial malignancies has been established in vivo and in vitro in multiple cell types (McCawley and Matrisian 2001; Picard et al. 1986; Camps et al. 1990). These studies suggest that changes in epithelial–stromal signaling can lead to tumor development and progression.

Experimental Assessment of the Tumor–Stromal Interaction Requires Physiological Models of Tumor Invasion

A summary of tumor–stromal interactions necessitates a discussion of inherent limitations of experimental models used to study this phenomenon. Cytokines act over very narrow distances, in concert with multiple factors and at low concentrations, which makes assessment of expression and interpretation of in vitro phenotypes difficult. Although this can be generally said of in vitro work, observations made on the microenvironment in vitro poorly recapitulate the three-dimensional, multicellular, hypoxic, and vascular nature of the in vivo tumors. For this reason, therapeutic implications of in vitro studies should be interpreted with caution. Furthermore, as will be discussed later, the value of mouse models when assessing the tumor microenvironment is also of limited translational benefit based on the differences in gene expression between humans and mice, particularly with respect to MMPs (e.g., there is no murine equivalent of MMP-1).

Failure of in vitro experiments to predict in vivo results when assessing the tumor microenvironment is probably related to several factors including (1) an inability to recapitulate the elements of the tumor ECM in which the tumor cells reside, (2) failure to put all of the cell types that compose the complex tumor environment within the in vitro model, (3) failure to generate the three-dimensional complex structure in which tumors reside, and (4) use of serum free media or supplemented media that does not recapitulate the well vascularized conditions typically found in tumor including the ability to generate hydrostatic pressure, hypoxia, and pH specifically associated with the tumor environment. These limitations of in vitro systems and the need to isolate specific factors in order to identity therapeutic targets make studying the microenvironment particularly difficult.

In vitro assays used to assess tumor cell invasion or migration often fail to provide a physiological or anatomic barrier against tumor cell invasion. Most in vitro assays use Matrigel (Becton, Dickinson and Company, Franklin Lakes, NJ) or type I collagen. Matrigel is extracted from Engelbreth–Holm–Swarm mouse sarcoma cells and is composed of proteins most commonly associated with the basement membrane such as laminin and type IV collagen (Senger et al. 1997). However, data obtained from tumor cells traversing such a barrier in vitro should be interpreted with caution since neither the composition nor assembly of the Matrigel can be translated to human tumor cell invasion. Although these matrices are expedient and inexpensive, other matrices, such as commercially available cadaver dermis, should also be considered (Rosenthal et al. 1999). Examination of experimental details is often required to determine if physiological models were used to assess tumor phenotypes during the studies of tumor–stromal interactions.

Genetic Alterations in Tumor Associated Stroma

It is generally accepted that tumors arise from genetic changes within the normal mucosal squamous cell epithelium. However, the possibility of genetic mutations within the stroma has also recently been identified in head and neck cancer (Weber et al. 2007; Lu et al. 2006). This concept is supported by the high rate of second primaries associated with the generalized epithelial changes, referred to as field cancerization. It is possible that the tumor microenvironment generated by the stroma is in part responsible for this field cancerization (the tumor microenvironment refers to the generalized milieu which the tumor cell develops that includes both fibroblast and tumor cell and intraepithelial cell derived factors, and it also includes the tumor oxygenation and other generalized factors present within the tumor). Supporting this hypothesis is the evidence that the stroma may undergo distinct changes that lead to the elaboration of growth factors and other cytokines which promote epithelial tumor progression and metastasis. It has been previously demonstrated that carcinoma associated fibroblasts undergo genetic alterations that can potentially transform the premalignant epithelium to cancer in breast cancer and pancreatic cancer(Fukino et al. 2007; Kurose et al. 2001; Moinfar et al. 2004). Although the great majority of loss of heterozygosity (LOH), a measure of cellular gene altera-tions associated with tumor progression, is noted within the epithelial compartment as compared to the stroma compartment (Fukino et al. 2007; Kurose et al. 2001), it has been reported primarily in breast cancer that a high frequency of LOH is found within mammary stromal cells (Moinfar et al. 2000, 2004; Gocht et al. 1999).

Significantly, it has recently been shown that microenvironmental genomic alterations are associated with smoking in HNSCC (Fukino et al. 2007). A micro-dissection of tumor stroma from head and neck cancer and compartment specific frequency of LOH was determined in this study, and it was found that tumor associated stroma from smokers had a high degree of genetic changes and a correlation could be found between tumor aggressiveness and five specific genetic loci. In fact, there were three stroma specific loci that were associated with regional nodal metastasis as well as tumor size. Although this study assessed genetic changes in stromal and tumor cells in smokers and nonsmokers, other cancer types have been linked to genetic alterations associated with other environmental changes. For example, hypoxia conditions within the tumor can increase the number of genetic mutations (Mabjeesh and Amir 2007).

These studies suggest that the stromal elements within head and neck squamous cell tumors may have specific sites of genetic alterations that are associated with a clinically aggressive phenotype. Furthermore, this work implies that the genetic changes that occur within the epithelial cells also occur within the tumor associated stroma. With respect to changes in stroma in smokers who have undergone generalized epithelial changes (field cancerization), it is possible to hypothesize that genetically altered stromal cells gradually displace the normal stroma and promote epithelial proliferation and dysplasia. In this model, the stroma becomes the tumor promoting element.

Fibroblasts Promote a Malignant Environment

Fibroblasts are known to provide a favorable tumor microenvironment for tumor growth. The most striking evidence for this is when normal dermal fibroblasts are co-injected with head and neck cancer cells in immunodeficient mice. Simply by the addition of an equal number of fibroblasts, the tumor cells grow significantly faster and initiate earlier (Fig. 12.1) (Rosenthal et al. 2006). Although CAFs are

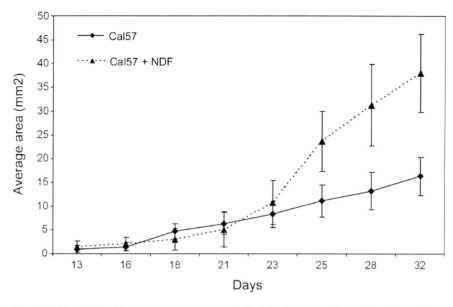

Fig. 12.1 Normal fibroblasts promote tumor growth. Co-injecting normal dermal fibroblasts (NDFs) with tumor cells causes increased tumor growth. Cal57 HNSCC tumor cells (2.5×10^5) were injected with ($n = 10$) and without ($n = 20$) NDFs (5×10^5) in the bilateral flanks of severe combined immunodeficient mice. Cal57 cells tumor show an increase in tumor area when co-injected with NDFs ($p = 0.0001$, *bars* = SEM)

considered to have the potential to induce more aggressive tumor formation, co-injection of primary CAF cultures does not accelerate tumor growth compared to co-injection with normal dermal fibroblasts (NDFs) (Rosenthal, unpublished data). It is clear that proliferation of fibroblasts within the tumor occurs in response to the tumor, and such proliferation has been compared to a wounding or chronic inflammation response (Micke and Ostman 2005). Although the comparison of wound healing as supporting tumor growth has certain clinical correlates, these are unusual. One example is that highly malignant SCC can arise from areas of previous trauma such as dermal scars. Another example is the association of cancer with autoimmune disease such as inflammatory bowel disease, in which chronic inflammation can result in a malignant tumor.

CAFs have been well described pathologically as large spindle like cells that express vimentin and alpha smooth muscle actin are generally termed myofibroblasts. Although it is likely that CAFs control the tumor microenvironment by secretion of multiple growth factors, it is unclear if CAFs are a distinct entity. Studies presented earlier suggest that genetic changes do occur in the CAFs, but isolation and analysis of carcinoma associated fibroblasts require that they be able to be cultured and retain their phenotype in vitro for analysis of growth factor expression and phenotypic changes.

CAFS are best described in breast cancer where the stroma support is known to be critical for the development and progression of tumor. But, it remains unclear if CAFs can be cultured from HNSCC tumors and subsequently induce a malignant phenotype. CAFs have been shown to induce malignant changes in SV-40 immortalized benign prostatic epithelial cells in vivo (Olumi et al. 1999). These findings suggested that fibroblasts isolated from prostate cancer, but not benign prostatic tissue, could induce differentiation in SV-40 immortalized benign prostatic prostate cells and induced dramatic growth within the renal capsule of nude mice. However, these prostatic tumor xenografts were performed in the renal capsule of immunodeficient mice which is an unusual tumor microenvironment and may not be generalizable to other biological sites. Studies in breast cancer have identified a similar phenomenon (Orimo et al. 2005). CAFs have been shown to initiate tumor progression in a murine model of breast cancer (Barcellos-Hoff 2005; Barcellos-Hoff and Brooks 2001). One study demonstrated that removing epithelial cells from the mammary fat pad of mice and irradiating and then retransplanting them result in changes in the stroma that then can transform the transplanted epithelial cells in these mice. A significantly higher number of tumors form in mice that had irradiated stromal tissue (Barcellos-Hoff and Ravani 2000). This study suggests that radiation can have a carcinogenic effect on the stromal tissue. Of course, it is unclear which cell type (fibroblast or epithelial cells or other) was tumor promoting within this in vivo setting. Aside from these two organs, however, there has been limited evidence to suggest that carcinoma associated fibroblast comprise a distinct entity, which can transform epithelial cells.

Tumor Derived Growth Factors Influence Stromal Formation

The elaboration of stromal derived cytokines has been found to affect tumor growth, angiogenesis, and immune functions within the tumor. The cytokines most commonly associated with head and neck cancer include interleukin 4 (IL-4), IL-6, IL-8, IL-10, IL-1β, granulocyte–macrophage colony-stimulating factor (GM-CSF), vascular endothelial growth factor (VEGF), prostaglandin E2, and basic fibroblast growth factor (bFGF) (Pries et al. 2006; Pries and Wollenberg 2006; Lewis et al. 2006). Other growth factors that promote tumor growth and invasion include transforming growth factor beta (TGFβ) (Hagedorn et al. 1999; Gruss et al. 2003; Rosenthal et al. 2004a), transforming growth factor alpha (TGFα) (Grandis et al. 1998; Dumont and Arteaga 2002) and hepatocyte growth factor/scatter factor (HGF/SF) (Pries et al. 2006; Pries and Wollenberg 2006). These cytokines and growth factors are mechanisms by which tumor cells recruit the surrounding stroma to promote growth through induction of neovascularization, immune suppression, and invasion/metastasis. These growth factors are often responsible for multiple effects. For example, VEGF-A expression is known to trigger angiogenesis, but another subtype of VEGF, VEGF-C, is associated with lymphangiogenesis and increased rates of lymph node metastasis, suggesting a dual role of these growth factors in metastasis and angiogenesis (O-Charoenrat et al. 2001a). This review will focus on the role of MMPs as a paradigm for tumor stromal interactions, as the complex roles of immunosuppression, angiogenesis, and growth stimulated by elaboration of these growth factors are beyond the scope of this chapter.

Assessment of Stromal Components in HNSCC

Although generally assumed to be a significant component of most HNSCC, the percent of stroma within HNSCC has not been defined. Despite a significant increase in data to suggest that the stromal component and the inflammatory infiltrate promote tumor cell invasion in multiple tumor types (Olumi et al. 1999; Pauli and Knudson 1988; Rofstad 2000), including head and neck cancer (Rosenthal et al. 2004b), tumor associated stroma has not been well characterized. The relative expression of transcripts or protein between tumors will vary greatly depending on the relative percent of stroma or the extent of inflammatory cells. Therefore, accurate classification of samples is particularly important when using molecular techniques that are dependent on the stromal composition: molecular characterization of tumors by immunohistochemistry, microarray analysis, or proteomics requires a consistent definition of the sample.

To better characterize the stromal and inflammatory component of oral cavity tumors, we have examined the histology of tumors from previously untreated oral cavity SCC patients in order to improve the understanding of the variations of the stroma in head and neck cancer. TNM stage, survival, and histology were assessed on a retrospective cohort of 54 patients with untreated oral tongue SCC (Rosenthal, unpublished data). Analysis was performed to grade the inflammatory infiltrate and the percent of the tumor mass composed of stroma based on review of hematoxylin-eosin-stained specimens. The relative composition of the tumor associated macrophages in the epithelial and stromal components of the tumor was assessed by immunohistochemical staining of tumors using CD68. In this analysis, the stromal portion represented 8–74% of the tumor mass, with an average of 36.5%. Within that stromal component, an average of 49% of stroma was composed of inflammatory infiltrate (range, 6–94%). The classification of tumors based on inflammatory infiltrate could be divided into low (<30%), intermediate (30–50%), and high (>50%). This classification results in roughly equal distribution of the tumors (Fig. 12.2). Despite the even distribution between groups, the group with the high inflammatory infiltrate had the poorest survival ($p = 0.21$, two-tailed chi-square test).

Analysis of tumor associated macrophages by CD68 immunostaining of tumor specimens demonstrated that the macrophages are not evenly distributed throughout the tumor mass (Fig. 12.3). There was a nonsignificant correlation between the tumor associated macrophage composition in the epithelial component as compared with the stromal component. As more attention is given to the role of these cells in the development of head and neck cancer (Marcus et al. 2004), these data suggest that localization of these cells and other inflammatory cells within the tissue mass may be important for accurate data analysis.

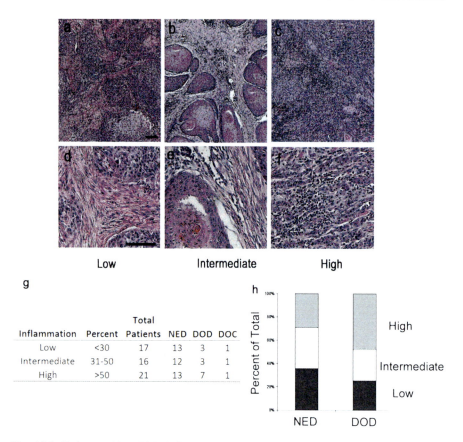

Fig. 12.2 Patients with a high inflammatory infiltrate demonstrated had worse treatment outcomes ($p = 0.21$). The inflammatory infiltrate was assessed in 54 patients with greater than 2 year follow-up and classified as low (**a, d**), intermediate (**b, e**), or high (**c, f**). Patients were evenly distributed (**g**), but the outcome was not (**g, h**). Bar is 100 μm

In summary, the amount of stroma and inflammatory infiltrate within oral tongue SCC specimens varies widely, with an average of 36.5%. The high percent of nontumor cells within the HNSCC tumor mass supports the concept of identifying molecularly targeted, antistromal cytostatic agents for therapy to be used in combination with cytotoxic therapies.

Role of Proteases in Tumor–Stromal Interaction

Mechanisms by which cancer cells invade the basement membrane and ECM remain undefined. Proteases are thought to regulate tumor cell migration and metastasis by cleavage of growth factors, cell adhesion molecules, other proteases,

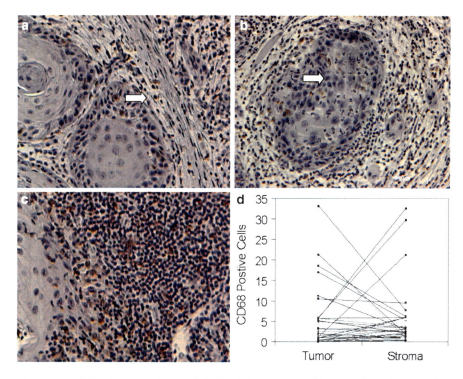

Fig. 12.3 Variation in macrophage distribution between nests of tumor cells and surrounding stromal cells. Immunohistochemical analysis of CD68 reactivity (*arrows* demonstrate CD68 positive cells) in HNSCC primary tumors (**a–c**) demonstrating even distribution throughout the tumor mass and stroma (**a, b**) and uneven distribution with greater CD68 positive staining in the stroma (**c**). A poor correlation was seen between CD68 reactive cells in the tumor compartment were compared with the number of cells counted in the stromal compartment (**d**), suggesting that the macrophages are not evenly distributed throughout the tumor

and ECM macromolecules (Pauli and Knudson 1988; Liotta 1986). These proteases can be roughly broken into two groups: MMPs and serine proteases.

Serine proteases have been implicated in the process of tumor cell extravasation into the lymphatic and circulatory system. Plasmin is a circulating protease responsible for degradation of intraluminal thrombi and is formed by activation of plasminogen by plasminogen activators (tissue type plasminogen activators [tPA] and urokinase-type PA [uPA]). Because plasmin is found to be overexpressed in tumors and uPA receptors expressed on tumor cells are known to bind uPA to the cell surface, this protease is thought to influence tumor cell migration by the degradation of fibrin and other matrix components as well as activation of MMPs. By binding to the cell surface, uPA receptors are likely to focus uPA proteolysis to the peritumor microenvironment.

Matrix metalloproteinases are a family of over 25 Zn^{2+}-dependent matrix-degrading enzymes that are secreted as inactive zymogens that have been implicated throughout the temporal progression of tumorigenesis and are expressed in most cell types in the tumor mass. Although multiple proteases have been implicated in tumor cell invasion, malignant progression of oral cavity SCC (OSCC) is most commonly associated with elevated expression of MMPs (Rosenthal et al. 1999; O-Charoenrat et al. 2001b; Imanishi et al. 2000; Yoshizaki et al. 1997; Kurahara et al. 1999).

The importance of MMPs in HNSCC has been established over the past 20 years since their discovery in cancer and their role in tumor invasion (Liotta and Kohn 2001). Initially classified as just as cleaving ECM components, the proteolytic targets of MMPs have been expanded to include other proteases, protease inhibitors, clotting factors, chemotactic molecules, growth factors, cell-surface receptors, and adhesion molecules (Egeblad and Werb 2002). The importance of MMPs in epithelial tumor formation has been demonstrated by upregulation and downregulation studies (Coussens et al. 2000; Thomasset et al. 1998; Sternlicht et al. 1999). In HNSCC, advanced-stage disease and nodal status have been correlated with immunopositivity for MT1-MMP, MMP1, MMP2, and MMP9 (Imanishi et al. 2000; Yoshizaki et al. 1997; Mueller et al. 2001; Werner et al. 2002; Johansson et al. 1997).

Evaluation of MMPs usually requires assessment of their endogenous inhibitors, tissue inhibitors of metalloproteinases (TIMPs). TIMPs are known to be potent inhibitors of MMPs in vitro, although their in vivo role is not well understood. TIMP-1 and TIMP-2, but not TIMP-3, are consistently measured in HNSCC. In fact, the expression of TIMP-1 in tumors (and in one case TIMP-2) positively correlates with metastatic disease (O-Charoenrat et al. 2001b; Kurahara et al. 1999; Ondruschka et al. 2002). Other physiological MMP inhibitors have been identified in tumors, including RECK (REversion-inducing-Cystein-rich protein with Kazal motifs), which is a membrane bound MMP inhibitor (MT1-MMP activity and MMP9 expression) that was recently identified (Oh et al. 2001; Sasahara et al. 2002; Herold et al. 2002). Expression of endogenous MMP inhibitors, such as TIMPs and RECK, in tumors has not been clearly demonstrated to have a protective effect in human cancers.

Role of MT1-MMP in Carcinoma Associated Fibroblasts

Experimental models of tumor invasion suggest that MMPs mediate HNSCC tumor cell invasion, and the supporting evidence includes the following: (1) in vitro invasion and growth is arrested by MMP inhibitors (MMPI) (Rosenthal et al. 1999; O-Charoenrat et al. 2002) and (2) HNSCC tumor cell growth and metastasis are reduced in vivo by synthetic and endogenous MMPIs (Katori et al. 2002). Although many MMPs have been identified, MT1-MMP, also known as MMP-14, is thought to be a critical enzyme in HNSCC tumorigenesis and invasion because it can

(1) degrade type I collagen and fibrin, (2) alter cell–cell adhesion (Kajita et al. 2001), and (3) convert pro-MMP-2 to its active form (Pei and Weiss 1996; Aznavoorian et al. 2001; Hotary et al. 2000, 2002). Identified on the membranes of both tumor cells and peritumoral fibroblasts, MT1-MMP expression has been correlated with an aggressive pattern of invasive and ECM degradation in HNSCC (Kurahara et al. 1999; Okada et al. 1995; Chenard et al. 1999). In vitro data suggest that not only does MT1-MMP regulate HNSCC invasion (Rosenthal et al. 1999), but also its expression correlates positively with poor patient outcomes (Imanishi et al. 2000; Yoshizaki et al. 1997; Kurahara et al. 1999; Mueller et al. 2001). Elevated MT1-MMP expression in OSCC has been shown to positively correlate with an aggressive pattern of invasion, poor survival, and lymph node metastasis (O-Charoenrat et al. 2001b; Imanishi et al. 2000; Yoshizaki et al. 1997; Janot et al. 1996).

MT1-MMP is converted to its active form by furin, an intracellular proprotein convertase. Increased activity of furin in OSCC is associated with more aggressiveness in vitro and in vivo tumor activity (Bassi et al. 2001, 2003). In vitro data similarly suggest that overexpression of MT1-MMP promotes OSCC tumor cell invasion (Rosenthal et al. 1999; Pauli and Knudson 1988). As previously mentioned, MT1-MMP plays a critical role in tumor cell invasion and angiogenesis through several known mechanisms: (1) activation of MMP2 (72-kDa type IV collagenase) in SCC (Imanishi et al. 2000; Jiang and Pei 2003), (2) cleavage of the cell adhesion molecule CD44 from the cell surface (Hotary et al. 2002; Jiang et al. 2001), (3) degradation of type I collagen and fibrin substrates (Kajita et al. 2001; Mori et al. 2002), and (4) enabling cell survival in three dimensional matrices (Hotary et al. 2003). TIMPs and RECK are endogenous inhibitors of MT1-MMP and MMP2 (Rhee and Coussens 2002; Heppner et al. 1996; Sutinen et al. 1998), whose role in tumor cell invasion is unclear. TIMP1 and TIMP2 have been found to positively correlate with metastatic disease, and the ratio of MMP to TIMPs has been found to influence the ability of TIMPs to modulate MMP catalytic activity (O-Charoenrat et al. 2001b; Kurahara et al. 1999; Ondruschka et al. 2002). RECK has only recently been identified, and the function of this membrane bound molecule to influence cancer cell invasion remains to be fully elucidated (Oh et al. 2001; Rhee and Coussens 2002; Noda et al. 2003; Span et al. 2003).

Recognition that CAFs synthesize most of the peritumoral MMPs by in situ hybridization in breast cancer (Heppner et al. 1996; O-Charoenrat et al. 2000) led to similar observations in other tumors (McCawley and Matrisian 2001; Matrisian et al. 1994; Bodey et al. 2001), including HNSCC (Sutinen et al. 1998; Tsukifuji et al. 1999). This suggested that tumor cell–related factors induce MMP expression in the surrounding fibroblasts. Although the mechanism by which tumor cells provide instructive signals to fibroblasts is largely unknown, multiple tumor-secreted growth factors and cytokines have been implicated in peritumoral MMP regulation. Tumor cells' induction of MMP expression in stromal tissues can be considered an archetype for tumor–stromal interactions. In a recent study, immunolocalization of MT1-MMP using three monoclonal antibodies with distinct epitopes identified MT1-MMP exclusively in the surrounding stromal cells (Chenard et al. 1999). Although studies have demonstrated that MT1-MMP correlates with poor outcome in

HNSCC and localizes to fibroblasts in vivo, the mechanism by which tumor cells promote MT1-MMP and other MMP expression in surrounding fibroblasts has been partially elucidated by studies of EMMPRIN.

EMMPRIN Modulates Stromal MMP Expression

EMMPRIN has been recognized as a critical modulator of tumor–stromal interaction and is highly expressed in HNSCC. EMMPRIN, also known as CD147, was initially isolated by Biswas et al. and was labeled "tumor collagenase stimulating factor" (Biswas et al. 1995). The cDNA for human EMMPRIN encodes 269 amino acid residues that include a cytoplasmic domain, a transmembrane domain, and two domains that are characteristic of the immunoglobulin superfamily. Although the receptor for EMMPRIN is unknown, it is thought to act as its own receptor. Overexpression of CD147 has been identified in multiple tumor types but has the highest expression in HNSCC and pancreatic cancer (Riethdorf et al. 2006). EMMPRIN has been isolated from bone marrow metastasis in breast cancer and lung cancer patients and is thought to be a critical mediator of head and neck invasion in metastasis (Klein et al. 2002).

Expression of EMMPRIN as determined by immunohistochemical analysis is upregulated in HNSCC human tumors and dysplastic epithelium as compared with normal mucosa (Polette et al. 1997). Development of HNSCC is typically preceded by transition of normal mucosa to dysplastic epithelium, which is clinically identified as an area of leukoplakia or erythroplakia. In normal mucosa, EMMPRIN expression is limited to the basal layer, but spreads to superficial layers as the epithelium becomes more dysplastic (Vigneswaran et al. 2006). EMMPRIN expression levels positively correlated with degree of dysplasia, and high levels of expression heralds the development of frank SCC (Vigneswaran et al. 2006).

EMMPRIN expression has been correlated with metastasis and tumor progression in multiple other tumor types (Cheng et al. 2006; Jin et al. 2006), including HNSCC (Rosenthal et al. 2003; Bordador et al. 2000). Overexpression of EMMPRIN in breast cancer cell lines results in accelerated in vivo growth (Tang et al. 2005), and this effect was also shown to be largely fibroblast dependent in HNSCC cell lines (Rosenthal et al. 2006). Analysis of individual metastatic tumor cells isolated from the bone marrow of patients with epithelial malignancies identified EMMPRIN as the most frequently expressed gene (Klein et al. 2002). Xenografted breast cancer cell lines overexpressing EMMPRIN demonstrated significantly enhanced tumor growth (Tang et al. 2005) and distant metastasis (Zucker et al. 2001) when compared with control vector transfected tumor cells. This has similarly been demonstrated in xenografted HNSCC cell lines (Rosenthal et al. 2006). These results suggest that EMMPRIN would be an outstanding therapeutic target in HNSCC.

EMMPRIN is expressed on the cell surface of tumor cells in HNSCC and promotes MMP expression in surrounding fibroblasts. Although well recognized as a critical molecule in the progression, growth, and metastasis of HNSCC, the mechanism by which EMMPRIN recruits fibroblasts and promotes these effects remains largely unknown. EMMPRIN exists primarily on the cell surface of tumor cells, but relatively small levels of EMMPRIN are released from the tumor cell surface, most likely through microvesicle shedding. EMMPRIN has been found to stimulate fibroblast and endothelial cell expression of MMP1, MMP2, MMP3, and MT1-MMP in cancer (Caudroy et al. 2002; Braundmeier et al. 2006; Dalberg et al. 2000). This effect has been shown to occur in dose-dependent manner for multiple tumor types using recombinant and isolated protein (Guo et al. 1997; Taylor et al. 2002). EMMPRIN functions to stimulate surrounding stromal elements such as fibroblasts and endothelial cells, but because the receptor for EMMPRIN has not been identified, its paracrine and autocrine effects have not been fully elucidated. However, EMMPRIN-mediated collagen degradation has been shown to be dependent on MMPs derived from fibroblasts, rather than tumor cells (Zhang et al. 2006). Despite its label as an inducer of MMPs, this may not reflect its primary role in tumor development, which has recently been shown to be MMP independent in melanoma tumor growth (Table 12.1).

Tumor cell derived EMMPRIN has recently been shown to stimulate angiogenesis (Tang et al. 2005). Angiogenesis is present in most malignant tumors and is defined by an increase in the density of small capillaries (Hanahan and Folkman 1996). It is critical for tumor formation and is recognized as a potential therapeutic target (McDonald et al. 2004) in multiple cancer types. However, accurate therapeutic targeting requires an improved understanding of the steps leading to neovascularization. Tumor cells' recruitment of endothelial cells into the tumor is dependent upon the elaboration of cytokines within the tumor microenvironment. EMMPRIN stimulates VEGF expression in fibroblasts, which then acts to recruit endothelial cells. Using breast cancer cell lines engineered to express variable levels of EMMPRIN, it was shown that fibroblasts and endothelial cells express VEGF in response to EMMPRIN stimulation (Tang et al. 2005). Xenografts of these same cells result in accelerated growth in vivo and are associated with increased capillary density and elevated VEGF levels (Tang et al. 2005; Zucker et al. 2001). Although it has recently been shown that EMMPRIN stimulates expression of VEGF, other potential mechanisms of EMMPRIN-mediated tumor growth are likely.

Therapies directed against early tumor development and arresting local tumor invasion are critical in HNSCC because these patients have poor survival rates and a high second primary tumor rate. HNSCC most commonly arises in patients with a history of smoking and alcohol consumption. After initial presentation, patients have a 5–7% second primary rate per year because diffuse carcinogenic changes occur throughout the upper areodigestive tract (Scherubl et al. 2002; Casiglia and Woo 2001; Leon et al. 2001). Furthermore, they are at high risk for other respiratory malignancies and gastrointestinal and uroepithelial cancers (Leon et al. 2001; Kuriakose et al. 2002). Because of the high rate of second primaries and local-regional recurrence, these patients are ideal candidates for preventative therapies directed at inhibiting early tumor progression and local tumor invasion.

Evidence outlined above suggests one mechanism by which tumor cells harness peritumor fibroblast-mediated ECM degradation is through cell-surface

Table 12.1 Source of expression of proteases and growth factors within the tumor mass

Factor	Expression in tumor	Expression in stroma	References
EMMPRIN (CD147)	+		Polette et al. (1997)
MMPs			
MMP-1	+	++	Mueller and Fusenig (2002), Birkedal-Hansen (1995), Ala-aho et al. (2004), and Muller et al. (1993)
MMP-2	+	++	O-Charoenrat et al. (2001b), Heppner et al. (1996), Patel et al. (2005), and Arenas-Huertero et al. (1999)
MMP-3	+	++	Egeblad and Werb (2002), Heppner et al. (1996), and Stamenkovic (2000)
MMP-7	+		Egeblad and Werb (2002), Heppner et al. (1996), Fingleton et al. (2001), and Cunha and Matrisian (2002)
MMP-8		+	Lynch and Matrisian (2002) and DeClerck et al. (2004)
MMP-9	+	++	Coussens et al. (2000), Kurahara et al. (1999), Egeblad and Werb (2002), Mueller and Fusenig (2002), and Patel et al. (2005)
MMP-10	+	++	O-Charoenrat et al. (2001b)
MMP-11	+	++	O-Charoenrat et al. (2001b) and Heppner et al. (1996)
MMP-13	+	++	Heppner et al. (1996), Mueller and Fusenig (2002), Ala-aho et al. (2004), and Mandic et al. (2002)
MT1-MMP (MMP14)	++	+	Rosenthal et al. (1999, 2004b), Kurahara et al. (1999), and Tokumaru et al. (2000)
MMP inhibitors			
TIMP-1	+	++	Heppner et al. (1996)
TIMP-2		+	Stetler-Stevenson (2008) and Stetler-Stevenson and Seo (2005)
TIMP-3		+	Kishnani et al. (1995) and Uria et al. (1994)
RECK	+	+	Li et al. (2007) and Clark et al. (2007)
Growth factors			
VEGF	+	++	Micke and Ostman (2005), Fukumura et al. (1998), and Guidi et al. (1996)
TGF-β	+		Micke and Ostman (2005)
PDGF	+		Micke and Ostman (2005)
HGF/SF		+	Micke and Ostman (2005)

EMMPRIN extracellular matrix metalloproteinase inducer; *MMP* matrix metalloproteinase; *TIMP* tissue inhibitors of metalloproteinases; *RECK* reversion-inducing-cystein-rich protein with Kazal motifs; *VEGF* vascular endothelial growth factor; *TGF-β* transforming growth factor beta; *PDGF* platelet derived growth factor; *HGF* hepatocyte growth factor. + = expression; ++ = higher expression

expression of EMMPRIN. Although tumor metastasis is enhanced in tumor cells overexpressing EMMPRIN in vivo, the significance of MMP recruitment in fibroblasts remains unclear. It is unknown if EMMPRIN expression is able to transform normal epithelial cells or to alter the invasive phenotype in HNSCC tumor cells. Understanding the significance of EMMPRIN in HNSCC tumor invasion may lead to new pharmacological agents or a better therapeutic design and use of MMP inhibitors as anticancer agents.

Clinical Implications of MMPs in Cancer and the Failure of Clinical Trials

Localization of the expression and identification of the role of MMPs in HNSCC are critical to improve results from previous broad spectrum MMP inhibitor trials. Initial trials of MMP inhibitors in phase II and III clinical trials proved to be complicated by reversible musculoskeletal pain as a side effect and poor clinical efficacy that failed to limit tumor progression in patients with late-stage tumors. Hindsight has provided many reasons for their clinical failure, including the importance of targeting specific MMPs (Coussens et al. 2002). Understanding the role of MT1-MMP and its localization within the tumor microenvironment may lead to chemopreventive treatment of patients with premalignant disease to prevent the development of an invasive cancer.

Phase II trials were largely omitted from the development process, and several drugs went directly to large-scale randomized trials that compared cytostatic MMP inhibitors (MMPIs) with cytotoxic therapies. Unfortunately, no significant benefit in survival or disease progression was found in patients with advanced-stage pancreatic, gastric, breast, nonsmall cell lung, and prostate cancer (Sparano et al. 2004; Evans et al. 2001; Bramhall et al. 2002a). There were some more promising clinical trial results in gastric cancer and nonsmall cell lung cancer (Latreille et al. 2003; Bramhall et al. 2002b). Patients with limited musculoskeletal symptoms have improved survival in recent studies (Sparano et al. 2004). There are no published data on clinical trials with MMPIs in head and neck cancer, but results in other cancers imply that broad spectrum inhibitors will have limited clinical benefit due to the dose-limiting musculoskeletal symptoms. Perhaps, addition of MMPIs to conventional chemotherapy agents with nonoverlapping toxicities or radiation will be better tolerated by patients, allowing for combination therapy (Douillard et al. 2004).

The failure of MMPIs in clinical trials remains baffling in light of the overwhelming preclinical data to support in vivo antitumor activity. While it is possible that MMPIs simply are ineffective in human cancers, analysis of the MMPI clinical trials has identified some possible reasons for their failure. First, promising results in the laboratory reflect the failure of mouse models of human cancer to predict clinical benefit when assessing MMPIs. Although most novel therapeutic agents are subject to the same mouse model limitation, in the case of MMP investigations, it may be especially true because of the stromal source of the MMPs and the difference between human biology and mouse MMP biology (mice do not have a gene equivalent for MMP-1). Second, preclinical data that were available were not incorporated into the design of clinical trials; preclinical mouse data suggested that MMP inhibition was far more efficient at preventing metastasis rather than reducing tumor size (Sledge et al. 1995). Third, the potential of MMPIs to inhibit intratumoral MMPs at the administered concentrations remains unknown. Dosing was dependent on musculoskeletal side effects rather than tissue penetration or inhibition of catalytic activity. However, recent studies show that the serum levels of MMP inhibitors are sufficient to inhibit MMP activity in vitro at the administered dose (Sparano et al. 2004). Fourth, limited information was available about specific MMP expression within tumors at the time of trial design. The specific MMP profile of different tumor types is highly variable.

The only U.S. Food and Drug Administration (FDA)-approved MMPI is doxycycline hyclate (Periostat). This agent is an MMP-1 inhibitor used as an adjunct to prevent periodontitis despite the fact that it has no antibacteria activity. As a collagenase inhibitor, it prevents host derived MMPs from cleaving tooth-supporting ECM molecules. Although enthusiasm for cancer is limited, there are currently multiple MMPIs under evaluation for treatment of psoriasis, acne, arthritis, cancer, and congestive heart failure (Peterson 2004). As a cell surface expressed protein, MT1-MMP would make an ideal target for antibody based therapies, but attempts to generate a human specific anti-MT1-MMP antibody-for therapy have not been successful owing to unclear reasons.

Acknowledgment This work was supported by grants from the American Head and Neck Society and the National Cancer Institute (NCI K08CA102154).

References

Ala-aho R, Ahonen M, George SJ et al (2004) Targeted inhibition of human collagenase-3 (MMP-13) expression inhibits squamous cell carcinoma growth in vivo. Oncogene 23(30):5111–5123

Almholt K, Johnsen M (2003) Stromal cell involvement in cancer. Recent Results Cancer Res 162:31–42

Arenas-Huertero FJ, Herrera-Goepfert R, Delgado-Chavez R et al (1999) Matrix metalloproteinases expressed in squamous cell carcinoma of the oral cavity: correlation with clinicopathologic features and neo-adjuvant chemotherapy response. J Exp Clin Cancer Res 18(3):279–284

Aznavoorian S, Moore BA, Alexander-Lister LD, Hallit SL, Windsor LJ, Engler JA (2001) Membrane type I-matrix metalloproteinase-mediated degradation of type I collagen by oral squamous cell carcinoma cells. Cancer Res 61(16):6264–6275

Barcellos-Hoff MH (2005) Integrative radiation carcinogenesis: interactions between cell and tissue responses to DNA damage. Semin Cancer Biol 15(2):138–148

Barcellos-Hoff MH, Brooks AL (2001) Extracellular signaling through the microenvironment: a hypothesis relating carcinogenesis, bystander effects, and genomic instability. Radiat Res 156(5 Pt 2):618–627

Barcellos-Hoff MH, Ravani SA (2000) Irradiated mammary gland stroma promotes the expression of tumorigenic potential by unirradiated epithelial cells. Cancer Res 60(5):1254–1260

Bassi DE, Mahloogi H, Al-Saleem L, Lopez De Cicco R, Ridge JA, Klein-Szanto AJ (2001) Elevated furin expression in aggressive human head and neck tumors and tumor cell lines. Mol Carcinog 31(4):224–232

Bassi DE, Mahloogi H, Lopez De Cicco R, Klein-Szanto A (2003) Increased furin activity enhances the malignant phenotype of human head and neck cancer cells. Am J Pathol 162(2):439–447

Birkedal-Hansen H (1995) Proteolytic remodeling of extracellular matrix. Curr Opin Cell Biol 7(5):728–735

Biswas C, Zhang Y, DeCastro R et al (1995) The human tumor cell-derived collagenase stimulatory factor (renamed EMMPRIN) is a member of the immunoglobulin superfamily. Cancer Res 55(2):434–439

Bodey B, Bodey B Jr, Groger AM, Siegel SE, Kaiser HE (2001) Invasion and metastasis: the expression and significance of matrix metalloproteinases in carcinomas of the lung. In Vivo 15(2):175–180

Bordador LC, Li X, Toole B et al (2000) Expression of emmprin by oral squamous cell carcinoma. Int J Cancer 85(3):347–352

Bramhall SR, Schulz J, Nemunaitis J, Brown PD, Baillet M, Buckels JA (2002a) A double-blind placebo-controlled, randomised study comparing gemcitabine and marimastat with gemcitabine and placebo as first line therapy in patients with advanced pancreatic cancer. Br J Cancer 87(2):161–167

Bramhall SR, Hallissey MT, Whiting J et al (2002b) Marimastat as maintenance therapy for patients with advanced gastric cancer: a randomised trial. Br J Cancer 86(12):1864–1870

Braundmeier AG, Fazleabas AT, Lessey BA, Guo H, Toole BP, Nowak RA (2006) Extracellular matrix metalloproteinase inducer regulates metalloproteinases in human uterine endometrium. J Clin Endocrinol Metab 91(6):2358–2365

Camps JL, Chang SM, Hsu TC et al (1990) Fibroblast-mediated acceleration of human epithelial tumor growth in vivo. Proc Natl Acad Sci USA 87(1):75–79

Casiglia J, Woo SB (2001) A comprehensive review of oral cancer. Gen Dent 49(1):72–82

Caudroy S, Polette M, Nawrocki-Raby B et al (2002) EMMPRIN-mediated MMP regulation in tumor and endothelial cells. Clin Exp Metastasis 19(8):697–702

Chenard MP, Lutz Y, Mechine-Neuville A et al (1999) Presence of high levels of MT1-MMP protein in fibroblastic cells of human invasive carcinomas. Int J Cancer 82(2):208–212

Cheng MF, Tzao C, Tsai WC et al (2006) Expression of EMMPRIN and matriptase in esophageal squamous cell carcinoma: correlation with clinicopathological parameters. Dis Esophagus 19(6):482–486

Clark JC, Thomas DM, Choong PF, Dass CR (2007) RECK-a newly discovered inhibitor of metastasis with prognostic significance in multiple forms of cancer. Cancer Metastasis Rev 26(3–4):675–683

Coussens LM, Tinkle CL, Hanahan D, Werb Z (2000) MMP-9 supplied by bone marrow-derived cells contributes to skin carcinogenesis. Cell 103(3):481–490

Coussens LM, Fingleton B, Matrisian LM (2002) Matrix metalloproteinase inhibitors and cancer: trials and tribulations. Science 295(5564):2387–2392

Crowe DL, Hacia JG, Hsieh CL, Sinha UK, Rice H (2002) Molecular pathology of head and neck cancer. Histol Histopathol 17:909–914

Cunha GR, Matrisian LM (2002) It's not my fault, blame it on my microenvironment. Differentiation 70(9–10):469–472

Dalberg K, Eriksson E, Enberg U, Kjellman M, Backdahl M, Gelatinase A (2000) membrane type 1 matrix metalloproteinase, and extracellular matrix metalloproteinase inducer mRNA expression: correlation with invasive growth of breast cancer. World J Surg 24(3):334–340

DeClerck YA, Mercurio AM, Stack MS et al (2004) Proteases, extracellular matrix, and cancer: a workshop of the path B study section. Am J Pathol 164(4):1131–1139

Douillard JY, Peschel C, Shepherd F et al (2004) Randomized phase II feasibility study of combining the matrix metalloproteinase inhibitor BMS-275291 with paclitaxel plus carboplatin in advanced non-small cell lung cancer. Lung Cancer 46(3):361–368

Dumont N, Arteaga CL (2002) The tumor microenvironment: a potential arbitrator of the tumor suppressive and promoting actions of TGFbeta. Differentiation 70(9–10):574–582

Egeblad M, Werb Z (2002) New functions for the matrix metalloproteinases in cancer progression. Nat Rev Cancer 2(3):161–174

Elenbaas B, Weinberg RA (2001) Heterotypic signaling between epithelial tumor cells and fibroblasts in carcinoma formation. Exp Cell Res 264:169–184

Evans JD, Stark A, Johnson CD et al (2001) A phase II trial of marimastat in advanced pancreatic cancer. Br J Cancer 85(12):1865–1870

Fingleton B, Vargo-Gogola T, Crawford HC, Matrisian LM (2001) Matrilysin [MMP-7] expression selects for cells with reduced sensitivity to apoptosis. Neoplasia 3(6):459–468

Fukino K, Shen L, Patocs A, Mutter GL, Eng C (2007) Genomic instability within tumor stroma and clinicopathological characteristics of sporadic primary invasive breast carcinoma. JAMA 297(19):2103–2111

Fukumura D, Xavier R, Sugiura T et al (1998) Tumor induction of VEGF promoter activity in stromal cells. Cell 94(6):715–725

Gocht A, Bosmuller HC, Bassler R et al (1999) Breast tumors with myofibroblastic differentiation: clinico-pathological observations in myofibroblastoma and myofibrosarcoma. Pathol Res Pract 195(1):1–10

Grandis JR, Melhem MF, Gooding WE et al (1998) Levels of TGF-alpha and EGFR protein in head and neck squamous cell carcinoma and patient survival. J Natl Cancer Inst 90(11):824–832

Gruss CJ, Satyamoorthy K, Berking C et al (2003) Stroma formation and angiogenesis by overexpression of growth factors, cytokines, and proteolytic enzymes in human skin grafted to SCID mice. J Invest Dermatol 120(4):683–692

Guidi AJ, Abu-Jawdeh G, Tognazzi K, Dvorak HF, Brown LF (1996) Expression of vascular permeability factor (vascular endothelial growth factor) and its receptors in endometrial carcinoma. Cancer 78(3):454–460

Guo H, Zucker S, Gordon MK, Toole BP, Biswas C (1997) Stimulation of matrix metalloproteinase production by recombinant extracellular matrix metalloproteinase inducer from transfected Chinese hamster ovary cells. J Biol Chem 272(1):24–27

Hagedorn H, Sauer U, Schleicher E, Nerlich A (1999) Expression of TGF-beta 1 protein and mRNA and the effect on the tissue remodeling in laryngeal carcinomas. Anticancer Res 19(5B):4265–4272

Hanahan D, Folkman J (1996) Patterns and emerging mechanisms of the angiogenic switch during tumorigenesis. Cell 86(3):353–364

Heppner KJ, Matrisian LM, Jensen RA, Rodgers WH (1996) Expression of most matrix metalloproteinase family members in breast cancer represents a tumor-induced host response. Am J Pathol 149(1):273–282

Herold C, Reck T, Fischler P et al (2002) Prognosis of a large cohort of patients with hepatocellular carcinoma in a single European centre. Liver 22(1):23–28

Hotary K, Allen E, Punturieri A, Yana I, Weiss SJ (2000) Regulation of cell invasion and morphogenesis in a three-dimensional type I collagen matrix by membrane-type matrix metalloproteinases 1, 2, and 3. J Cell Biol 149(6):1309–1323

Hotary KB, Yana I, Sabeh F et al (2002) Matrix metalloproteinases (MMPs) regulate fibrin-invasive activity via MT1-MMP-dependent and -independent processes. J Exp Med 195(3):295–308

Hotary KB, Allen ED, Brooks PC, Datta NS, Long MW, Weiss SJ (2003) Membrane type I matrix metalloproteinase usurps tumor growth control imposed by the three-dimensional extracellular matrix. Cell 114(1):33–45

Imanishi Y, Fujii M, Tokumaru Y et al (2000) Clinical significance of expression of membrane type 1 matrix metalloproteinase and matrix metalloproteinase-2 in human head and neck squamous cell carcinoma. Hum Pathol 31(8):895–904

Janot F, Klijanienko J, Russo A et al (1996) Prognostic value of clinicopathological parameters in head and neck squamous cell carcinoma: a prospective analysis. Br J Cancer 73(4):531–538

Jiang A, Pei D (2003) Distinct roles of catalytic and pexin-like domains in MT-MMP mediated proMMP-2 activation and collagenolysis. J Biol Chem 278(40):38765–38771

Jiang A, Lehti K, Wang X, Weiss SJ, Keski-Oja J, Pei D (2001) Regulation of membrane-type matrix metalloproteinase 1 activity by dynamin-mediated endocytosis. Proc Natl Acad Sci USA 98(24):13693–13698

Jin JS, Yao CW, Loh SH, Cheng MF, Hsieh DS, Bai CY (2006) Increasing expression of extracellular matrix metalloprotease inducer in ovary tumors: tissue microarray analysis of immunostaining score with clinicopathological parameters. Int J Gynecol Pathol 25(2):140–146

Johansson N, Airola K, Grenman R, Kariniemi AL, Saarialho-Kere U, Kahari VM (1997) Expression of collagenase-3 (matrix metalloproteinase-13) in squamous cell carcinomas of the head and neck. Am J Pathol 151(2):499–508

Kajita M, Itoh Y, Chiba T et al (2001) Membrane-type 1 matrix metalloproteinase cleaves CD44 and promotes cell migration. J Cell Biol 153(5):893–904

Katori H, Baba Y, Imagawa Y et al (2002) Reduction of in vivo tumor growth by MMI-166, a selective matrix metalloproteinase inhibitor, through inhibition of tumor angiogenesis in squamous cell carcinoma cell lines of head and neck. Cancer Lett 178(2):151–159

Kishnani NS, Staskus PW, Yang T-T, Masiarz FR, Hawkes SP (1995) Identification and characterization of human tissue inhibitor of metalloproteinase-3 and detection of three additional metalloproteinase inhibitor activities in extracellular matrix. Matrix Biol 14(6):479–488

Klein CA, Seidl S, Petat-Dutter K et al (2002) Combined transcriptome and genome analysis of single micrometastatic cells. Nat Biotechnol 20(4):387–392

Kurahara S, Shinohara M, Ikebe T et al (1999) Expression of MMPS, MT-MMP, and TIMPs in squamous cell carcinoma of the oral cavity: correlations with tumor invasion and metastasis. Head Neck 21(7):627–638

Kuriakose MA, Loree TR, Rubenfeld A et al (2002) Simultaneously presenting head and neck and lung cancer: a diagnostic and treatment dilemma. Laryngoscope 112(1):120–123

Kurose K, Hoshaw-Woodard S, Adeyinka A, Lemeshow S, Watson PH, Eng C (2001) Genetic model of multi-step breast carcinogenesis involving the epithelium and stroma: clues to tumour-microenvironment interactions. Hum Mol Genet 10(18):1907–1913

Latreille J, Batist G, Laberge F et al (2003) Phase I/II trial of the safety and efficacy of AE-941 (Neovastat) in the treatment of non-small-cell lung cancer. Clin Lung Cancer 4(4):231–236

Leon X, Quer M, Orus C, del Prado Venegas M (2001) Can cure be achieved in patients with head and neck carcinomas? The problem of second neoplasm. Expert Rev Anticancer Ther 1(1):125–133

Lewis AM, Varghese S, Xu H, Alexander HR (2006) Interleukin-1 and cancer progression: the emerging role of interleukin-1 receptor antagonist as a novel therapeutic agent in cancer treatment. J Transl Med 4:48

Li SL, Gao DL, Zhao ZH et al (2007) Correlation of matrix metalloproteinase suppressor genes RECK, VEGF, and CD105 with angiogenesis and biological behavior in esophageal squamous cell carcinoma. World J Gastroenterol 13(45):6076–6081

Liotta LA (1986) Tumor invasion and metastases – role of the extracellular matrix: Rhoads Memorial Award lecture. Cancer Res 46(1):1–7

Liotta LA, Kohn EC (2001) The microenvironment of the tumour-host interface. Nature 411(6835):375–379

Lu SL, Herrington H, Reh D et al (2006) Loss of transforming growth factor-beta type II receptor promotes metastatic head-and-neck squamous cell carcinoma. Genes Dev 20(10):1331–1342

Lynch CC, Matrisian LM (2002) Matrix metalloproteinases in tumor-host cell communication. Differentiation 70(9–10):561–573

Mabjeesh NJ, Amir S (2007) Hypoxia-inducible factor (HIF) in human tumorigenesis. Histol Histopathol 22(5):559–572

Mandic R, Dunne AA, Eikelkamp N et al (2002) Expression of MMP-3, MMP-13, TIMP-2 and TIMP-3 in the VX2 carcinoma of the New Zealand white rabbit. Anticancer Res 22(6A):3281–3284

Marcus B, Arenberg D, Lee J et al (2004) Prognostic factors in oral cavity and oropharyngeal squamous cell carcinoma. Cancer 101(12):2779–2787

Matrisian LM, Wright J, Newell K, Witty JP (1994) Matrix-degrading metalloproteinases in tumor progression. Princess Takamatsu Symp 24:152–161

McCawley LJ, Matrisian LM (2001) Tumor progression: defining the soil round the tumor seed. Curr Biol 11(1):R25–R27

McDonald DM, Teicher BA, Stetler-Stevenson W et al (2004) Report from the society for biological therapy and vascular biology faculty of the NCI workshop on angiogenesis monitoring. J Immunother 27(2):161–175

Micke P, Ostman A (2005) Exploring the tumour environment: cancer-associated fibroblasts as targets in cancer therapy. Expert Opin Ther Targets 9(6):1217–1233

Moinfar F, Man YG, Arnould L, Bratthauer GL, Ratschek M, Tavassoli FA (2000) Concurrent and independent genetic alterations in the stromal and epithelial cells of mammary carcinoma: implications for tumorigenesis. Cancer Res 60(9):2562–2566

Moinfar F, Kremser ML, Man YG, Zatloukal K, Tavassoli FA, Denk H (2004) Allelic imbalances in endometrial stromal neoplasms: frequent genetic alterations in the nontumorous normal-appearing endometrial and myometrial tissues. Gynecol Oncol 95(3):662–671

Mori H, Tomari T, Koshikawa N et al (2002) CD44 directs membrane-type 1 matrix metalloproteinase to lamellipodia by associating with its hemopexin-like domain. EMBO J 21(15):3949–3959

Mueller MM, Fusenig NE (2002) Tumor-stroma interactions directing phenotype and progression of epithelial skin tumor cells. Differentiation 70(9–10):486–497

Mueller MM, Peter W, Mappes M et al (2001) Tumor progression of skin carcinoma cells in vivo promoted by clonal selection, mutagenesis, and autocrine growth regulation by granulocyte colony-stimulating factor and granulocyte-macrophage colony-stimulating factor. Am J Pathol 159(4):1567–1579

Muller D, Wolf C, Abecassis J et al (1993) Increased stromelysin 3 gene expression is associated with increased local invasiveness in head and neck squamous cell carcinomas. Cancer Res 53(1):165–169

Noda M, Oh J, Takahashi R, Kondo S, Kitayama H, Takahashi C (2003) RECK: a novel suppressor of malignancy linking oncogenic signaling to extracellular matrix remodeling. Cancer Metastasis Rev 22(2–3):167–175

O-Charoenrat P, Rhys-Evans P, Modjtahedi H, Court W, Box G, Eccles S (2000) Overexpression of epidermal growth factor receptor in human head and neck squamous carcinoma cell lines correlates with matrix metalloproteinase-9 expression and in vitro invasion. Int J Cancer 86(3):307–317

O-Charoenrat P, Rhys-Evans P, Eccles SA (2001a) Expression of vascular endothelial growth factor family members in head and neck squamous cell carcinoma correlates with lymph node metastasis. Cancer 92(3):556–568

O-Charoenrat P, Rhys-Evans PH, Eccles SA (2001b) Expression of matrix metalloproteinases and their inhibitors correlates with invasion and metastasis in squamous cell carcinoma of the head and neck. Arch Otolaryngol Head Neck Surg 127(7):813–820

O-Charoenrat P, Rhys-Evans P, Eccles S (2002) A synthetic matrix metalloproteinase inhibitor prevents squamous carcinoma cell proliferation by interfering with epidermal growth factor receptor autocrine loops. Int J Cancer 100(5):527–533

Oh J, Takahashi R, Kondo S et al (2001) The membrane-anchored MMP inhibitor RECK is a key regulator of extracellular matrix integrity and angiogenesis. Cell 107(6):789–800

Okada A, Bellocq JP, Rouyer N et al (1995) Membrane-type matrix metalloproteinase (MT-MMP) gene is expressed in stromal cells of human colon, breast, and head and neck carcinomas. Proc Natl Acad Sci USA 92(7):2730–2734

Olumi AF, Grossfeld GD, Hayward SW, Carroll PR, Tlsty TD, Cunha GR (1999) Carcinoma-associated fibroblasts direct tumor progression of initiated human prostatic epithelium. Cancer Res 59(19):5002–5011

Ondruschka C, Buhtz P, Motsch C et al (2002) Prognostic value of MMP-2, -9 and TIMP-1,-2 immunoreactive protein at the invasive front in advanced head and neck squamous cell carcinomas. Pathol Res Pract 198(8):509–515

Orimo A, Gupta PB, Sgroi DC et al (2005) Stromal fibroblasts present in invasive human breast carcinomas promote tumor growth and angiogenesis through elevated SDF-1/CXCL12 secretion. Cell 121(3):335–348

Patel BP, Shah PM, Rawal UM et al (2005) Activation of MMP-2 and MMP-9 in patients with oral squamous cell carcinoma. J Surg Oncol 90(2):81–88

Pauli BU, Knudson W (1988) Tumor invasion: a consequence of destructive and compositional matrix alterations. Hum Pathol 19(6):628–639

Pei D, Weiss SJ (1996) Transmembrane-deletion mutants of the membrane-type matrix metallopro-teinase-1 process progelatinase A and express intrinsic matrix-degrading activity. J Biol Chem 271(15):9135–9140

Peterson JT (2004) Matrix metalloproteinase inhibitor development and the remodeling of drug discovery. Heart Fail Rev 9(1):63–79

Picard O, Rolland Y, Poupon MF (1986) Fibroblast-dependent tumorigenicity of cells in nude mice: implication for implantation of metastases. Cancer Res 46(7):3290–3294

Polette M, Gilles C, Marchand V et al (1997) Tumor collagenase stimulatory factor (TCSF) expression and localization in human lung and breast cancers. J Histochem Cytochem 45(5):703–709

Ponec M, Hoekman K, Lowik C (1991) Cell-cell communication: parathyroid hormone-like protein production by squamous carcinoma cells is modulated by fibroblasts. A possible mechanism in the development of humoral hypercalcemia of malignancy. Curr Probl Dermatol 20:1–10

Pries R, Wollenberg B (2006) Cytokines in head and neck cancer. Cytokine Growth Factor Rev 17(3):141–146

Pries R, Nitsch S, Wollenberg B (2006) Role of cytokines in head and neck squamous cell carcinoma. Expert Rev Anticancer Ther 6(9):1195–1203

Rhee JS, Coussens LM (2002) RECKing MMP function: implications for cancer development. Trends Cell Biol 12(5):209–211

Riethdorf S, Reimers N, Assmann V et al (2006) High incidence of EMMPRIN expression in human tumors. Int J Cancer 119(8):1800–1810

Rofstad EK (2000) Microenvironment-induced cancer metastasis. Int J Radiat Biol 76(5):589–605

Rosenthal EL, Hotary K, Bradford C, Weiss SJ (1999) Role of membrane type 1-matrix metallo-proteinase and gelatinase A in head and neck squamous cell carcinoma invasion in vitro. Otolaryngol Head Neck Surg 121(4):337–343

Rosenthal EL, Shreenivas S, Peters GE, Grizzle WE, Desmond R, Gladson CL (2003) Expression of extracellular matrix metalloprotease inducer in laryngeal squamous cell carcinoma. Laryngoscope 113(8):1406–1410

Rosenthal E, McCrory A, Talbert M, Young G, Murphy-Ullrich J, Gladson C (2004a) Elevated expres-sion of TGF-beta1 in head and neck cancer-associated fibroblasts. Mol Carcinog 40(2):116–121

Rosenthal EL, McCrory A, Talbert M, Carroll W, Magnuson JS, Peters GE (2004b) Expression of proteolytic enzymes in head and neck cancer-associated fibroblasts. Arch Otolaryngol Head Neck Surg 130(8):943–947

Rosenthal EL, Vidrine DM, Zhang W (2006) Extracellular matrix metalloprotease inducer stimulates fibroblast-mediated tumor growth in vivo. Laryngoscope 116(7):1086–1092

Sasahara RM, Brochado SM, Takahashi C et al (2002) Transcriptional control of the RECK metastasis/angiogenesis suppressor gene. Cancer Detect Prev 26(6):435–443

Scherubl H, Scherer H, Hoffmeister B (2002) Head and neck cancer. N Engl J Med 346(18):1416–1417

Senger DR, Claffey KP, Benes JE, Perruzzi CA, Sergiou AP, Detmar M (1997) Angiogenesis promoted by vascular endothelial growth factor: regulation through alpha1beta1 and alpha-2beta1 integrins. Proc Natl Acad Sci USA 94(25):13612–13617

Skobe M, Fusenig NE (1998) Tumorigenic conversion of immortal human keratinocytes through stromal cell activation. Proc Natl Acad Sci USA 95(3):1050–1055

Sledge GW Jr, Qulali M, Goulet R, Bone EA, Fife R (1995) Effect of matrix metalloproteinase inhibitor batimastat on breast cancer regrowth and metastasis in athymic mice. J Natl Cancer Inst 87(20):1546–1550

Span PN, Sweep CG, Manders P, Beex LV, Leppert D, Lindberg RL (2003) Matrix metallopro tei-nase inhibitor reversion-inducing cysteine-rich protein with Kazal motifs: a prognostic marker for good clinical outcome in human breast carcinoma. Cancer 97(11):2710–2715

Sparano JA, Bernardo P, Stephenson P et al (2004) Randomized phase III trial of marimastat versus placebo in patients with metastatic breast cancer who have responding or stable disease after first-line chemotherapy: Eastern Cooperative Oncology Group trial E2196. J Clin Oncol 22(23):4683–4690

Stamenkovic I (2000) Matrix metalloproteinases in tumor invasion and metastasis. Semin Cancer Biol 10(6):415–433

Sternlicht MD, Lochter A, Sympson CJ et al (1999) The stromal proteinase MMP3/stromelysin-1 promotes mammary carcinogenesis. Cell 98(2):137–146

Stetler-Stevenson WG (2008) The tumor microenvironment: regulation by MMP-independent effects of tissue inhibitor of metalloproteinases-2. Cancer Metastasis Rev 27(1):57–66

Stetler-Stevenson WG, Seo DW (2005) TIMP-2: an endogenous inhibitor of angiogenesis. Trends Mol Med 11(3):97–103

Sutinen M, Kainulainen T, Hurskainen T et al (1998) Expression of matrix metalloproteinases (MMP-1 and -2) and their inhibitors (TIMP-1, -2 and -3) in oral lichen planus, dysplasia, squamous cell carcinoma and lymph node metastasis. Br J Cancer 77(12):2239–2245

Tang Y, Nakada MT, Kesavan P et al (2005) Extracellular matrix metalloproteinase inducer stimulates tumor angiogenesis by elevating vascular endothelial cell growth factor and matrix metalloproteinases. Cancer Res 65(8):3193–3199

Taylor PM, Woodfield RJ, Hodgkin MN et al (2002) Breast cancer cell-derived EMMPRIN stimulates fibroblast MMP2 release through a phospholipase A(2) and 5-lipoxygenase catalyzed pathway. Oncogene 21(37):5765–5772

Thomasset N, Lochter A, Sympson CJ et al (1998) Expression of autoactivated stromelysin-1 in mammary glands of transgenic mice leads to a reactive stroma during early development. Am J Pathol 153(2):457–467

Tokumaru Y, Fujii M, Otani Y et al (2000) Activation of matrix metalloproteinase-2 in head and neck squamous cell carcinoma: studies of clinical samples and in vitro cell lines co-cultured with fibroblasts. Cancer Lett 150(1):15–21

Tsukifuji R, Tagawa K, Hatamochi A, Shinkai H (1999) Expression of matrix metalloproteinase-1, -2 and -3 in squamous cell carcinoma and actinic keratosis. Br J Cancer 80(7):1087–1091

Uria JA, Ferrando AA, Velasco G, Freije JM, Lopez-Otin C (1994) Structure and expression in breast tumors of human TIMP-3, a new member of the metalloproteinase inhibitor family. Cancer Res 54(8):2091–2094

Vigneswaran N, Beckers S, Waigel S et al (2006) Increased EMMPRIN (CD 147) expression during oral carcinogenesis. Exp Mol Pathol 80(2):147–159

Weber F, Xu Y, Zhang L et al (2007) Microenvironmental genomic alterations and clinicopathological behavior in head and neck squamous cell carcinoma. JAMA 297(2):187–195

Werner JA, Rathcke IO, Mandic R (2002) The role of matrix metalloproteinases in squamous cell carcinomas of the head and neck. Clin Exp Metastasis 19(4):275–282

Yoshizaki T, Sato H, Maruyama Y et al (1997) Increased expression of membrane type 1-matrix metalloproteinase in head and neck carcinoma. Cancer 79(1):139–144

Zhang W, Matrisian LM, Holmbeck K, Vick CC, Rosenthal EL (2006) Fibroblast-derived MT1-MMP promotes tumor progression in vitro and in vivo. BMC Cancer 6:52

Zucker S, Hymowitz M, Rollo EE et al (2001) Tumorigenic potential of extracellular matrix metalloproteinase inducer. Am J Pathol 158(6):1921–1928

Chapter 13
Chemokines and Their Receptors in Oral Cancer Metastasis

Yvonne K. Mburu and Robert L. Ferris

Abstract In oral cancers, a high degree of local invasion and metastases to the regional cervical lymph nodes is observed. Distant metastases occur at a low rate and are rarely observed until late in the disease. The underlying mechanism(s) of this site-specific metastasis has been the subject of numerous studies. Chemokine receptors have been described as being important in the metastatic process of these tumors given that the lymph nodes, which represent a key site of metastasis, also happen to be an abundant source of the chemokine ligands for oral cancer tumor-associated chemokine receptors. We review our current understanding of the role that chemokines, and their receptors play in the dissemination of metastatic disease in oral cancers while highlighting their importance to the overall survival and migratory ability of these tumors. Ongoing advances in our knowledge of cell migration and tumor metastasis continue to present opportunities for the development of prognostic markers and therapeutic intervention.

Introduction

Chemokines are small proinflammatory "chemotactic cytokines" that mediate the selective recruitment and directional migration of leukocytes to inflammatory sites. They are typically induced by inflammatory cytokines, growth factors, and pathogenic stimuli and signal through seven-transmembrane G-protein-coupled (chemokine) receptors (Rossi and Zlotnik 2000). Chemokines are structurally classified into four highly conserved groups based on the position of the first two N-terminal cysteine residues (C, CC, CXC, CX_3C) (Zlotnik and Yoshie 2000). Chemokine receptors are also subdivided into these four families based on the family to which their cognate ligands belong (Table 13.1).

Since chemokines were discovered over 20 years ago, they have been studied extensively, more so with regard to their role in cell motility. However, the promiscuity

R.L. Ferris (✉)
Hillman Cancer Center, Research Pavilion 1.19d, Pittsburgh, PA, 15213, USA
e-mail: ferrisrl@msx.upmc.edu

J. Myers (ed.), *Oral Cancer Metastasis*,
DOI 10.1007/978-1-4419-0775-2_13, © Springer Science+Business Media, LLC 2010

Table 13.1 Chemokine receptors and their ligands

Family	Chemokine receptor	Chemokine ligands
C	XCR1	XCL1, XCL2
CC	CCR1	CCL3, CCL5, CCL6, CCL7, CCL9/10, CCL13, CCL14, CCL15, CCL16, CCL23
	CCR2	CCL2, CCL6, CCL7, CCL8, CCL12, CCL13, CCL27
	CCR3	CCL5, CCL6, CCL7, CCL8, CCL11, CCL13, CCL15, CCL24, CCL26, CCL27, CCL28
	CCR4	CCL17, CCL22
	CCR5	CCL3, CCL4, CCL5, CCL8,
	CCR6	CCL20
	CCR7	CCL19, CCL21
	CCR8	CCL1
	CCR9	CCL25
	CCR10	CCL27, CCL28
CXC	CXCR1	CXCL1, CXCL6, CXCL7, CXCL8
	CXCR2	CXCL1, CXCL2, CXCL3, CXCL5, CXCL6, CXCL7, CXCL8
	CXCR3	CXCL9, CXCL10, CXCL11
	CXCR4	CXCL12
	CXCR5	CXCL13
	CXCR6	CXCL16
CX_3C	CX_3CR1	CX_3CL1

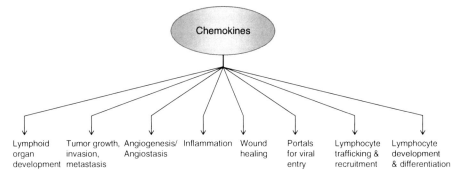

Fig. 13.1 Chemokines control various cellular processes

of ligand–receptor interactions in vivo coupled with functional redundancies of some chemokines and their receptors has slowed the progress in understanding how they are expressed and functioning. The naming of chemokines by the multiple groups that identified them has contributed to the confusion, although this problem has now been alleviated by adopting a numbering system that relies on the classification of the four structural families (Zlotnik and Yoshie 2000). Nevertheless, the interest in understanding chemokines has been fueled by the finding that these molecules are expressed by not only lymphocytes but also many other cell types, and they control numerous physiological and pathological processes, including the metastasis of neoplastic cells to distant organs (Fig. 13.1). Recent reviews have alluded to the contribution by an inflammatory tumor environment by promoting angiogenesis, tumor growth, invasion, and metastasis and the crucial role played by cytokines and chemokines in inflammation-associated tumorigenesis (Lu et al. 2006).

Involvement of Chemokines in Metastasis

The pathological mechanisms of tumor metastasis are poorly understood. However, the wealth of the scientific literature has led to a general consensus that the propensity of a tumor to metastasize is a nonrandom process that depends on its interactions with the homeostatic factors that facilitate its continued proliferation and survival. In truth, this idea was first introduced cohesively by Stephen Paget in the late nineteenth century when he published the "seed and soil" hypothesis (Paget 1889). He studied hundreds of autopsy records from patients with different types of tumors and observed that there was a predisposition of tumors to migrate to specific organs.

> The evidence seems to me irresistible that in cancer of the breast, the bones suffer in a special way, which cannot be explained by any theory of embolism alone. Some bones suffer more than others; the disease has its "seats of election". (Paget 1889)

He went on to propose the idea that certain tumor cells (the seed) migrated selectively toward organ microenvironments which facilitated their relentless growth (the soil). Each organ microenvironment, therefore, must possess certain unique "signatures" that qualify it as a suitable site for the migrating tumor cell to colonize successfully. This view is now widely accepted, and three contemporary theories have been postulated to explain the "homing" of cancer cells toward specific organ sites (Liotta 2001). The "organ selection" theory proposes that tumors emigrate from the primary site and spread through the circulation and/or lymphatics to a similar extent in all tissues, but the presence of appropriate growth factors in the target organs determines whether the invading tumor cells will establish successful metastases. The "adhesion" theory proposes that tissue-specific adhesion molecules expressed on the endothelial surfaces of target organs are responsible for anchoring migrating tumor cells and setting up a premetastatic niche that develops into a secondary tumor. The "chemoattraction" theory proposes that malignant cells expressing functional chemokine receptors can respond to organ-specific chemoattractant molecules and migrate directionally along chemokine gradients to set up site-specific metastases in the target organ(s). Such chemotactic migration of tumors would mirror the physiologic mechanisms of lymphocyte homing into lymphoid organs.

The observation that organs representing key sites of metastasis also happen to be abundant sources of the chemokine ligands for certain tumor-associated chemokine receptors has piqued interest in this theory. Initial evidence for the involvement of chemokines in metastasis was presented in a seminal article by Muller et al., who demonstrated that CXCR4 and CCR7 expression in breast cancer cell lines resulted in metastases to organs that express high amounts of the respective cognate ligands, CXCL12 and CCL19/21 (Muller et al. 2001). Other groups have confirmed these findings, including work by Wiley et al. showing that transfection of CCR7 into a murine melanoma cell line was sufficient to result in a significant increase in lymph node metastasis in vivo (Wiley et al. 2001). Moreover, it has been shown that the neutralization of such chemokine receptor–ligand interactions results in a marked inhibition of metastases, suggesting that such an avenue might represent a potential target for clinical intervention. Thus, chemokine receptor-expressing tumors are capable of responding to environmental cues intended for immune cells and mimicking physiologic mechanisms of leukocyte migration to further their own migration and colonization of secondary microenvironments (Fig. 13.2).

In oral cancers, a high degree of local invasion and metastases to the regional cervical lymph nodes is observed. Distant metastases occur at a low rate and are rarely observed until late in the disease. The underlying mechanism(s) of this site-specific metastasis has been the subject of numerous studies. In particular, the chemokine receptors CXCR4 and CCR7 have been described as being important in the metastatic process of these tumors. This chapter aims to review our current understanding of the role that chemokines and their receptors play in the dissemination of metastatic disease in oral cancers while highlighting their importance to the overall survival and migratory ability of these tumors. Ongoing advances in our knowledge of cell migration and tumor metastasis continue to present opportunities for the development of prognostic markers and therapeutic intervention.

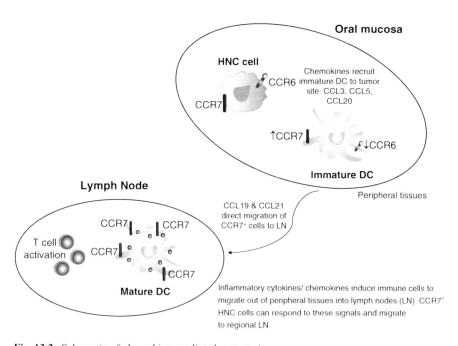

Fig. 13.2 Schematic of chemokine-mediated metastasis

Chemokine Expression Patterns in Oral Cancer

As in numerous other malignancies, various chemokines and their receptors have been found to be overexpressed in oral cancers. Indeed, multiple chemokine-receptor interactions are likely to be important in oral cancer progression, although it is not clear whether they can act in synergy. The chemokine ligand CCL2 is expressed in esophageal squamous cell carcinoma (SCC) and was reported to play a role in macrophage infiltration and the enhancement of tumor vascularity (Ohta et al. 2002). The expression of CXCL1 [found to be expressed in melanoma (Dhawan and Richmond 2002)] was studied in oral SCC and found to be overexpressed in 40% of the cases examined (Shintani et al. 2004). This expression was correlated with tumor angiogenesis, leukocyte infiltration, and nodal metastasis. In another study utilizing microarray analysis, gene expression was compared between synchronous primary and metastatic head and neck SCC. Among other genes, the chemokines CXCL5 and CXCL8 were found significantly upregulated in metastatic SCC (Miyazaki et al. 2006a). The targeting of CXCL5 in these cells using RNA interference resulted in decreased proliferation of cells, impaired ability to migrate and invade in vitro, and inhibited tumor formation in vivo, suggesting that CXCL5 is intimately involved in these tumorigenic properties (Miyazaki et al. 2006b). On the other hand, CXCL8 (a well characterized proangiogenic chemokine) was shown to upregulate matrix metalloproteinase (MMP)-7 secretion, thereby, contributing to oral SCC invasion and migration by facilitating the degradation of the basement membrane (Watanabe et al. 2002).

Chemokine receptor expression has also been investigated in oral cancers. CXCR4 has been found upregulated in oral SCC as compared with normal epithelium and signaling with its cognate ligand CXCL12 is suggested to be important for the establishment of lymph node metastasis in oral SCC (Delilbasi et al. 2004; Uchida et al. 2003; Ishikawa et al. 2006), as discussed in detail below. Another study comparing the expression of various chemokine receptors in autologous primary and metastatic SCC cell lines found that CCR6 is selectively expressed in primary tumors while CCR7 appears to be upregulated significantly in metastatic SCC tumors (Wang et al. 2004). Further studies have implicated CCR7 expression in the lymph node metastasis of SCC.

In light of the variable and often heterogeneous patterns of chemokine expression that have been observed on tumor cells, the mechanisms that are responsible for reprogramming malignant cells to express functional chemokine receptors need to be further examined. Given the degree to which metastatic tumors differ both genotypically and phenotypically from their parental primary tumors, it is generally agreed upon that tumor environmental factors must play a key role in shaping the repertoire of receptor expression on the evolving neoplasm. Whether these receptor changes occur at the primary tumor site or at the secondary tumor site remains to be investigated (Bernards and Weinberg 2002; Hynes 2003). Studies on the activation of CXCR4 expression have demonstrated that hypoxic conditions or mutations that result in the accumulation of the hypoxia-inducible factor (HIF) can lead to the upregulation of CXCR4 (Staller et al. 2003; Schioppa et al. 2003; Burger and Kipps 2006). This provides a likely mechanism for the expression of CXCR4 on patient tumors which are often hypoxic due to poor blood supply. The stimulation of endothelins in breast cancer has also been suggested to induce CCR7 through the activation of HIF-1 (Wilson et al. 2006). Autocrine signaling through the vascular endothelial growth factor has also been shown to induce the expression of CXCR4 in breast cancer cells (Bachelder et al. 2002). Furthermore, the activation of the nuclear transcription factor nuclear factor kappa B (NF-κB) has been reported to be important for the induction of CXCR4 and CCR7 expression, both of which are NF-κB target genes (Helbig et al. 2003; Kulbe et al. 2005; Richmond 2002; Mburu et al. 2006). Epigenetic modifications that result in alterations in gene activity have also been reported to be responsible for CXCR4 and CCR7 upregulation in melanoma (Mori et al. 2005).

In summary, the chemokines CXCR4 and CCR7 are the most widely studied examples of chemokine receptors involved in metastasis and provide the most compelling data. Not surprisingly, the ligands for these receptors are expressed in the lymph nodes which are key sites for oral cancer metastasis. The rest of this chapter will be devoted to highlighting our understanding of these chemokine receptors and their overall significance to oral cancer progression and metastasis.

Role of CXCR4 in Oral Cancer Metastasis

CXCR4 is the most commonly overexpressed chemokine in human cancers. Its expression has been described in at least 23 different human malignancies, including breast cancer, colorectal cancer, cervical cancer, melanoma, and SCCs (Balkwill 2004a, b), and has been associated with tumor progression and poor prognosis in these malignancies. Although CXCR4 can sometimes be found expressed at very low levels in some normal tissues, its overexpression in various cancers has resulted in a vigorous scientific effort to understand its regulation and function in tumor cells.

As earlier described, CXCR4 has been found to be frequently overexpressed in oral SCC and has been significantly associated with various clinicopathological factors including lymph node metastasis (70% of cases examined), tumor recurrence (74%), and mode of invasion, where its expression was strongly associated with grade-4 diffuse type invasion (85%) (Almofti et al. 2004). Notably, there was no association between CXCR4 expression and age, sex, or tumor size. In addition and likely as a result of the aforementioned factors, the overall prognosis for patients with CXCR4-positive tumors remains poorer than that of patients with CXCR4-negative tumors. In another study, transfection of CXCR4 into an oral SCC cell line with poor metastatic potential generated a highly metastatic cell line that was found to frequently metastasize to the cervical lymph nodes but not to distant organs of an orthotopic mouse model (Uchida et al. 2004). These nodal metastases could be inhibited by the use of mitogen activated protein (MAP) kinase inhibitors, or by phosphatidylinosotol 3 kinase (PI3K) inhibitors, suggesting that the CXCR4/CXCL12 signaling axis was important for the establishment of these metastases.

While the significance of CXCR4 expression on a tumor cannot be overstated, it is also becoming increasingly clear that the expression of CXCL12 by tumors may be important in determining the overall prognosis. A recent study found that the 5-year survival of patients with CXCL12-positive tumors was significantly lower (25%) than that of patients with CXCL12-negative tumors (71%) (Uchida et al. 2007). In this study, cases of secondary lung metastasis were reported in patients with CXCL12-positive tumors. In examining the factors that determine regional vs. distant CXCR4-mediated metastasis in oral SCC, the role of autocrine and paracrine secretion of the CXCL12 ligand was analyzed. A CXCR4-positive oral SCC cell line transfected to express CXCL12 was reported to have more metastatic foci and heavier lymph node metastases in an orthotopic mouse model than the parental CXCL12-negative cell line. Furthermore, intravenous inoculation of the tumor cells (hence, seeding of lung tumors) resulted in numerous metastatic nodules in the lungs with CXCL12-positive tumors while few (*if any*) were observed from CXCL12-negative tumors. These findings suggest that autocrine CXCR4/CXCL12 signaling is responsible for the establishment of distant metastases due to the acquisition of an aggressive metastatic potential. Notably, the use of a CXCR4 antagonist inhibited the in vitro motility of tumors, significantly reduced the in vivo formation of metastatic nodules and prolonged the survival of tumor-bearing mice.

Further studies have examined this CXCR4/CXCL12 signaling axis, and the role it plays in the stimulation of other intracellular signaling pathways that are important for cell motility. Studies from various tumor models suggest that chemokines may facilitate the metastasis of tumors by inducing the expression of MMPs and collagenases. Indeed, CXCR4 stimulation by its ligand CXCL12 in head and neck SCC has been demonstrated to increase cell adhesion and activate the secretion of MMP-9, a key component in the degradation of ECM proteins (Samara et al. 2004). Moreover, CXCR4/CXCL12 signaling in oral SCC cells has also been associated with the induction of the epithelial–mesenchymal transition, a critical event occasionally observed prior to tumor invasion by which the cells acquire a more aggressive phenotype by exhibiting reduced cell–cell adhesion and increased motility. This transition was dependent on the PI3K signaling pathway (Onoue et al. 2006).

Role of CCR7 in Oral Cancer Metastasis

The distinct migration pattern of oral cancers into regional tumor-draining lymph nodes raised a particular interest in examining the role of CCR7 and its ligands in metastasis. A recent study on dendritic cell (DC) migration indicated that CCR7 appears to be a stronger mediator of lymph node homing than CXCR4 (Humrich et al. 2006) providing impetus to further explore the involvement of the CCR7 in metastasis of oral cancers to regional lymph nodes. Indeed, CCR7 has been associated with lymph node homing of several malignancies including breast cancer, melanoma, gastric cancer, esophageal cancer, and head and neck SCC (Muller et al. 2001; Wiley et al. 2001; Wang et al. 2004; Mashino et al. 2002; Ding et al. 2003). High CCR7 expression in esophageal SCC tumors was correlated with clinicopathological characteristics such as tumor depth, TNM stage, lymphatic invasion, and lymph node metastasis (Ding et al. 2003). Not surprisingly, esophageal carcinoma patients with CCR7-positive tumors were reported to have significantly poorer prognosis than those with CCR7-negative tumors.

In head and neck SCC cell lines, the transcriptional expression of various chemokine receptors (CCR1 to CCR10 and CXCR1 to CXCR5) was examined using real-time polymerase chain reaction (PCR). Though there was some appreciable albeit inconsistent expression of the other chemokine receptors, CCR7 was the only chemokine receptor that was found to be consistently upregulated in metastatic tumors as compared with the autologous primary tumors (Wang et al. 2004). This trend was mirrored in patient tissue biopsies using immunohistochemical staining. In this study, surface chemokine expression on primary tumors was found to be predominantly $CCR6^+$ $CCR7^{low}$ while their metastatic counterparts were $CCR6^-$ $CCR7^{high}$. This receptor expression is reminiscent of the response of immune cells to inflammatory stimuli: peripheral immature DCs express CCR6 but lose this receptor upon antigen uptake and maturation and upregulate CCR7 which facilitates emigration from peripheral sites and trafficking into the lymph nodes. That these head and neck SCC cells can mimic the differentiation, and migration pattern of DCs is noteworthy and calls for further investigation into the inflammatory signaling mechanisms involved.

CCR7 expression has been reported to protect circulating $CD8^+$ T cells from apoptosis (Kim et al. 2005). Likewise, our studies have shown that CCR7 expression in head and neck SCC mediates pro-survival and invasive pathways through PI3K activation (Wang et al. 2005a) (Fig. 13.3). Autocrine CCR7 activation has been identified in head and neck SCC cell lines. Indeed, the autocrine and paracrine activation of CCR7 may promote tumor aggressiveness by maintaining basal activation of these survival and invasive pathways (Wang et al. 2008). Recent data suggest that CCR7-mediated pro-survival pathways may be responsible for the resistance of head and neck SCCs to platinum-based chemotherapies, thereby, associating CCR7 expression with aggressive, recurrent tumors.

In our studies, we have also investigated the in vivo role of the CCR7-CCL19/21 signaling axis in tumor progression by utilizing *plt* mice. The *plt* mutation results in the loss of expression of CCL19 and CCL21-ser in the secondary lymphoid organs and, therefore, an inability to recruit $CCR7^+$ cells to these organs. When a $CCR7^+$ murine oral SCC cell line was implanted in *plt* mice, we observed a lower rate of tumor growth and a lower ultimate tumor burden as compared with Balb/c littermates, suggesting that CCR7 stimulation by its ligands was important for tumor progression (Wang et al. 2008). Whether this *plt* mutation leads to decreased lymphatic invasion of tumors and fewer lymph node metastases is still under

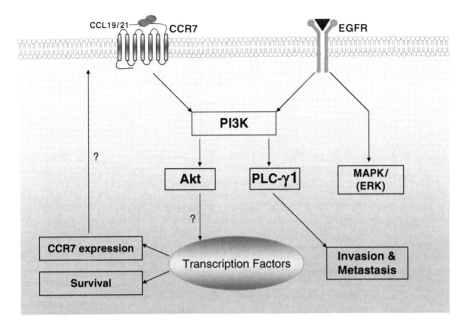

Fig. 13.3 CCR7 signaling mediates survival and invasive pathways through PI3K

investigation. However, the data support that CCR7 signaling contributes to tumor survival and proliferation. It is also worth noting that the elevated expression of CCR7 ligands has been correlated with the presence of CCR7+ tumors (Wang et al. 2005b; Takeuchi et al. 2004).

In yet another study, when chemokine expression in SCC was compared with adenoid cystic carcinoma (ACC), head and neck SCC were found to consistently upregulate CCR7 and CXCR5 mRNA (Muller et al. 2006). In cell lines, CCR7 was only detectable intracellularly whereas surface expression was evident in tissue sections examined by immunohistochemistry. On the other hand, CXCR4 was found to be predominantly expressed in ACC as opposed to SCC tumors. This was consistent with the tendency for ACC to metastasize to distant sites such as the lung and liver (Fordice et al. 1999), both abundant sources of CXCL12.

The discordant findings from different groups based on the expression of CXCR4 and CCR7 in head and neck SCC may reflect differences in the histological phenotypes and clinical characteristics of head and neck carcinomas in general. However, it also emphasizes the importance of examining patient tissue biopsies to corroborate findings from cultured cell lines, and reinforces the need to investigate the mechanisms that induce chemokine expression in SCCs. We cannot rule out the concomitant expression of these chemokine receptors, and it is indeed likely that multiple chemokine-receptor interactions are important at various stages in SCC progression and metastasis.

Conclusion

Current treatment modalities for oral SCC have established fairly good locoregional control. However, the progression to metastatic disease remains the major hurdle in the overall tumor control and patient survival. As reviewed in this chapter, chemokines and their receptors can act at multiple points on the path to malignancy. Based on their involvement in tumor proliferation, invasion and metastasis, and the efficacies observed in preclinical cancer models using chemokine-based immunotherapy, a new paradigm for cancer therapy emerges. Targeting this chemokine ligand/receptor axis and neutralizing the tumor-chemokine networks could provide exciting new therapeutic options in oral SCC and a range of other malignancies.

References

Almofti A, Uchida D, Begum NM, Tomizuka Y, Iga H, Yoshida H, Sato M (2004) The clinicopathological significance of the expression of CXCR4 protein in oral squamous cell carcinoma. Int J Oncol 25:65–71

Bachelder RE, Wendt MA, Mercurio AM (2002) Vascular endothelial growth factor promotes breast carcinoma invasion in an autocrine manner by regulating the chemokine receptor CXCR4. Cancer Res 62:7203–7206

Balkwill F (2004a) Cancer and the chemokine network. Nat Rev Cancer 4:540

Balkwill F (2004b) The significance of cancer cell expression of the chemokine receptor CXCR4. Semin Cancer Biol 14:171–179

Bernards R, Weinberg RA (2002) Metastasis genes: A progression puzzle. Nature 418:823

Burger JA, Kipps TJ (2006) CXCR4: A key receptor in the crosstalk between tumor cells and their microenvironment. Blood 107:1761–1767

Delilbasi CB, Okura M, Iida S, Kogo M (2004) Investigation of CXCR4 in squamous cell carcinoma of the tongue. Oral Oncol 40:154–157

Dhawan P, Richmond A (2002) Role of CXCL1 in tumorigenesis of melanoma. J Leukoc Biol 72:9–18

Ding Y, Shimada Y, Maeda M, Kawabe A, Kaganoi J, Komoto I, Hashimoto Y, Miyake M, Hashida H, Imamura M (2003) Association of CC chemokine receptor 7 with lymph node metastasis of esophageal squamous cell carcinoma. Clin Cancer Res 9:3406–3412

Fordice J, Kershaw C, El-Naggar A, Goepfert H (1999) Adenoid cystic carcinoma of the head and neck: predictors of morbidity and mortality. Arch Otolaryngol Head Neck Surg 125:149–152

Helbig G, Christopherson KW II, Bhat-Nakshatri P, Kumar S, Kishimoto H, Miller KD, Broxmeyer HE, Nakshatri H (2003) NF-{kappa} B promotes breast cancer cell migration and metastasis by inducing the expression of the chemokine receptor CXCR4. J Biol Chem 278:21631–21638

Humrich JY, Humrich JH, Averbeck M, Thumann P, Termeer C, Kampgen E, Schuler G, Jenne L (2006) Mature monocyte-derived dendritic cells respond more strongly to CCL19 than to CXCL12: consequences for directional migration. Immunology 117:238–247

Hynes RO (2003) Metastatic potential: Generic predisposition of the primary tumor or rare, metastatic variants – or both? Cell 113:821–823

Ishikawa T, Nakashiro K-I, Hara S, Klosek SK, Li C, Shintani S, Hamakawa H (2006) CXCR4 expression is associated with lymph-node metastasis of oral squamous cell carcinoma. Int J Oncol 28:61–66

Kim JW, Ferris RL, Whiteside TL (2005) Chemokine C receptor 7 expression and protection of circulating CD8+ T lymphocytes from apoptosis. Clin Cancer Res 11:7901–7910

Kulbe H, Hagemann T, Szlosarek PW, Balkwill FR, Wilson JL (2005) The inflammatory cytokine tumor necrosis factor-{alpha} regulates chemokine receptor expression on ovarian cancer cells. Cancer Res 65:10355–10362

Liotta LA (2001) Cancer: An attractive force in metastasis. Nature 410:24–25

Lu H, Ouyang W, Huang C (2006) Inflammation, a key event in cancer development. Mol Cancer Res 4:221–233

Mashino K, Sadanaga N, Yamaguchi H, Tanaka F, Ohta M, Shibuta K, Inoue H, Mori M (2002) Expression of chemokine receptor CCR7 is associated with lymph node metastasis of gastric carcinoma. Cancer Res 62:2937–2941

Mburu YK, Wang J, Wood MA, Walker WH, Ferris RL (2006) CCR7 mediates inflammation-associated tumor progression. Immunol Res 36:61–72

Miyazaki H, Patel V, Wang H, Ensley JF, Gutkind JS, Yeudall WA (2006a) Growth factor-sensitive molecular targets identified in primary and metastatic head and neck squamous cell carcinoma using microarray analysis. Oral Oncol 42:240–256

Miyazaki H, Patel V, Wang H, Edmunds RK, Gutkind JS, Yeudall WA (2006b) Down-regulation of CXCL5 inhibits squamous carcinogenesis. Cancer Res 66:4279–4284

Mori T, Kim J, Yamano T, Takeuchi H, Huang S, Umetani N, Koyanagi K, Hoon DSB (2005) Epigenetic up-regulation of C–C chemokine receptor 7 and C–X–C chemokine receptor 4 expression in melanoma cells. Cancer Res 65:1800–1807

Muller A, Homey B, Soto H, Ge N, Catron D, Buchanan ME, McClanahan T, Murphy E, Yuan W, Wagner SN, Barrera JL, Mohar A, Verastegui E, Zlotnik A (2001) Involvement of chemokine receptors in breast cancer metastasis. Nature 410:50–56

Muller A, Sonkoly E, Eulert C, Gerber PA, Kubitza R, Schirlau K, Franken-Kunkel P, Poremba C, Snyderman C, Klotz LO, Ruzicka T, Bier H, Zlotnik A, Whiteside TL, Homey B, Hoffmann TK (2006) Chemokine receptors in head and neck cancer: association with metastatic spread and regulation during chemotherapy. Int J Cancer 118:2147–2157

Ohta M, Kitadai Y, Tanaka S, Yoshihara M, Yasui W, Mukaida N, Haruma K, Chayama K (2002) Monocyte chemoattractant protein-1 expression correlates with macrophage infiltration and tumor vascularity in human esophageal squamous cell carcinomas. Int J Cancer 102:220–224

Onoue T, Uchida D, Begum NM, Tomizuka Y, Yoshida H, Sato M (2006) Epithelial-mesenchymal transition induced by the stromal cell-derived factor-1/CXCR4 system in oral squamous cell carcinoma cells. Int J Oncol 29:1133–1138

Paget S (1889) The distribution of secondary growths in cancer of the breast. Lancet 1:571–573

Richmond A (2002) NF-[kappa]B chemokine gene transcription and tumour growth. Nat Rev Immunol 2:664–674

Rossi D, Zlotnik A (2000) The biology of chemokines and their receptors. Annu Rev Immunol 18:217–242

Samara GJ, Lawrence DM, Chiarelli CJ, Valentino MD, Lyubsky S, Zucker S, Vaday GG (2004) CXCR4-mediated adhesion and MMP-9 secretion in head and neck squamous cell carcinoma. Cancer Lett 214:231–241

Schioppa T, Uranchimeg B, Saccani A, Biswas SK, Doni A, Rapisarda A, Bernasconi S, Saccani S, Nebuloni M, Vago L, Mantovani A, Melillo G, Sica A (2003) Regulation of the chemokine receptor CXCR4 by hypoxia. J Exp Med 198:1391–1402

Shintani S, Ishikawa T, Nonaka T, Li C, Nakashiro K-i, Wong DTW, Hamakawa H (2004) Growth-regulated oncogene-1 expression is associated with angiogenesis and lymph node metastasis in human oral cancer. Oncology 66:316–322

Staller P, Sulitkova J, Lisztwan J, Moch H, Oakeley EJ, Krek W (2003) Chemokine receptor CXCR4 downregulated by von Hippel–Lindau tumour suppressor pVHL. Nature 425:307–311

Takeuchi H, Fujimoto A, Tanaka M, Yamano T, Hsueh E, Hoon DS (2004) CCL21 chemokine regulates chemokine receptor CCR7 bearing malignant melanoma cells. Clin Cancer Res 10:2351–2358

Uchida D, Begum N-M, Almofti A, Nakashiro K-i, Kawamata H, Tateishi Y, Hamakawa H, Yoshida H, Sato M (2003) Possible role of stromal-cell-derived factor-1/CXCR4 signaling on lymph node metastasis of oral squamous cell carcinoma. Exp Cell Res 290:289–302

Uchida D, Begum N-M, Tomizuka Y, Bando T, Almofti A, Yoshida H, Sato M (2004) Acquisition of lymph node, but not distant metastatic potentials, by the overexpression of CXCR4 in human oral squamous cell carcinoma. Lab Invest 84:1538–1546

Uchida D, Onoue T, Tomizuka Y, Begum NM, Miwa Y, Yoshida H, Sato M (2007) Involvement of an autocrine stromal cell derived factor-1/CXCR4 system on the distant metastasis of human oral squamous cell carcinoma. Mol Cancer Res 5:685–694

Wang J, Xi L, Hunt JL, Gooding W, Whiteside TL, Chen Z, Godfrey TE, Ferris RL (2004) Expression pattern of chemokine receptor 6 (CCR6) and CCR7 in squamous cell carcinoma of the head and neck identifies a novel metastatic phenotype. Cancer Res 64:1861–1866

Wang J, Zhang X, Thomas SM, Grandis JR, Wells A, Chen ZG, Ferris RL (2005a) Chemokine receptor 7 activates phosphoinositide-3 kinase-mediated invasive and prosurvival pathways in head and neck cancer cells independent of EGFR. Oncogene 24:5897–5904

Wang J, Xi L, Gooding W, Godfrey TE, Ferris RL (2005b) Chemokine receptors 6 and 7 identify a metastatic expression pattern in squamous cell carcinoma of the head and neck. Adv Otorhinolaryngol 62:121–133

Wang J, Seethala R, Zhang Q, Gooding W, van Waes C, Hasegawa H, Ferris RL (2008) Autocrine and paracrine chemokine receptor 7 (CCR7) activation in head and neck cancer: Implications for therapy. J Natl Cancer Inst 100:502–512

Watanabe H, Iwase M, Ohashi M, Nagumo M (2002) Role of interleukin-8 secreted from human oral squamous cell carcinoma cell lines. Oral Oncol 38:670–679

Wiley HE, Gonzalez EB, Maki W, Wu M-t, Hwang ST (2001) Expression of CC chemokine receptor-7 and regional lymph node metastasis of B16 murine melanoma. J Natl Cancer Inst 93:1638–1643

Wilson JL, Burchell J, Grimshaw MJ (2006) Endothelins induce ccr7 expression by breast tumor cells via endothelin receptor A and hypoxia-inducible factor-1. Cancer Res 66:11802–11807

Zlotnik A, Yoshie O (2000) Chemokines: A new classification system and their role in immunity. Immunity 12:121–127

Chapter 14
Hypoxia, Angiogenesis, and Oral Cancer Metastasis

Quynh-Thu Le, Donald Courter, and Amato Giaccia

Abstract With the improvements in the diagnosis and management of head and neck cancer (HNC), there appears to be a shift in the pattern of failure. Better locoregional control is now achievable with combined modality therapy, and this has translated into a higher rate of observed distant metastasis. A similar shift in the pattern of failure over time has also been noted in oral cavity cancers. In addition, patients who develop distant metastasis have an extremely poor prognosis, with only few long-term survivors. A better understanding of the molecular pathways governing tumor dissemination is critical for the treatment and prevention of metastases in oral cavity cancers. Both tumor hypoxia and angiogenesis have been implicated in the development of distant metastasis in solid cancers, specifically HNC. Both processes mediate the induction of several genes that have been shown to modulate cellular properties critical for tumor dissemination. In this chapter, we review the role of hypoxia and angiogenesis in the development of metastasis, with a focus on oral cavity cancer.

Introduction

With the improvements in the diagnosis and management of head and neck cancers (HNC), there appears to be a shift in the pattern of failure (Argiris et al. 2003). Combined modality therapy has greatly improved the ability to control the tumor locally. As locoregional control has improved, the ability to prevent distant metastatic spread is becoming increasingly important (Brockstein et al. 2004). A similar shift in the pattern of failure over time has also been reported in oral cavity cancers (Kowalski et al. 2005). In addition, patients who develop distant metastasis have an extremely poor prognosis, with only few patients surviving long-term despite

Q.-T. Le (✉)
Department of Radiation Oncology, Stanford University, 875 Blake Wilbur Dr, MC 5847, Stanford, CA, 94305-5847, USA
e-mail: qle@stanford.edu

J. Myers (ed.), *Oral Cancer Metastasis*,
DOI 10.1007/978-1-4419-0775-2_14, © Springer Science+Business Media, LLC 2010

aggressive salvage therapies (Kowalski et al. 2005; Liao et al. 2007). A better way to address this dilemma is to identify patients who are prone to develop distant spread as early as possible and to treat them with novel targeted therapy to prevent tumor dissemination. A better understanding of the molecular pathways or factors governing tumor metastasis in oral cavity cancer is critical for such strategies.

Hypoxia or a reduction of the tissue oxygen tension is a common microenvironmental factor in solid tumors. Poorly oxygenated regions develop within cancers due to aberrant blood vessel formation, fluctuations in blood flow, and inability of the existing tumor vasculature to meet the oxygen demands of rapid tumor expansion (Brown and Giaccia 1998). That hypoxia exists in human tumors was first noted in 1955 by Thomlinson and Gray (1955). It was subsequently shown that hypoxia limited the response of tumor cells to traditional treatment such as radiation and chemotherapy, and these findings resulted in the devotion of substantial laboratory and clinical efforts to overcome this phenomenon (Brown and Giaccia 1998; Kennedy et al. 1980). In addition to modulating treatment responses, tumor hypoxia has also been implicated in the development of distant metastasis. Clinical studies have suggested that it is an important microenvironmental determinant for tumor cell dissemination distantly (Brizel et al. 1996; Nordsmark et al. 2001). Laboratory investigations show that adaptation of tumor cells to an anaerobic environment can be achieved through the transcriptional induction of genes involved in angiogenesis, survival, and tissue invasion – cellular processes critical for the development of metastasis (Harris 2002; Le et al. 2004). We have previously reviewed the relationship between hypoxic gene expression and solid tumor metastasis (Le et al. 2004). In this chapter, we discuss the relationships between hypoxia, angiogenesis, and metastasis in HNC in general and, where data are available, in oral cavity cancers specifically. As most data published in the literature have mainly related hypoxia and angiogenesis to overall patient prognosis in HNC rather than discuss their impact on nodal or distant metastasis, we will first cover the role of these two microenvirnomental factors on the overall treatment outcomes in head and neck and oral cavity cancers and, where available, their impact on tumor metastasis.

Hypoxia and Prognosis in Head and Neck Cancers

Head and neck cancers were of the first few tumors that were shown to harbor hypoxia using the Polarographic needle electrodes (pO_2 histograph, Eppendorf, Hamburg, Germany) (Lartigau et al. 1993). Using this device, a sensing electrode, mounted on the tip of a needle, is advanced automatically via a step motor through the tissue taking readings rapidly (within 1.4 s) to avoid changes in oxygen tension resulting from pressure artifacts or tissue damage caused by the needle. A histogram of oxygen tensions can then be generated from multiple points along different tracks through the tissue. An example of measurements made in an oral tongue cancer, the involved neck node, and the adjacent normal subcutaneous tissue from

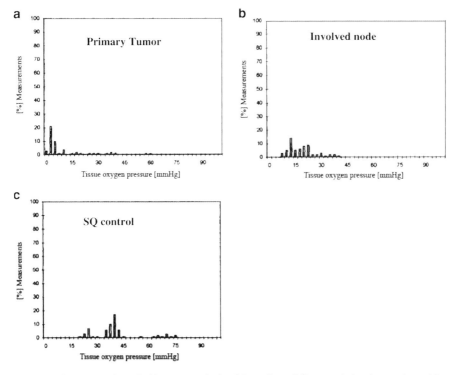

Fig. 14.1 Representative pO_2 histograms obtained from three different subsites in a patient with a T3N2b oral tongue cancer. The y-axis on the histogram shows the percentage of the total pO_2 measurements obtained in each site (usually 60–70 measurements). (**a**) The primary oral tongue cancer. (**b**) A metastatic neck node. (**c**) Subcutaneous tissue from the contralateral uninvolved neck

the same patient is shown in Fig. 14.1. The normal tissues show a typical Gaussian distribution of oxygen tensions with a median between 40 and 60 mmHg, whereas tumors and their involved nodes invariably show a lower oxygen tension distribution. Gatenby et al. first reported that HNC with lower pO_2 had poorer radiation response than those with higher pO_2 (Gatenby et al. 1988). Since then, several studies have confirmed that low tumoral pO_2, defined by either the median value or the hypoxic proportion (% readings below 2.5 [HP2.5] or 5 mm Hg [HP5]), correlates with treatment outcomes in HNC patients treated with radiation or chemoradiotherapy (Rudat et al. 2000; Brizel et al. 1999; Nordsmark and Overgaard 2000; Rudat et al. 2001). One study also found that tumor pO_2 predicted for pathologically persistent neck nodes in patients undergoing a neck dissection for clinical N2-3 necks after the chemoradiation treatment (Brizel et al. 2004). Pooled data in 397 HNC patients provided definitive evidence that tumor pO_2 is an independent predictor for survival (Nordsmark et al. 2005). In this study, HP2.5 was the only independent prognostic factor for survival. Patients with HP2.5 $\leq$ 19 % faired significantly better than those with HP2.5 > 19% ($p = 0.0006$).

Other studies, using different methods to measure tumor hypoxia, reported similar findings. Evans et al. used EF5 [2-(2-nitro-1H-imidazol-1-yl)-N-(2,2,3,3,3-pentaflouropropyl) acetamide], a nitroimidazole-based injectable reporter drug to assess hypoxia in 22 HNC patients, of which 15 were from oral cavity subsites (Evans et al. 2007). EF5 forms stable adducts with intracellular macromolecules only in hypoxic regions (<10 mm Hg), and detection of these adducts with antibodies can provide information on the relative oxygenation at cellular resolution (Ljungkvist et al. 2007; Evans and Koch 2003). They reported that patients with an EF5 binding pattern that corresponded to severe hypoxia had shorter event-free survival than others (Evans et al. 2007). Similar findings were reported for pimonidazole (1-[(2-hydroxy-3-piperidinyl)propyl]-2-nitroimidazole hydrochloride), an analog of EF5, in another group of HNC patients. High pimonidazole staining correlated with a higher risk of locoregional relapse in patients treated with radiotherapy alone but not in patients treated with radiotherapy plus carbogen and nicotinamide, which are used to modulate tumor hypoxia (Kaanders et al. 2002).

Hypoxia in Oral Cavity Cancers and Metastasis

Although promising, reported studies to date had included tumors from all head and neck subsites and none had focused directly on oral cavity cancers. In addition, the pattern of relapse was not described in most of these series. We measured tumor pO_2 in 21 patients with oral cavity primary tumors: 11 in the oral tongue, six in the floor of mouth, three in the lip, and one in the hard palate. Table 14.1 shows the demographic and pO_2 data for these individual patients. Figure 14.2 shows that the median pO_2 measurements in the tumor were significantly lower than those obtained from the control subcutaneous tissues in the same patients. Of these patients, five developed eventual distant metastasis. There was a trend for higher HF2.5 in the five patients who developed distant metastasis (average HF2.5 of 39% +/− 14) when compared with those who did not (average HF2.5 of 22% +/− 7); however, the difference was not statistically significant ($p=0.26$).

Similar findings have been reported for tumor hypoxia in other solid cancers. Brizel et al. showed that patients with hypoxic soft tissue sarcomas (median $pO_2 < 10$ mmHg) had a significantly higher risk of lung metastasis and lower disease-free survival when compared to those with less hypoxic tumors (Brizel et al. 1996). These data were subsequently confirmed by Nordsmark et al., who found an association between low tumor pO_2 and increased risk of distant spread in 28 patients with soft tissue sarcomas (Nordsmark et al. 2001). Another connection between tumor hypoxia as measured by the polarographic needle electrode came from Fyles et al., who reported a lower progression-free survival rate in node-negative cervical cancer patients with hypoxic tumors (higher HP5) when compared to those with better oxygenated tumors and that most of the failures occurred outside the pelvis, consistent with enhanced distant tumor dissemination with hypoxia (Fyles et al. 2002).

Table 14.1 Characteristics of 21 patients with oral cavity tumors with tumor pO_2 measurements

Pt No	Gender	Age	Tumor site	T-stage	N-stage	Treatment	Med tumor pO_2 (mm Hg)	HP2.5 (%)	HP5 (%)	SQ pO_2 (mm Hg)	Distant metastasis
1	M	56	FOM	1	0	S	19.13	0	18	ND	No
2	F	45	FOM	2	0	S+RT	2.99	31	83	ND	No
3	M	80	FOM	4	0	S	2.12	53.33	85	ND	No
4	M	57	FOM	4	2b	CRT	21.02	0.00	0.02	58.29	No
5	M	61	FOM	3	2c	CRT	1.7	67	96	ND	No
6	M	44	FOM	2	0	S	15.9	0	0	ND	No
7	F	80	Oral tongue	2	0	S	6.96	0	42	49.54	No
8	F	94	Oral tongue	2	0	S	41.98	2.53	6.33	ND	No
9	F	36	Oral tongue	3	0	S+RT	9.16	0	0	ND	No
10	M	67	Oral tongue	4	0	S+RT	4.2	31	53	41.1	No
11	F	50	Oral tongue	4	1	S	11.35	0	0	58.69	No
12	M	41	Oral tongue	4	1	CRT	28.36	0	0	62.29	No
13	M	55	Oral tongue	2	3	CRT	8.60	20	44	28.02	No
14	M	60	Oral tongue	3	2b	CRT	14.69	18.37	26.53	49.81	Yes
15	M	36	Oral tongue	4	2c	CRT	10.57	33	43	40.84	Yes
16	M	57	Oral tongue	4	2c	CRT	8.06	2	32	86.74	Yes
17	M	34	Oral tongue	2	0	S+RT	3	75	90	37.25	Yes
18	F	93	Hard palate	2	2c	S+RT	1.53	65.1	98.8	42.27	No
19	F	63	Lip	0	2c	S+RT	8.05	26.3	35.7	ND	No
20	F	78	Lip	0	2a	S+RT	0	63.49	77.78	61.41	No
21	M	54	Lip	1	3	S+RT	0.5	65.1	66.7	36.4	Yes

Pt patient, *No* number, *M* Male, *F* females, *FOM* floor of mouth, *S* surgery, *RT* radiation therapy, *CRT* chemoradiotherapy, *SQ* subcutaneous, *ND* Not done

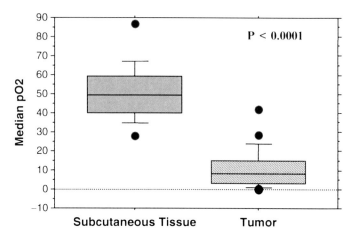

Fig. 14.2 Box plots showing the distribution of the median pO$_2$ measurements in the tumors or involved cervical nodes vs. the subcutaneous normal tissues in 21 patients with oral cavity cancers

Relationship Between Certain Hypoxia Induced Proteins and Outcomes

Hypoxia-Related Proteins Detectable in Tumor Tissues

Adaptation of cells to an anaerobic environment is achieved by the transcriptional induction of genes that are involved in glycolysis, hematopoiesis, angiogenesis, invasive capacity, and regulating vascular tone, as well as a number of other functions (Giaccia et al. 2003). Perhaps the earliest insight into the transcriptional regulation of gene expression by hypoxia came from studies on erythropoietin (EPO) gene regulation. In the early 1990s, several groups demonstrated that the hypoxic inducibility of the EPO gene was due in part to a hypoxia response element (HRE), 5'-ACGTG-3', localized in its 3' flanking region (Semenza et al. 1991; Imagawa et al. 1991). The transcription factor that bound this HRE was designated the hypoxia inducible factor-1 (HIF-1) and is composed of two subunits, an oxygen sensitive HIF-1α subunit, and a constitutively expressed HIF-1β subunit (Wang and Semenza 1995). Since then, HIF1 has been shown to regulate several genes that have been implicated in tumor progression and treatment resistance (Harris 2002; Le et al. 2004). HIF-1 and several of its downstream targets such as Glut-1 (glucose transporter-1), carbonic anhydrase IX (CA IX), and vascular endothelial growth factor (VEGF) have been widely investigated as prognostic markers in HNC with mixed results. Table 14.2 summarizes representative large clinical series (>50 patients) that focused on the prognostic significance of HIF-1, CA IX, and Glut-1 for HNC. Studies that contained oral cavity cancers were included. It is by no mean an exhaustive list, but it does show that in general, elevated expression of these markers portends poorer outcomes in patients treated with either nonsurgical or surgical therapies.

Table 14.2 Relationship between treatment outcomes and the expression of HIF-1, CA IX & Glut-1 hypoxia-induced proteins as reported in selective head and neck cancer studies.

Author	Hypoxia marker	# Pts (% OC)	Treatment	Survival
HIF markers				
Beasley et al. (2002)	HIF-1α	69 (39%)	S	↑ DFS, OS with ↑HIF1-α (Multivariate)
Kyzas et al. (2005b)	HIF-1α, VEGF	81 (27%)	S	↓ OS with ↑ VEGF, but not with HIF-1α (Univariate)
Winter et al. (2006)	HIF-2α, CA IX	140 (34%)	S	↓CSS & DFS with ↑ HIF-1α (multivariate): model improved with addition of HIF-2α; model not significant for CA IX
Koukourakis et al. (2006)	HIF-2α, CA IX	198 (17%)	RT (CHART vs. conventional)	↓ LRC & OS for both ↑ HIF-2α & CA IX (Multivariate)
CA IX only				
Beasley et al. (2001)	CA IX	79 (39%)	Surgery	Not assessed
Jonathan et al. (2006)	CAIX, Glut-1, Glut-3	58 (9%)	RT + ARCON	↑ LRC & MFS with ↑ CA IX & Glut-3 (Univariate)
De Schutter et al. (2005)	CA IX, Glut-1	67 (3%)	RT ± C	↓ LRC & DFS only with ↑CA IX +Glut-1 when grouped together but not individually (multivariate)
Glut-1 only				
Oliver et al. (2004)	Glut-1	54 (100%)	S	↓ LRC, FFR, CSS with ↑ Glut-1 (Univariate)
Kunkel et al. (2003)	Glut-1	118 (100%)	S ± RT	↓ OS with ↑ Glut-1 (multivariate)

Pt patients, *OC* oral cavity, *S* surgery, *RT* radiotherapy, *C* chemotherapy, *ARCON* carbogen and nicotidamide, *CHART* continuous hyperfractionated accelerated radiotherapy; *LRC* locoregional control, *DFS* disease-free survival, *OS* overall survival, *CSS* cancer specific survival, *LRC* locoregional control, *MFS* metastasis-free survival, *FFR* freedom from relapse

Within this group, very few studies reported data on nodal relapse or distant metastasis. Oliver et al. reported that intense Glut-1 staining was associated with a higher risk of regional relapse but not local relapse in 54 patients with oral cavity tumors (Oliver et al. 2004). Similarly, Jonathan et al. showed that higher pretreatment expression of Glut-1 was associated with an increased risk of distant relapse in 58 HNC patients treated with accelerated radiation therapy with carbogen and nicotidamide (ARCON therapy); 9% of these patients had oral cavity primaries (Jonathan et al. 2006).

Other endogenous tissue markers that have been studied in relation to hypoxia include VEGF, ephrin A1, lysyl oxidase (LOX), and galectin-1 (Le et al. 2005; Le et al. 2007; Erler et al. 2006; Linderholm et al. 2003). Data on VEGF and Ephrin A1 are discussed below in the angiogenesis section. Our group has identified LOX and galectin-1 as hypoxia induced proteins (Le et al. 2005; Erler et al. 2006). LOX is an amine oxidase that crosslinks collagens and elastins in the extracellular matrix. We have shown that LOX expression was associated with tumor hypoxia in patients with breast and head and neck cancers. Specifically, high LOX expression levels in the primary tumor before treatment correlated with a reduction in metastasis-free and overall survival in 101 HNC patients, of which 13% had oral cavity primaries (Erler et al. 2006). We demonstrated that LOX inhibition by different means, including genetic (LOX shRNA), chemical (beta-aminoproprionitrile), or antibody (anti-LOX blocking antibody), eliminated the formation of metastases in an orthotopic breast cancer model, and this occurred through the prevention of cell invasion and deterrence of metastatic growth (Erler et al. 2006).

Using surface enhanced laser desorption ionization time of flight (SELDI-TOF) mass spectrometry on HNC cell lines, we identified galectin-1 as a hypoxia-induced protein, whose secretion is strongly enhanced by the hypoxia exposure (Le et al. 2005). Previous data suggested that galectin-1, a beta-galactoside binding protein, is a novel regulator of the antitumor immune response. It has been shown to inhibit T-cell effector function by promoting T-cell apoptosis, blocking T-cell activation, and inhibiting secretion of pro-inflammatory cytokines (Rabinovich et al. 1999; Rubinstein et al. 2004; Chung et al. 2000). We, therefore, studied galectin-1 expression in a HNC tissue microarray and investigated its relationship with tumor hypoxia and intratumoral immune surveillance as measured by the level of T-lymphocytes in the tumor (Le et al. 2005). We found a significant direct correlation between galectin-1 and CA IX staining (a marker for hypoxia, $p=0.01$) and a strong inverse correlation between galectin-1 and CD3 staining, a pan T-cell marker ($p=0.01$). In addition, expressions of Galectin-1 and CD3 were significant predictors for overall survival on multivariate analysis and galectin-1 staining intensity predicted specifically for nodal failure (Fig. 14.3) but not for local or distant relapses. The direct relationship between galectin-1 and hypoxia and the inverse relationship between galectin-1 and T-cell levels in the tumor suggest a novel mechanism of how hypoxia can influence tumor progression and therapeutic response by affecting the secretion of proteins that modulate immune privilege.

The advantage of using hypoxia-induced proteins to assess prognosis is that the levels of these proteins can be determined on archival materials, thereby allowing

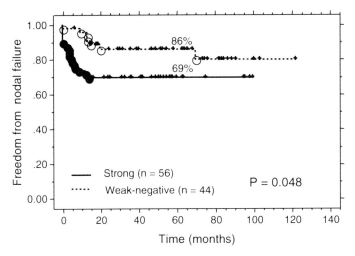

Fig. 14.3 Kaplan Meier curves showing freedom from nodal failure by Galectin-1 staining intensity in 100 HNC patients

rapid correlation to treatment outcomes. In addition, it requires neither the injection of foreign material nor any additional invasive procedure beyond a biopsy at diagnosis. It is also inexpensive and does not require any dedicated equipment or expertise for analysis. A significant drawback to these approaches is that these proteins can be regulated by factors other than hypoxia. For example, HIF-1α expression can be influenced by several nonhypoxic stimuli including nitric oxide, cytokines (interleukin [IL]-1β and tumor necrosis factor [TNF]-α), trophic stimuli (serum, insulin, insulin-like-growth factors), and oncogenes (e.g., p53, Vsrc, phosphate and tensin homolog [PTEN]) (Stroka et al. 2001; Zundel et al. 2000; Zelzer et al. 1998; Zhong et al. 2000). Comparison of the staining patterns between endogenous and injectable markers for hypoxia such as pimonidazole showed that the former, in general, stained more diffusely and closer to the blood vessels than the latter, suggesting other modes of induction and activation at a wider range of oxygen concentration (Kaanders et al. 2002; Janssen et al. 2002). In addition, there is minimal correlation between the intensity of endogenous marker staining and tumor pO_2. In the most rigorous studies in which tumor biopsies were performed along the paths of the polarographic electrode and stained for HIF-1α, CA IX, and Glut-1, there was no observed correlation between any staining parameter and measured pO_2 (Mayer et al. 2004, 2005a, b). These discrepancies make it less desirable to use an individual hypoxia inducible protein alone to identify patients with hypoxic tumors.

To circumvent this dilemma, suggestions have been made to combine several hypoxia-regulated proteins together to improve specificity for hypoxic tumor identification. For example, gene expression analysis has been used to generate a hypoxia gene signature or a hypoxia metagene to predict treatment outcomes in several solid tumors, including HNC (Chi et al. 2006; Winter et al. 2007). Using gene expression profiling of 59 HNCs, Winter et al. generated a hypoxia metagene by identifying genes whose expression was clustered with 10 known hypoxia regulated genes (Winter et al. 2007). They found that this metagene was able to predict recurrence-free survival in an independent HNC data set as well as overall survival in another breast cancer series. We have also used a combination of gene expression and proteomic analyses to identify novel hypoxia induced proteins. After confirming their hypoxic inducibility in cell lines and animal models, we investigated their utility in combination with CA IX to predict outcomes by staining the previously described HNC tissue array with known tumor pO_2. These studies resulted in a panel of four hypoxia markers (CA IX, LOX, Galectin-1, and Ephrin A1) that can be used to predict treatment outcomes in terms of cancer-specific survival (Le et al. 2007). These endogenous hypoxia signatures, though promising, need to be validated in larger independent data sets.

Secreted Hypoxia Related Protein Detectable in the Blood

A major focus of research in our group is to identify secreted markers of hypoxia that can be rapidly and inexpensively measured in the blood. Even though several hypoxia-induce proteins are secreted, only a few of them have levels detected in the blood due to either protein sequestration locally as in the case of galectin-1 (Le et al. 2005) or the current lack of a sensitive method (such as an enzyme-linked immunosorbent assay [ELISA]-based assay) to quantify their circulating levels as in LOX. The plasminogen activator inhibitor-1 (PAI-1) and its related family member such as urokinase-type plasminogen activator (uPA) and urokinase plasminogen activator receptors (uPAR) are hypoxia inducible genes whose proteins are secreted (Koong et al. 2000; Sprague et al. 2007). In vitro studies have shown that the levels of these secreted proteins are increased by hypoxia and reoxygenation in HNC cell lines (Schilling et al. 2007; Sprague et al. 2006). However, there are no published data on the circulating levels of these markers in HNC patients. We have analyzed plasma samples from the 27 HNC patients enrolled in a study at our institution and found that none of these three factors had circulating levels which correlated with either tumor pO_2 or treatment outcomes (unpublished data). Figure 14.4 shows that although patients with hypoxic tumors had higher plasma PAI-1 levels than those with less hypoxic tumors, there was a significant overlap between the two populations, and the results were not statistically significant.

Two markers that have been tested clinically with mixed results are VEGF and osteopontin (OPN). Although circulating VEGF levels were elevated in cancer patients (Riedel et al. 2000; Salven et al. 1997) and in those with acute hypoxia such as obstructive apnea (Imagawa et al. 2001), the relationship between tumor hypoxia and systemic VEGF levels is unclear. Dunst et al. found that serum VEGF levels independently correlated with hypoxic tumor subvolume in 56 HNC patients (Dunst et al. 2001). However, it also correlated with total tumor volume, hemoglobin level, and platelet counts. They did not report on the clinical significance of serum VEGF levels in terms of treatment outcomes. In contrast, we did not find a

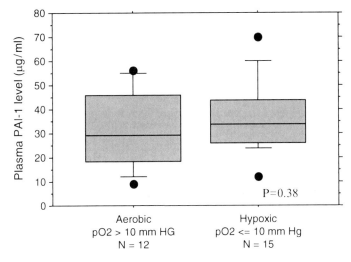

Fig. 14.4 Box plots showing a lack of relationship between tumor pO_2 and plasma PAI-1 levels in 27 HNC patients

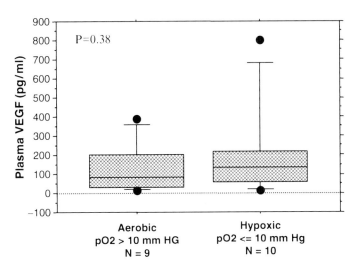

Fig. 14.5 Box plots showing a lack of relationship between tumor pO_2 and plasma VEGF levels in 19 HNC patients

direct relationship between plasma VEGF and tumor pO_2 in the first 19 HNC patients in our study (unpublished observations, Fig. 14.5). We did, however, find a small, but significant, relationship between OPN level and tumor pO_2 in our HNC patient cohort, of which 22% had oral cavity primary tumors (Le et al. 2003). This was confirmed by Nordsmark et al. (2007) In addition, plasma OPN was an independent and significant predictor for treatment outcomes in these patients.

A prospective validation study using a different cohort of HNC patients, of which 19% had oral cavity primaries, confirmed the prognostic significance of OPN, using the predefined cut point of 450 ng/ml from the prior study (Petrik et al. 2006). These results were validated by the Danish Head and Neck Cancer (DAHANCA) group in a larger group of HNC patients treated with radiation therapy +/– nimorazole, a hypoxic cell radiosensititizer (Overgaard et al. 2005). Intriguingly, only patients with high pretreatment circulating OPN levels benefited from nimorazole, whereas those with low to intermediate levels did not, suggesting that OPN may be used to select patients for hypoxia targeting. Further validation of this marker is ongoing in another set of HNC patients treated with or without tirapazamine (TPZ), a hypoxic cell cytotoxin. Since OPN is a secreted phosphoglycoprotein that has been implicated in tumor transformation and progression, specifically mediating nodal and distant metastasis in breast cancers (Singhal et al. 1997; Allan et al. 2006), we also analyzed pattern of relapse based on OPN status. In the entire cohort of 140 HNCs, pattern of relapse studies suggested that higher OPN levels was associated with a higher risk of local and nodal relapse (Petrik et al. 2006). However, in a small subset of patients with oral cavity primary, there was a trend for more distant relapse with higher OPN levels, though the difference was not statistically significant (Fig. 14.6).

Advantages of secreted markers for hypoxia is that they are noninvasive, easy to measure, and inexpensive and allow for serial measurements through the course of therapies. However, they do have the same drawbacks faced by endogenous tissue markers, including the lack of method standardization and regulation by factors other than hypoxia. In addition, spatial information is lost and contributions from noncancerous tissues and other pathological processes such as inflammation cannot be ruled out. For example, Jablonska et al. showed that the polymorphonuclear

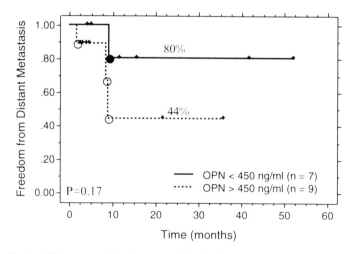

Fig. 14.6 Kaplan Meier curves showing a trend for higher risk of distant metastasis by plasma Osteopontin levels in 16 patients with oral cavity cancers

leukocytes (PMN) derived from oral cavity cancer patients secreted more VEGF than those from healthy control subjects (Jablonska et al. 2002). Moreover, the level of VEGF secretion from PMN was correlated with tumor classification and was improved after therapy. On the basis of this experience, we recommend that one or multiple molecular markers be combined with another approach of assessing hypoxia such as imaging be used to define a tumor as being hypoxic.

Angiogenesis and Prognosis in Head and Neck Cancer

Vascular Endothelial Growth Factor

Angiogenesis, the growth of new blood vessels, plays an important role in tumor progression and metastasis. For solid tumors to grow and metastasize, an adequate blood supply is essential. Vascular development and factors that regulate it have, therefore, been extensively studied in many tumor sites, including oral cavity cancers. Several studies have shown an increase in the number of small blood vessels in oral cavity cancers when they transitioned from normal mucosa to dysplasia to invasive tumors (Pazouki et al. 1997; Lopez de Cicco R et al. 2004). Similarly, multiple studies have shown that microvessel density count, based on CD31, CD34, or factor VIII staining, was associated with more advanced stage, specifically with more nodal metastasis at presentation (Ascani et al. 2005; Penfold et al. 1996; Gleich et al. 1997).

   Formation of the new blood vessels in cancer is mediated by different molecular pathways. Perhaps the most important pathway involved in tumor angiogenesis is the VEGF family of growth factors, of which $VEGF_{165}$ is the predominant isoform produced by tumor cells (Ferrara et al. 2003). VEGF receptors (VEGFRs), which are receptor tyrosine kinases (RTKs), exist in 3 known isoforms: VEGFR-1, VEGFR-2, and VEGFR-3 (Barbera-Guillem et al. 2002). VEGFR-2 is the main form that is found on the tumor vasculature. There is ample preclinical and clinical evidence that activation of the VEGF pathway is a major contributor to tumor angiogenesis and growth in solid tumors (Dvorak et al. 1999). Most tumor cells produce high levels of VEGF, and VEGFRs are expressed in tumor-associated endothelial cells. VEGF and VEGFR2 expressions are enhanced by hypoxia and are often elevated in regions of tumor necrosis (Ziemer et al. 2001). Various antagonists of VEGF have been shown to delay tumor growth. For example, tumor angiogenesis and subsequent tumor growth are inhibited in vivo by antibodies directed against VEGF (Presta et al. 1997). Similarly, soluble VEGF receptor ectodomains suppressed the growth of tumors in vivo (Goldman et al. 1998). Phase III clinical trials have shown that the addition of bevacizumab, a monoclonal antibody against VEGF, to conventional chemotherapy resulted in increased survival in patients with metastatic colorectal and non-small cell lung cancers (Hurwitz et al. 2004; Sandler et al. 2006). The use of multikinase inhibitors with anti-VEGFR2 activities resulted in a higher response rate and longer progression-free survival in patients with metastatic renal cells carcinomas when compared with placebos or conventional therapy (Motzer et al. 2007; Escudier et al. 2007).

The role of VEGF in tumor metastasis and outcomes has not been as clearly defined for oral cavity cancers as for other solid tumors. Most reported studies evaluated VEGF expression in tumors from different head and neck subsites, and only very few focused directly on oral cavity primaries. Table 14.3 is a summary of selective studies reported in the literature. As shown, several studies came from the same group and presumably overlapped with one another. In addition, patient populations are heterogeneous, different antibodies are used, and the staining criteria are variable from study to study. Nevertheless, most studies suggest that VEGF expression is a prognostic factor for survival or relapse on univariate but not multivariate analysis. This is consistent with the findings from a meta-analysis, which showed that VEGF positivity appeared to be associated with worse overall survival, though some modest biases cannot be excluded (Kyzas et al. 2005a). Only one study related VEGF expression to the risk of distant metastasis. Smith et al. reported on 56 oral cavity and oropharyngeal cancer patients, of which over half had oral cavity primaries (Smith et al. 2000). They found that tumors with strong-intense VEGF staining were more likely on univariate analysis to have distant recurrence. The risk of distant metastasis was 12% for VEGF-negative tumors compared with 43% for VEGF-positive tumors (relative risk: 4.62; p value 0.006). A multivariate analysis was not performed for distant metastasis. In summary, the presented data suggest that VEGF expression in oral cavity cancers is associated with a higher risk of nodal metastasis at presentation and an enhanced chance of tumor relapse after treatment; however, its relationship to distant metastasis is unclear in this setting.

Eph Receptors and Ephrin Ligands

Eph RTKs and their ligands, the ephrins, have emerged as important mediators of vascular remodeling during embryonic development and disease. This family, which consists of at least 16 receptors and nine ligands, is the largest family of RTKs (Heroult et al. 2006). One unique aspect of Eph receptors is that they interact with cell surface-bound ephrin ligands rather than soluble ligands. Ephrin ligands are attached to the cell membrane either through a glycosylphosphatidyl inositol (GPI) anchor or a transmembrane domain (Cheng et al. 2002). In general, GPI anchored-ephrin A ligands bind preferentially to EphA receptors, and transmembrane anchored-ephrin B ligands bind to EphB receptors. However, within each (A or B) subclass, receptor–ligand interactions are highly promiscuous and in vivo interactions likely occur where a receptor and ligand of the same subclass are co-expressed. Another distinct feature of the Eph receptor–ligand interaction is the bi-directional signaling that can be propagated downstream of the Eph receptors as well as downstream of their ligands upon receptor–ligand association (Bruckner et al. 1997; Holland et al. 1996). Activation of both Eph receptors and ligands has

Table 14.3 Relationship between VEGF expression and treatment outcomes as reported in selective head and neck cancer studies

Author	# Pts(% OC)	Site	Antibody	Positive criteria	Univariate	Multivariate
Smith et al. (2000)	56(57%)	OC & OP	JH121	Strong-intense staining	↓ LC, DM, DFS, OS	↓ DFS, OS
Kyzas et al. (2005c)	67(30%)	HNC	JH121	≥20% + cytoplasmic staining	↓ OS	↓ OS for OC/LX only
Eisma et al. (1997)	63 (NS)	HNC	Goat antihuman	NS	↓ FFR for + Factor VIII	ND
Maeda et al. (1998)	45(100%)	OC only	Rabbit polyclonal (Santa Cruz)	≥5% + tumor cell staining	↓ OS	ND
Eisma et al. (1999)	33(NS)	HNC	Rabbit polyclonal	NS	↓ FFR	ND
Kyzas et al.(2005b)	81(27%)	HNC	JH121	≥20% + cytoplasmic staining	↓ OS	ND
Tse et al. (2007)	164 (49%)	HNC	Santa Cruz Ab, Not otherwise specified	≥5% tumor cells with strong staining	↓ DFS, OS	↓ DSF, OS

OC oral cavity, *OP* oropharynx, *HNC* head and neck cancers, *LC* local control, *DM* distant metastasis, *DFS* disease-free survival, *OS* overall survival, *LX* larynx, *FFR* freedom from relapse. *NS* not stated, *ND* not done, *Ab* antibody

been shown to regulate integrin-dependent cell adhesion, resulting in changes in the actin cytoskeleton, cell attachment, and migration (Heroult et al. 2006).

Although initially characterized in the central nervous system, recent studies have suggested key roles for the ephrins and their receptors in angiogenesis and vascular development during embryogenesis. Targeted disruption of ephrin B2, EphB2/EphB3 or EphB4 resulted in embryonic lethality due to defects in primary capillary network remodeling and subsequent patterning defects in the embryonic vasculatures (Adams et al. 1999; Gerety et al. 1999; Wang et al. 1998). More recently, the Eph receptors and ephrin ligands have been implicated in tumor growth, progression, and metastasis. The expressions of ephrin A1, ephrin B2, EphA2, and EphB2–4 are induced in several solid tumors (Heroult et al. 2006). Recent evidences have linked EphA2 and its ligand, ephrin A1, to tumor angiogenesis. Both molecules have been shown to be widely expressed in the tumor parenchyma and tumor endothelial cells (Ogawa et al. 2000). EphA2 deficient mice displayed less vascular remodeling in response to soluble ephrin A1-Fc ligand as well as impaired tumor angiogenesis in response to ephrin A1 expressing tumors in xenografts (Brantley-Sieders et al. 2004, 2005). Knocking down ephrin A1 expression in metastatic mammary tumor cells resulted in less tumor-induced endothelial cell migration in vitro and microvascular density in vivo (Brantley-Sieders et al. 2006). Conversely, overexpression of ephrin A1 in a nonmetastatic breast cancer cell line enhanced microvessel density and vascular recruitment with an associated increase in VEGF secretion. Knocking down ephrin A1 expression by small interfering RNA resulted in significantly less lung metastasis in an orthotopic breast cancer model without affecting the tumor volume, invasion, and lung colonization (Brantley-Sieders et al. 2006). These data strongly implicate the role of EphA receptors and their ligands in solid tumor angiogenesis and metastasis.

The regulation of these molecules is being elucidated. Expression of certain EphA receptors and Ephrin A1 are induced by various growth factors and cytokines, including TNF-α, lipopolysaccharides (LPS), IL-1β, and VEGF (Cheng et al. 2002). Tumor hypoxia is a microenvironmental regulator of these molecules (Denko et al. 2003). In a mouse skin flap model of hypoxia, both ephrin A1 and its receptor were induced in the hypoxic skin and the induction appeared to be modulated by HIF-1α as small interfering RNA to HIF-1α abrogated this hypoxic induction (Vihanto et al. 2005). In a gene array analysis, EphA1 was found to be positively correlated with increasing necrosis in human glioblastomas and was found to be localized to the perinecrotic areas on immuhistochemical staining (Raza et al. 2004). We performed gene expression studies on several solid cancer cell lines, including HNC, and found that ephrin A1 mRNA was highly induced by hypoxia (Denko et al. 2003). More importantly, we found that ephrin A1 was one of the four hypoxia markers that could be used to stratify prognosis in a group of HNC patients (Le et al. 2007). A pattern of failure study suggested that strong ephrin A1 staining was associated with a higher risk of distant metastasis (Fig. 14.7), but not with local or nodal relapse. Further work confirming this observation in a larger patient group is on going.

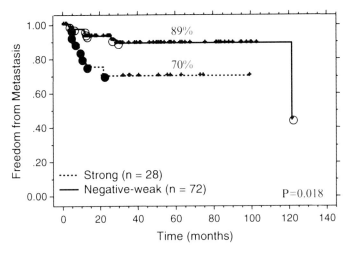

Fig. 14.7 Kaplan Meier curves showing freedom from distant metastasis by Ephrin A1 staining intensity in 100 HNC patients

In addition to ephrin A1, the only other family member of this group that has been studied in HNC is EphB4 (Masood et al. 2006). Its expression was found to be higher in HNC tumors compared with matched normal tissues and correlated directly with higher stage and nodal metastasis. Knocking down EphB4 expression with either siRNA or phosphorothioate-modified antisense oligonucleotides (AS-ODN) resulted in increased tumor cell apoptosis, decreased cell migration and invasion in vitro, and smaller tumor size in vivo. In addition, AS-ODN-treated tumors had significantly less microvessel density than controls, which were untreated tumors. Although the reported data on the ephrins and their receptors are intriguing, no reported study has specifically evaluated the expression of these markers in oral cavity cancers. Similarly, no studies have assessed their role in tumor progression and metastasis in oral cavity primaries. This exciting unexplored area is ready for further study as reagents are now becoming available.

Conclusion

In this chapter, we have summarized the role of hypoxia and angiogenesis in oral cavity cancer metastasis and identified potential targets for risk stratification as well as for therapeutic intervention. The major challenge is how to translate these findings into the clinical setting. For the first step, some of the novel tissue hypoxia markers for metastasis such as LOX and ephrin A1 need to be validated in larger and more uniformly treated oral cavity cancer patients. Similar validation studies are also necessary for circulating markers such as OPN. Once confirmed, targeted treatments will need to be generated and tested in new HNC animal models that resemble the actual oral cavity tumors in their natural environment rather than the current artificial xenograft system. Testing of these new leads from the laboratory will require well-conducted clinical trials with innovative designs that incorporate serial novel noninvasive surrogate endpoints such as molecular makers or imaging methods. As oncologists, our responsibility is to support these trials in order to decrease metastasis and to improve survival in our patients.

References

Adams RH, Wilkinson GA, Weiss C et al (1999) Roles of ephrinB ligands and EphB receptors in cardiovascular development: demarcation of arterial/venous domains, vascular morphogenesis, and sprouting angiogenesis. Genes Dev 13:295–306

Allan AL, George R, Vantyghem SA et al (2006) Role of the integrin-binding protein osteopontin in lymphatic metastasis of breast cancer. Am J Pathol 169:233–246

Argiris A, Haraf DJ, Kies MS et al (2003) Intensive concurrent chemoradiotherapy for head and neck cancer with 5-Fluorouracil- and hydroxyurea-based regimens: reversing a pattern of failure. Oncologist 8:350–360

Ascani G, Balercia P, Messi M et al (2005) Angiogenesis in oral squamous cell carcinoma. Acta Otorhinolaryngol Ital 25:13–17

Barbera-Guillem E, Nyhus JK, Wolford CC et al (2002) Vascular endothelial growth factor secretion by tumor-infiltrating macrophages essentially supports tumor angiogenesis, and IgG immune complexes potentiate the process. Cancer Res 62:7042–7049

Beasley NJ, Wykoff CC, Watson PH et al (2001) Carbonic anhydrase IX, an endogenous hypoxia marker, expression in head and neck squamous cell carcinoma and its relationship to hypoxia, necrosis, and microvessel density. Cancer Res 61:5262–5267

Beasley NJ, Leek R, Alam M et al (2002) Hypoxia-inducible factors HIF-1alpha and HIF-2alpha in head and neck cancer: relationship to tumor biology and treatment outcome in surgically resected patients. Cancer Res 62:2493–2497

Brantley-Sieders DM, Caughron J, Hicks D et al (2004) EphA2 receptor tyrosine kinase regulates endothelial cell migration and vascular assembly through phosphoinositide 3-kinase-mediated Rac1 GTPase activation. J Cell Sci 117:2037–2049

Brantley-Sieders DM, Fang WB, Hicks DJ et al (2005) Impaired tumor microenvironment in EphA2-deficient mice inhibits tumor angiogenesis and metastatic progression. Faseb J 19: 1884–1886

Brantley-Sieders DM, Fang WB, Hwang Y et al (2006) Ephrin-A1 facilitates mammary tumor metastasis through an angiogenesis-dependent mechanism mediated by EphA receptor and vascular endothelial growth factor in mice. Cancer Res 66:10315–10324

Brizel DM, Scully SP, Harrelson JM et al (1996) Tumor oxygenation predicts for the likelihood of distant metastases in human soft tissue sarcoma. Cancer Res 56:941–943

Brizel DM, Dodge RK, Clough RW et al (1999) Oxygenation of head and neck cancer: changes during radiotherapy and impact on treatment outcome. Radiother Oncol 53:113–117

Brizel DM, Prosnitz RG, Hunter S et al (2004) Necessity for adjuvant neck dissection in setting of concurrent chemoradiation for advanced head-and-neck cancer. Int J Radiat Oncol Biol Phys 58:1418–1423

Brockstein B, Haraf DJ, Rademaker AW et al (2004) Patterns of failure, prognostic factors and survival in locoregionally advanced head and neck cancer treated with concomitant chemoradiotherapy: a 9-year, 337-patient, multi-institutional experience. Ann Oncol 15:1179–1186

Brown JM, Giaccia AJ (1998) The unique physiology of solid tumors: opportunities (and problems) for cancer therapy. Cancer Res 58:1408–1416

Bruckner K, Pasquale EB, Klein R (1997) Tyrosine phosphorylation of transmembrane ligands for Eph receptors. Science 275:1640–1643

Cheng N, Brantley DM, Chen J (2002) The ephrins and Eph receptors in angiogenesis. Cytokine Growth Factor Rev 13:75–85

Chi JT, Wang Z, Nuyten DS et al (2006) Gene expression programs in response to hypoxia: Cell type specificity and prognostic significance in human cancers. PLoS Med 3:e47

Chung CD, Patel VP, Moran M et al (2000) Galectin-1 induces partial TCR zeta-chain phosphorylation and antagonizes processive TCR signal transduction. J Immunol 165:3722–3729

De Schutter H, Landuyt W, Verbeken E et al (2005) The prognostic value of the hypoxia markers CA IX and GLUT 1 and the cytokines VEGF and IL 6 in head and neck squamous cell carcinoma treated by radiotherapy +/– chemotherapy. BMC Cancer 5:42

Denko NC, Fontana LA, Hudson KM et al (2003) Investigating hypoxic tumor physiology through gene expression patterns. Oncogene 22:5907–5914

Dunst J, Stadler P, Becker A et al (2001) Tumor hypoxia and systemic levels of vascular endothelial growth factor (VEGF) in head and neck cancers. Strahlenther Onkol 177:469–473

Dvorak HF, Nagy JA, Feng D et al (1999) Vascular permeability factor/vascular endothelial growth factor and the significance of microvascular hyperpermeability in angiogenesis. Curr Top Microbiol Immunol 237:97–132

Eisma RJ, Spiro JD, Kreutzer DL (1997) Vascular endothelial growth factor expression in head and neck squamous cell carcinoma. Am J Surg 174:513–517

Eisma RJ, Spiro JD, Kreutzer DL (1999) Role of angiogenic factors: coexpression of interleukin-8 and vascular endothelial growth factor in patients with head and neck squamous carcinoma. Laryngoscope 109:687–693

Erler JT, Bennewith KL, Nicolau M et al (2006) Lysyl oxidase is essential for hypoxia-induced metastasis. Nature 440:1222–1226

Escudier B, Eisen T, Stadler WM et al (2007) Sorafenib in advanced clear-cell renal-cell carcinoma. N Engl J Med 356:125–134

Evans SM, Koch CJ (2003) Prognostic significance of tumor oxygenation in humans. Cancer Lett 195:1–16

Evans SM, Du KL, Chalian AA et al (2007) Patterns and levels of hypoxia in head and neck squamous cell carcinomas and their relationship to patient outcome. Int J Radiat Oncol Biol Phys 69:1024–1031

Ferrara N, Gerber HP, LeCouter J (2003) The biology of VEGF and its receptors. Nat Med 9:669–676

Fyles A, Milosevic M, Hedley D et al (2002) Tumor hypoxia has independent predictor impact only in patients with node-negative cervix cancer. J Clin Oncol 20:680–687

Gatenby RA, Kessler HB, Rosenblum JS et al (1988) Oxygen distribution in squamous cell carcinoma metastases and its relationship to outcome of radiation therapy. Int J Radiat Oncol Biol Phys 14:831–838

Gerety SS, Wang HU, Chen ZF et al (1999) Symmetrical mutant phenotypes of the receptor EphB4 and its specific transmembrane ligand ephrin-B2 in cardiovascular development. Mol Cell 4:403–414

Giaccia A, Siim BG, Johnson RS (2003) HIF-1 as a target for drug development. Nat Rev Drug Discov 2:803–811

Gleich LL, Biddinger PW, Duperier FD et al (1997) Tumor angiogenesis as a prognostic indicator in T2–T4 oral cavity squamous cell carcinoma: a clinical-pathologic correlation. Head Neck 19:276–280

Goldman CK, Kendall RL, Cabrera G et al (1998) Paracrine expression of a native soluble vascular endothelial growth factor receptor inhibits tumor growth, metastasis, and mortality rate. Proc Natl Acad Sci U S A 95:8795–8800

Harris AL (2002) Hypoxia – a key regulatory factor in tumour growth. Nat Rev Cancer 2:38–47

Heroult M, Schaffner F, Augustin HG (2006) Eph receptor and ephrin ligand-mediated interactions during angiogenesis and tumor progression. Exp Cell Res 312:642–650

Holland SJ, Gale NW, Mbamalu G et al (1996) Bidirectional signalling through the EPH-family receptor Nuk and its transmembrane ligands. Nature 383:722–725

Hurwitz H, Fehrenbacher L, Novotny W et al (2004) Bevacizumab plus irinotecan, fluorouracil, and leucovorin for metastatic colorectal cancer. N Engl J Med 350:2335–2342

Imagawa S, Goldberg MA, Doweiko J et al (1991) Regulatory elements of the erythropoietin gene. Blood 77:278–285

Imagawa S, Yamaguchi Y, Higuchi M et al (2001) Levels of vascular endothelial growth factor are elevated in patients with obstructive sleep apnea–hypopnea syndrome. Blood 98:1255–1257

Jablonska E, Piotrowski L, Jablonski J et al (2002) VEGF in the culture of PMN and the serum in oral cavity cancer patients. Oral Oncol 38:605–609

Janssen HL, Haustermans KM, Sprong D et al (2002) HIF-1A, pimonidazole, and iododeoxyuridine to estimate hypoxia and perfusion in human head-and-neck tumors. Int J Radiat Oncol Biol Phys 54:1537–1549

Jonathan RA, Wijffels KI, Peeters W et al (2006) The prognostic value of endogenous hypoxia-related markers for head and neck squamous cell carcinomas treated with ARCON. Radiother Oncol 79:288–297

Kaanders JH, Wijffels KI, Marres HA et al (2002) Pimonidazole binding and tumor vascularity predict for treatment outcome in head and neck cancer. Cancer Res 62:7066–7074

Kennedy KA, Teicher BA, Rockwell S et al (1980) The hypoxic tumor cell: a target for selective cancer chemotherapy. Biochem Pharmacol 29:1–8

Koong AC, Denko NC, Hudson KM et al (2000) Candidate genes for the hypoxic tumor phenotype. Cancer Res 60:883–887

Koukourakis MI, Bentzen SM, Giatromanolaki A et al (2006) Endogenous markers of two separate hypoxia response pathways (hypoxia inducible factor 2 alpha and carbonic anhydrase 9) are associated with radiotherapy failure in head and neck cancer patients recruited in the CHART randomized trial. J Clin Oncol 24:727–735

Kowalski LP, Carvalho AL, Martins Priante AV et al (2005) Predictive factors for distant metastasis from oral and oropharyngeal squamous cell carcinoma. Oral Oncol 41:534–541

Kunkel M, Reichert TE, Benz P et al (2003) Overexpression of Glut-1 and increased glucose metabolism in tumors are associated with a poor prognosis in patients with oral squamous cell carcinoma. Cancer 97:1015–1024

Kyzas PA, Cunha IW, Ioannidis JP (2005a) Prognostic significance of vascular endothelial growth factor immunohistochemical expression in head and neck squamous cell carcinoma: a meta-analysis. Clin Cancer Res 11:1434–1440

Kyzas PA, Stefanou D, Batistatou A et al (2005b) Hypoxia-induced tumor angiogenic pathway in head and neck cancer: an in vivo study. Cancer Lett 225:297–304

Kyzas PA, Stefanou D, Batistatou A et al (2005c) Prognostic significance of VEGF immunohistochemical expression and tumor angiogenesis in head and neck squamous cell carcinoma. J Cancer Res Clin Oncol 131:624–630

Lartigau E, Le Ridant AM, Lambin P et al (1993) Oxygenation of head and neck tumors. Cancer 71:2319–2325

Le QT, Sutphin PD, Raychaudhuri S et al (2003) Identification of osteopontin as a prognostic plasma marker for head and neck squamous cell carcinomas. Clin Cancer Res 9:59–67

Le QT, Denko NC, Giaccia AJ (2004) Hypoxic gene expression and metastasis. Cancer Metastasis Rev 23:293–310

Le QT, Shi G, Cao H et al (2005) Galectin-1: a link between tumor hypoxia and tumor immune privilege. J Clin Oncol 23:8932–8941

Le QT, Kong C, Lavori PW et al (2007) Expression and prognostic significance of a panel of tissue hypoxia markers in head-and-neck squamous cell carcinomas. Int J Radiat Oncol Biol Phys 69:167–175

Liao CT, Wang HM, Chang JT et al (2007) Analysis of risk factors for distant metastases in squamous cell carcinoma of the oral cavity. Cancer 110:1501–1508

Linderholm BK, Lindh B, Beckman L et al (2003) Prognostic correlation of basic fibroblast growth factor and vascular endothelial growth factor in 1307 primary breast cancers. Clin Breast Cancer 4:340–347

Ljungkvist AS, Bussink J, Kaanders JH et al (2007) Dynamics of tumor hypoxia measured with bioreductive hypoxic cell markers. Radiat Res 167:127–145

Lopez de Cicco R, Watson JC, Bassi DE et al (2004) Simultaneous expression of furin and vascular endothelial growth factor in human oral tongue squamous cell carcinoma progression. Clin Cancer Res 10:4480–4488

Maeda T, Matsumura S, Hiranuma H et al (1998) Expression of vascular endothelial growth factor in human oral squamous cell carcinoma: its association with tumour progression and p53 gene status. J Clin Pathol 51:771–775

Masood R, Kumar SR, Sinha UK et al (2006) EphB4 provides survival advantage to squamous cell carcinoma of the head and neck. Int J Cancer 119:1236–1248

Mayer A, Wree A, Hockel M et al (2004) Lack of correlation between expression of HIF-1alpha protein and oxygenation status in identical tissue areas of squamous cell carcinomas of the uterine cervix. Cancer Res 64:5876–5881

Mayer A, Hockel M, Vaupel P (2005a) Carbonic anhydrase IX expression and tumor oxygenation status do not correlate at the microregional level in locally advanced cancers of the uterine cervix. Clin Cancer Res 11:7220–7225

Mayer A, Hockel M, Wree A et al (2005b) Microregional expression of glucose transporter-1 and oxygenation status: lack of correlation in locally advanced cervical cancers. Clin Cancer Res 11:2768–2773

Motzer RJ, Hutson TE, Tomczak P et al (2007) Sunitinib versus interferon alfa in metastatic renal-cell carcinoma. N Engl J Med 356:115–124

Nordsmark M, Overgaard J (2000) A confirmatory prognostic study on oxygenation status and loco-regional control in advanced head and neck squamous cell carcinoma treated by radiation therapy. Radiother Oncol 57:39–43

Nordsmark M, Alsner J, Keller J et al (2001) Hypoxia in human soft tissue sarcomas: adverse impact on survival and no association with p53 mutations. Br J Cancer 84:1070–1075

Nordsmark M, Bentzen SM, Rudat V et al (2005) Prognostic value of tumor oxygenation in 397 head and neck tumors after primary radiation therapy. An international multi-center study. Radiother Oncol 77:18–24

Nordsmark M, Eriksen JG, Gebski V, Nordsmark M, Eriksen JG, Gebski V et al (2007) Differential risk assessments from five hypoxia specific assays: The basis for biologically adapted individualized radiotherapy in advanced head and neck cancer patients. Radiother Oncol 83:389–397

Ogawa K, Pasqualini R, Lindberg RA et al (2000) The ephrin-A1 ligand and its receptor, EphA2, are expressed during tumor neovascularization. Oncogene 19:6043–6052

Oliver RJ, Woodwards RT, Sloan P et al (2004) Prognostic value of facilitative glucose transporter Glut-1 in oral squamous cell carcinomas treated by surgical resection; results of EORTC Translational Research Fund studies. Eur J Cancer 40:503–507

Overgaard J, Eriksen JG, Nordsmark M et al (2005) Plasma osteopontin, hypoxia, and response to the hypoxia sensitiser nimorazole in radiotherapy of head and neck cancer: results from the DAHANCA 5 randomised double-blind placebo-controlled trial. Lancet Oncol 6:757–764

Pazouki S, Chisholm DM, Adi MM et al (1997) The association between tumour progression and vascularity in the oral mucosa. J Pathol 183:39–43

Penfold CN, Partridge M, Rojas R et al (1996) The role of angiogenesis in the spread of oral squamous cell carcinoma. Br J Oral Maxillofac Surg 34:37–41

Petrik D, Lavori PW, Cao H et al (2006) Plasma osteopontin is an independent prognostic marker for head and neck cancers. J Clin Oncol 24:5291–5297

Presta LG, Chen H, O'Connor SJ et al (1997) Humanization of an anti-vascular endothelial growth factor monoclonal antibody for the therapy of solid tumors and other disorders. Cancer Res 57:4593–4599

Rabinovich GA, Ariel A, Hershkoviz R et al (1999) Specific inhibition of T-cell adhesion to extracellular matrix and proinflammatory cytokine secretion by human recombinant galectin-1. Immunology 97:100–106

Raza SM, Fuller GN, Rhee CH et al (2004) Identification of necrosis-associated genes in glioblastoma by cDNA microarray analysis. Clin Cancer Res 10:212–221

Riedel F, Gotte K, Schwalb J et al (2000) Serum levels of vascular endothelial growth factor in patients with head and neck cancer. Eur Arch Otorhinolaryngol 257:332–336

Rubinstein N, Alvarez M, Zwirner NW et al (2004) Targeted inhibition of galectin-1 gene expression in tumor cells results in heightened T cell-mediated rejection; A potential mechanism of tumor-immune privilege. Cancer Cell 5:241–251

Rudat V, Vanselow B, Wollensack P et al (2000) Repeatability and prognostic impact of the pre-treatment pO(2) histography in patients with advanced head and neck cancer. Radiother Oncol 57:31–37

Rudat V, Stadler P, Becker A et al (2001) Predictive value of the tumor oxygenation by means of pO$_2$ histography in patients with advanced head and neck cancer. Strahlenther Onkol 177:462–468

Salven P, Manpaa H, Orpana A et al (1997) Serum vascular endothelial growth factor is often elevated in disseminated cancer. Clin Cancer Res 3:647–651

Sandler A, Gray R, Perry MC et al (2006) Paclitaxel-carboplatin alone or with bevacizumab for non-small-cell lung cancer. N Engl J Med 355:2542–2550

Schilling D, Bayer C, Geurts-Moespot A et al (2007) Induction of plasminogen activator inhibitor type-1 (PAI-1) by hypoxia and irradiation in human head and neck carcinoma cell lines. BMC Cancer 7:143

Semenza GL, Nejfelt MK, Chi SM et al (1991) Hypoxia-inducible nuclear factors bind to an enhancer element located 3' to the erythropoietin gene. Proc Natl Acad Sci USA 88:5680–5684

Singhal H, Bautista DS, Tonkin KS et al (1997) Elevated plasma osteopontin in metastatic breast cancer associated with increased tumor burden and decreased survival. Clin Cancer Res 3:605–611

Smith BD, Smith GL, Carter D et al (2000) Prognostic significance of vascular endothelial growth factor protein levels in oral and oropharyngeal squamous cell carcinoma. J Clin Oncol 18:2046–2052

Sprague LD, Mengele K, Schilling D et al (2006) Effect of reoxygenation on the hypoxia-induced up-regulation of serine protease inhibitor PAI-1 in head and neck cancer cells. Oncology 71:282–291

Sprague LD, Tomaso H, Mengele K et al (2007) Effects of hypoxia and reoxygenation on the expression levels of the urokinase-type plasminogen activator, its inhibitor plasminogen activator inhibitor type-1 and the urokinase-type plasminogen activator receptor in human head and neck tumour cells. Oncol Rep 17:1259–1268

Stroka DM, Burkhardt T, Desbaillets I et al (2001) HIF-1 is expressed in normoxic tissue and displays an organ-specific regulation under systemic hypoxia. Faseb J 15:2445–2453

Thomlinson RH, Gray LH (1955) The histological structure of some human lung cancers and the possible implications for radiotherapy. Br J Cancer 9:539–549

Tse GM, Chan AW, Yu KH et al (2007) Strong immunohistochemical expression of vascular endothelial growth factor predicts overall survival in head and neck squamous cell carcinoma. Ann Surg Oncol 14:3558–3565

Vihanto MM, Plock J, Erni D et al (2005) Hypoxia up-regulates expression of Eph receptors and ephrins in mouse skin. Faseb J 19:1689–1691

Wang GL, Semenza GL (1995) Purification and characterization of hypoxia-inducible factor 1. J Biol Chem 270:1230–1237

Wang HU, Chen ZF, Anderson DJ (1998) Molecular distinction and angiogenic interaction between embryonic arteries and veins revealed by ephrin-B2 and its receptor Eph-B4. Cell 93:741–753

Winter SC, Shah KA, Han C et al (2006) The relation between hypoxia-inducible factor (HIF)-1alpha and HIF-2alpha expression with anemia and outcome in surgically treated head and neck cancer. Cancer 107:757–766

Winter SC, Buffa FM, Silva P et al (2007) Relation of a hypoxia metagene derived from head and neck cancer to prognosis of multiple cancers. Cancer Res 67:3441–3449

Zelzer E, Levy Y, Kahana C et al (1998) Insulin induces transcription of target genes through the hypoxia-inducible factor HIF-1alpha/ARNT. Embo J 17:5085–5094

Zhong H, Chiles K, Feldser D et al (2000) Modulation of hypoxia-inducible factor 1alpha expression by the epidermal growth factor/phosphatidylinositol 3-kinase/PTEN/AKT/FRAP pathway in human prostate cancer cells: implications for tumor angiogenesis and therapeutics. Cancer Res 60:1541–1545

Ziemer LS, Koch CJ, Maity A et al (2001) Hypoxia and VEGF mRNA expression in human tumors. Neoplasia 3:500–508

Zundel W, Schindler C, Haas-Kogan D et al (2000) Loss of PTEN facilitates HIF-1-mediated gene expression. Genes Dev 14:391–396

Chapter 15
Cancer Stem Cells and Oral Cavity Cancer Metastasis

Mark Prince

Abstract Oral cavity squamous cell carcinoma is a common malignancy with a high propensity for the development of metastasis. Even early stage oral cavity tumors are frequently associated with metastasis to regional lymph nodes. Cancer stem cells have recently been isolated from head and neck squamous cell cancer and represent the critical population of cancer cells responsible for primary tumor growth. Cancer stem cells also likely represent the population of cancer cells responsible for resistance to therapy and regional and distant metastasis. The identification of this critical subpopulation of cancer cells will increase our ability to understand the mechanisms that which underlie the development of metastasis in head and neck cancer and holds promise for the development of new and more effective therapies for this devastating disease.

Introduction

Oral cavity cancer ranks as one of the ten most frequently diagnosed cancers in the world (Rodrigues et al. 1998), and the seventh most common cancer diagnosed in the United States (Jemal et al. 2004). After receiving standard therapy for their cancer, a subset of patients at each stage of disease develops cancer recurrence. Although nearly 90% of patients with stage I disease can be cured, nearly 10% will experience relapse and die from disease. For more advanced stages the proportion of patients whose disease relapses increases to 30% for stage II, 50% for stage III, and more than for 70% stage IV. These high failure rates occur in a large part due to the development of regional and distant metastatic disease. Progress in developing effective treatments and preventive strategies for head and neck squamous cell carcinoma (HNSCC) has been limited by our current level of understanding regarding how this cancer arises and which cells are involved in its development, progression and regional, and distant spread.

M. Prince (✉)
A. Alfred Taubman Health Care Center, 1500 East Medical Center Drive, Floor 1,
Reception: A, Ann Arbor, MI, 48109-5312, USA

J. Myers (ed.), *Oral Cancer Metastasis*,
DOI 10.1007/978-1-4419-0775-2_15, © Springer Science+Business Media, LLC 2010

The identification of subpopulations of cancer cells within HNSCC that may be responsible for tumor repopulation, metastasis and the failure of cell death pathways represents a major advance towards the development of improved treatment and increasing survival rates for patients diagnosed with this devastating disease. Cancer stem cells, which have recently been identified in a number of different types of solid tumors, including HNSCC, may play a key role in the development of regional and distant metastasis and resistance to therapy.

Metastasis of cancer cells from the primary tumor sites accounts for the majority of cancer mortality (Weigelt et al. 2005). Currently the role of cancer stem cells in the development of cancer metastasis is not well defined, although there are reasons to believe they may play a pivotal role (Croker and Allan 2008; Dalerba et al. 2007a). Normal stem cells are known to have the capacity to migrate and establish themselves in new locations. In order to survive and grow in a particular site, the stem cell needs to be supported by a specific stem cell niche. This niche is critical to stem cell maintenance and to the production of more differentiated progenitor cells (Morrison and Spradling 2008).

Similar to normal stem cells, cancer stem cells would be expected to require a specific niche in order to survive, multiply, and produce progenitor cancer cells. The exact mechanism by which normal stem cells are able to home to certain locations or tissue types is not yet fully understood but once more fully elucidated, may provide clues as to how cancer cells locate favorable sites in which to establish metastasis. The ability of circulating cancer cells to home to specific tissues and establish themselves within a supportive niche is critical to the successful establishment of a metastasis. It is likely that many of the same mechanisms which directs normal stem cell migration and maintenance play a role in cancer stem cell metastasis.

Stem Cells and Cancer Stem Cells

It has long been recognized that solid tumors, including HNSCC, are histologically heterogeneous and contain multiple diverse cell types including tumor cells, stromal cells, and infiltrating inflammatory cells. It is known that cancers contain subpopulations of cancer cells that may resemble the developmental hierarchy of normal tissues from which the cancer develops. Until recently, the importance of cancer cell subpopulations to tumor growth and development has been poorly understood (Lobo et al. 2007). The identification of a small subpopulation of highly tumorigenic cancer cells, which appear to be solely responsible for cancer growth and maintenance, has stimulated great interest in cancer stem cells and the "cancer stem cell model" of carcinogenesis (Lobo et al. 2007; Reya et al. 2001; Al-Hajj et al. 2004; Cho and Clarke 2008).

Adult stem cells have been identified in most human tissues, including bone marrow, brain, skin, gastrointestinal tract, liver, pancreas, lungs, breast, ovaries, prostate, and testis (Al-Hajj and Clarke 2004; Woodward et al. 2005; Li and Neaves 2006; Mimeault and Batra 2006). Adult stem cells are multipotent cells with the capacity to self renew that produce differentiated cell lineages (Al-Hajj and

Clarke 2004; Mimeault and Batra 2006; Reya and Clevers 2005; Fuchs et al. 2004). The stem cell is supported by a specific stem cell niche, which at least in part directs the stem cells' behavior and is vital to stem cell maintenance (Li and Neaves 2006; Mimeault and Batra 2006; Moore and Lemischka 2006). Interactions between the stem cells and their supporting cells occur through secreted factors and intercellular connections. The adult stem cells and their early progenitor cells perform the critical functions of tissue regeneration and repair.

Recently an accumulating body of evidence indicates that adult stem cells or their early progenitor cells play a role in carcinogenesis (Dalerba et al. 2007a; Clarke and Fuller 2006; Pardal et al. 2003; Wicha et al. 2006). Genetic and epigenetic changes in adult stem cells or their early progenitor cells may result in cancer initiation (Al-Hajj and Clarke 2004; Mimeault and Batra 2006; Reya and Clevers 2005; Bapat et al. 2005; Li et al. 2005; Kastan and Bartek 2004). These cells have been called cancer stem cells. A landmark study in human leukemia identified the leukemia initiating cells and stimulated further attempts to identify the cancer initiating cells in other cancer types (Bonnet and Dick 1997). Subsequent work has isolated highly tumorigenic subpopulations of cells, designated as cancer stem cells, in many solid tumor types. This work was performed initially in breast cancer followed by investigations of tumors of the brain, head and neck, lung, pancreas, prostate, and colon (Al-Hajj et al. 2003; Chiba et al. 2006; Collins et al. 2005; Dalerba et al. 2007b; Li et al. 2007; O'Brien et al. 2007; Prince et al. 2007; Singh et al. 2003, 2004). Similarities between the characteristics of normal stem cells and cancer cells are intriguing and suggest these cells share common genetic and molecular pathways that regulate their behavior.

According to the cancer stem cell theory of carcinogenesis, only the cancer stem cells have the ability to sustain cancer growth, and without cancer stem cells the cancer would stop growing and either remain quiescent or eventually regress. Three key characteristics define the cancer stem cell subpopulation (1) only a small portion of the cancer cells within a tumor have tumorigenic potential when transplanted into immune deficient mice, (2) the cancer stem cell subpopulation can be separated from the other cancer cells by distinctive cell surface markers, and (3) tumors resulting from the cancer stem cells contain the mixed tumorigenic and nontumorigenic cancer cells of the original tumor (Dalerba et al. 2007a).

Using methods similar to those used to identify the cancer stem cells from breast cancer, a highly tumorigenic subpopulation of cancer cells was isolated from HNSCC. HNSCC cells with high expression of the cell surface marker CD44 (CD44+) were found to be highly tumorigenic (Fig. 15.1). As few as 2×10^3 CD44+ HNSCC cells were able to generate new tumors when implanted into immunosuppressed mice. Additionally these cells could be passaged in an animal model and were capable of reproducing the original tumor heterogeneity. The CD44+ HNSCC cells have the characteristics that define the cancer stem cell subpopulation and represent only a small fraction of the total number of cells contained within the cancer (Prince et al. 2007). Cancer stem cells in HNSCC may have critical importance to our understanding of the development of regional and distant metastasis in this disease in addition to their importance in the primary tumor.

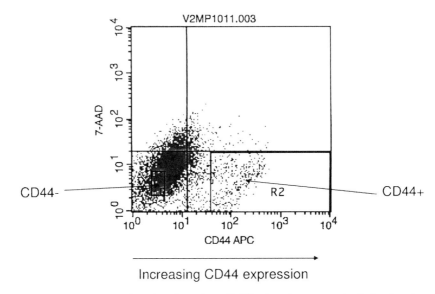

Increasing CD44 expression

Fig. 15.1 Flourescence-activated cell sorting (FACS) plot shows a patient's head and neck squamous cell carcinoma sorted for CD44 expression using flow cytometry. The cells contained in the area on the right are the CD44 positive cells that contain the cancer stem cell subpopulation

Cancer Stem Cells and Metastasis

Metastasis is a multistage process that involves the escape of cancer cells from the primary neoplasm followed by their dissemination through lymphatic vessels or the systemic circulation. Under the correct conditions, cancer cells can form micrometastases that develop into well-established cancer metastasis in distant tissues or organs. The steps required for a metastasis to become established in a new location include escape of cancer cells from the primary tumor with spread of the cells via the lymphatics or vascular channels and their survival in the circulation. This process is followed by adhesion and migration or extravasation of the cancer cells into the secondary tissue, and establishment the growth of a micrometastasis. Finally, the metastasis must establish a vascular supply which leads to the development of a macrometastasis (Pantel and Brakenhoff 2004; Chambers et al. 2002; MacDonald et al. 2002; Swartz and Skobe 2001; Woodhouse et al. 1997). The process of metastasis formation is remarkably similar to the migration and establishment of normal stem cells in new locations and suggests that the two processes may be related.

Normal stem cells have the intrinsic ability to migrate to specific locations where they can become established if local conditions are favorable. Cancer stem cells would be expected to maintain this ability and may then, under the correct conditions, be capable of forming a metastasis. The nonstem cell cancer cells, which do not even have the capacity to maintain the primary tumor, are highly unlikely to be the source of metastasis. The highly tumorigenic properties of the cancer stem cells suggest that they may be the critical population of cancer cells in the development of metastasis, just as they have been proven to be in primary tumor development and growth. The body of evidence supporting a role for cancer stem cells in the production of metastases is rapidly increasing.

Given the difficulty in completing the multistep process required to produce a metastasis, it is not surprising that the formation of metastasis is a highly inefficient process. Experimental studies have revealed that the early steps in the development of metastasis are efficient, with the majority of circulating cancer cells able to reach a secondary site. Only a small fraction of these cells, however, are able to create a micrometastasis, and an even smaller subset persist and are capable of developing into a macrometastasis (Pantel and Brakenhoff 2004; Luzzi et al. 1998; Cameron et al. 2000; Chambers et al. 2001; Weiss 1992) . Despite the fact that many cancer patients have hundreds or thousands of circulating cancer cells detectable in their bloodstream, only a very small fraction progress to form a macroscopic metastasis. This suggests that only a tiny fraction of the circulating cancer cells have an intrinsic metastatic potential, and that rarely do they manage to make their way to a location that can sustain their growth. This observation is consistent with the idea that only circulating cancer stem cells, which would make up a tiny proportion of the circulating cancer cells, have the potential to form macrometastasis (Fig. 15.2).

Several characteristics of cancer stem cells make them likely candidates to occupy and thrive in foreign tissues. The cancer stem cells, unlike the remainder of the cancer cells, have the unique ability to initiate and sustain cancer growth. It has been known for years that just one cell can initiate a metastatic lesion (Fidler and Talmadge 1986). However, it has also been observed that even with immortalized cancer cell lines large numbers of cells (in the range of 10^6) need to be injected to initiate a tumor in experimental animals, and only a very few of these cells have the potential to produce a metastasis (Chambers et al. 2002; Luzzi et al. 1998; Welch 1997). The stochastic theory of carcinogenesis predicts that every cancer cell has the potential to initiate a tumor but that very rare stochastic events control the progression to tumorigenic growth. The hierarchal theory of carcinogenesis predicts that only a subset of cells within a cancer are capable of initiating tumorigenic growth, which is in keeping with the current level of knowledge regarding cancer stem cells. It is logical to hypothesize that the cancer stem cell subpopulation contains the only cancer cells that are capable of producing a metastasis.

Researchers have begun to evaluate the cellular and molecular mechanisms that direct tissue specific metastasis. Results have shown that only a small subpopulation of breast cancer cells have a molecular profile that allows them to preferentially metastasize (Kang et al. 2003; Kang 2005; Minn et al. 2005; Kaplan et al. 2005). The molecular profile of tissue specific metastatic cancer cells can be distinguished from the overall molecular signatures of the cancer in general. It has not yet been determined if there is an overlap between the cancer stem cells and the population of cancer cells with a metastatic gene profile.

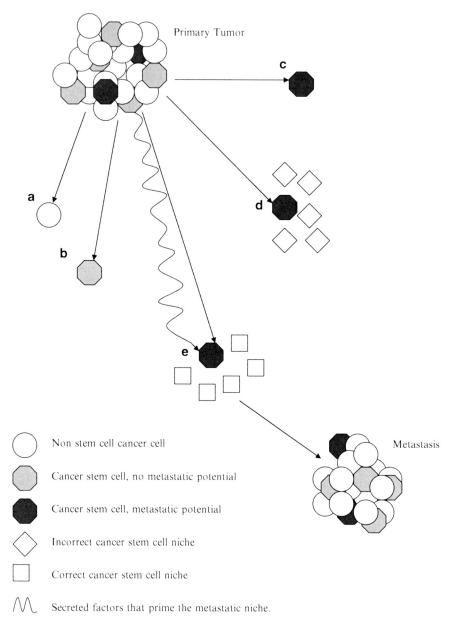

Fig. 15.2 Cancer stem cells in metastasis model. Schematic diagram representing a proposed relationship between noncancer stem cell cancer cells, the cancer stem cells, and the cancer stem cells with metastatic potential. The cancer stem cells represent only a small proportion of the primary tumor mass and cancer stem cells with metastatic potential represent even smaller sub-population of the cancer stem cells. (**a**) The noncancer stem cell cancer cells may be detected in the circulation or lymphatics but are not capable of forming a metastasis. (**b**) Cancer stem cells without metastatic potential, although capable of reproducing the original tumor, are not able to produce a metastasis. (**c, d**) Cancer stem cells with metastatic potential in the circulation which

The Cancer Stem Cell Niche and Metastasis

The factors that determine the balance between dormancy and proliferation with the development of a metastasis at a secondary site are not yet well understood. The identification of cancer stem cells suggests that one possible reason that cancer metastasis develops so infrequently, despite the frequently large number of circulating cancer cells, is that the majority of the cancer cells that escape into the circulation or lymphatics do not have the intrinsic ability to form a metastasis. It is highly likely that cancer stem cells or a subpopulation of cancer stem cells have the capacity to produce a metastasis, although this has yet to be proven. Even with this ability, however, if the cancer stem cell does not arrive in a location with a favorable supporting niche, a metastasis will not result and the cancer cells may remain quiescent or eventually die. The lack of a suitable niche or the lack of an intrinsic inability of the cancer cell to form a tumor might explain the observation of isolated cancer cells in remote locations that do not appear to result in metastasis.

The importance of the stem cell niche is well recognized for normal stem cells (Fuchs et al. 2004; Watt and Hogan 2000). Similar to normal stem cells, local conditions, the "niche," can also be predicted to be of great importance to cancer stem cell maintenance and growth. At the primary cancer site, it is apparent that a favorable cancer stem cell niche would exist, as this is the presumed normal location for the cells of origin of the cancer. At regional or distant metastatic sites, the cancer niche would either need to preexist or the cancer stem cells, the primary tumor, or accompanying supporting cells would need to act to create a favorable niche. It is possible that the niche is established by other cells prior to the arrival of the cancer stem cell. This effect might be regulated through circulating growth factors, cytokines, or hormones or by other noncancer stem cells that could prepare the location for the metastatic cancer stem cell. This is an area that requires a great deal of additional study.

The need for a specific niche to support normal stem cells was first suggested almost 30 years ago (Schofield 1978). Significant increases in our understanding of the structure and function of the stem cell niche have been made in the Drosophila model. For example, the BMP pathway and Jak–Stat pathways have been identified as critical signaling molecules that regulate self renewal in Drosophila germ line stem cells that are derived form the stem cell niche (Kiger et al. 2001; Song et al. 2004; Tulina and Matunis 2001; Morrison and Kimble 2006). These molecular pathways and others related to the normal stem cell maintenance and the stem cell niche, including the WNT and Notch signaling pathways, may be critical to cancer stem cells and to the development of metastasis (Lobo et al. 2007; Katoh and Katoh 2007; Gil et al. 2005). If confirmed, these pathways and others could prove to be

---

Fig. 15.2 (continued) do not establish themselves within a suitable niche cannot form metastasis. Cancer stem cells with metastatic potential not supported by a suitable niche may eventually die, may remain quiescent or may become active if the correct stimuli become available. (**e**) Cancer stem cells with metastatic potential that establish themselves in a secondary tissue with a suitable niche and under the influence of secreted stimulating factors can produce a metastasis

useful therapeutic targets to prevent the development of metastasis or eliminate them once they have been formed.

The stem cell niches for bone marrow, testis, intestine, and the neural system have been studied in mammals (Scadden 2006). Although stem cell niches vary from tissue to tissue, certain key factors seem to be conserved and as a result are potentially important in both normal and malignant stem cells. BMPs are an example of an important regulator of stem cell differentiation in mammals. They promote the differentiation of stem cells and are inhibited by Gremlin1, a secreted antagonist of the BMP pathway. Interestingly Gremlin1 has been found to be overexpressed by tumor stromal cells derived from basal cell cancer, but not in those derived from normal skin. BMP inhibits proliferation of basal cell cancer cells in culture, whereas Gremlin 1 enhances it (Sneddon et al. 2006). This finding reveals the importance of factors secreted by the niche to the tumor microenvironment. Secreted factors derived from the cancer stem cell niche would be expected to favorably prime the surrounding tissue to encourage the development of cancer metastasis. Interference with these exocrine signals could provide a novel method by which the successful implantation and growth of cancer stem cells at distant sites might be prevented.

The recruitment of circulating cancer cells at specific sites and metastasis formation may be influenced by the local dynamic microenvironment, including microvasculature endothelial cells, stromal fibroblasts, and osteoblasts that secrete soluble factors including chemokines. Kaplan et al provided major clues regarding the relationship of niche formation and metastasis development (Kaplan et al. 2005). In work that evaluated melanoma and lung cancer cells, bone marrow derived cells were found to be directed to future sites of metastasis prior to the arrival of cancer cells. This effect was found to be regulated by secreted factors contained in the cancer cell conditioned media. Removing the premetastasis niche factors almost completely eliminated the development of metastasis. This indicates the importance of the niche and provides evidence that interference with the preparation of the premetastasis cancer niche can inhibit the development of metastasis. If the specific factors that enable the development of metastasis in HNSCC can be identified, then this could lead to powerful new therapies to prevent the development of metastasis.

The fibroblasts associated with oral cavity cancer have been shown to be biologically distinct from normal fibroblasts (Liu et al. 2006). These fibroblasts have a specific and unique supporting function related to the cancer cells. Specialized supporting cells are also required in the normal stem cell niche and probably exist at metastatic sites, as an important part of the cancer stem cell niche, to support the development of a metastasis. Further study needs to be performed to see if biologic differences are evident in the supporting tissues associated with metastatic deposits when compared to normal tissue in the same organ. It can be anticipated that similar to the establishment and maintenance of normal stem cells in secondary tissues, the cancer stem cell niche, including supporting cells, will be a critical factor to the successful establishment of metastasis in cancer.

There is growing evidence that the primary tumor influences the development of metastasis by the secretion of various soluble cytokines and proteins that induce the formation of favorable conditions at potential sites of regional and distant metastasis. The release of the chemokine SDF-1 can contribute to the recruitment of circulating tumor cells that express the CXCR4 receptor to the specific metastatic site including lymph nodes and basement membrane (Kaplan et al. 2005; Kalluri and Zeisberg 2006; Balkwill 2004; Kucia et al. 2005; Engl et al. 2006). The preferential migration of CXCR4 positive prostate, breast, and small cell lung cancer cells to the microvasculature basement membrane and cancer cell adhesion to the extracellular matrix involves the SDF1–CXCR4 axis. Inhibition of prostate cancer cells movement towards the basement membrane by anti-CXCR4 antibody or the SDF1 inhibitor T140 supports the importance of the SDF1–CXCR4 axis to cancer cell migration (Engl et al. 2006; Hart et al. 2005).

Further study of CXCR4 indicates its critical role in cancer metastasis. Work with pancreatic cancer stem cells suggests that only a small subpopulation of all the cancer stem cells have metastatic potential, although all the pancreatic cancer stem cells retain the capacity to form primary tumors. Only CXCR4 positive pancreatic cancer stem cells are capable of producing both primary tumors and metastasis, whereas the other cancer stem cells are not able to reliably produce metastasis (Hermann et al. 2007). This is the first evidence that a subpopulation of cancer stem cells play a pivotal role in the development of cancer metastasis and that CXCR4 expression can be used to identify and select the cancer stem cells with metastatic potential from the other cancer stem cells. The role of CXCR4 expression in HNSCC cancer stem cells and metastasis is not yet known.

It is well established that certain types of cancers have organ specific preferences for metastatic growth. In the past, blood flow patterns were theorized to account for the pattern of metastasis development and a route for delivery of cancer cells (Chambers et al. 2002). A number of theories have challenged this hypothesis and propose that additional cellular and molecular level processes are required for cancer cells to home to and grow in their favored metastatic sites. The most important of these theories is the "seed and soil" theory of metastasis that proposes that cancer cells can only thrive in secondary sites that have the appropriate growth factors necessary for the particular type of cell (Hart 1982; Fidler 2001; Phadke et al. 2006). In addition to sustaining growth of metastatic cancer cells, the tissue microenvironment can also lead to dormancy through suppression of angiogenesis and alterations of growth-related signaling pathways (Holmgren et al. 1995; Hedley et al. 2006; Allan et al. 2006; El Saghir et al. 2005; Folkman 2002; Schirrmacher 2001).

Multiple events need to occur for a metastasis to successfully develop. A cancer stem cell with metastatic potential must leave the primary tumor, locate a secondary site with the correct cancer stem cell niche present, and settle there, and the necessary stimulating secreted factors must be present for a macrometastasis to develop (Fig. 15.2). It is vital that the role of cancer stem cells, the cancer stem cell niche, and secreted factors in the development of metastasis be clarified in order for us to develop effective strategies to prevent and treat metastasis.

Therapeutic Implications

The identification of cancer stem cells has required a change in our approach to cancer treatment and the evaluation of the efficacy of our therapies. Previously experimental assays and clinical evaluations of response to treatment have relied on measures of tumor shrinkage. Because the cancer stem cells make up only a small proportion of the cancer mass, even a large reduction in tumor size may not indicate eradication of the cancer stem cells, and failure to completely eliminate the cancer stem cells may result in tumor recurrence.

As the role of cancer stem cells and the cancer stem cell niche become more completely understood, new therapeutic options to prevent or eliminate metastasis will be developed. Directing therapy specifically against cancer stem cells has the potential to eradicate primary tumors and any metastasis that may be present. This treatment approach has the added challenge of identifying therapeutic agents that will target the cancer stem cells but not adversely affect normal stem cells. Understanding the niche that is required for metastasis to become established and to grow will enable us to design therapies which will target the cancer niche and eliminate the critical supporting role that it plays for metastatic cancer cells. As a preventative measure, developing drugs to block the secretion of factors by the primary tumor that "prime" a distant site for implantation may represent a strategy to prevent metastasis from arising.

Conclusions

The identification and characterization of cancer stem cells suggests that these cells may also be responsible for the development of metastasis. Because oral cavity cancers have a high propensity for metastasis, it is possible that tumors arising in this location have a high proportion of cancer stem cells that are capable of forming a metastasis by entering the lymphatics or circulation from this location and traveling to a location that is favorable for their establishment and growth. Through further research in this area, it is anticipated that we will better understand the role of head and neck cancer stem cells, secreted factors, and supporting cells of the stem cell niche in the development of oral cancer metastasis, and this will have a direct benefit to patients suffering from this disease.

Acknowledgment   Victoria Prince for help in creating the Metastasis Model figure.

References

Al-Hajj M, Clarke MF (2004) Self-renewal and solid tumor stem cells. Oncogene 23:7274–7282
Al-Hajj M, Wicha MS, Benito-Hernandez A, Morrison SJ, Clarke MF (2003) Prospective identification of tumorigenic breast cancer cells. Proc Natl Acad Sci U S A 100:3983–3988

Al-Hajj M, Becker MW, Wicha M, Weissman I, Clarke MF (2004) Therapeutic implications of cancer stem cells. Curr Opin Genet Dev 14:43–47

Allan AL, George R, Vantyghem SA, Lee MW, Hodgson NC, Engel CJ, Holliday RL, Girvan DP, Scott LA, Postenka CO et al (2006) Role of the integrin-binding protein osteopontin in lymphatic metastasis of breast cancer. Am J Pathol 169:233–246

Balkwill F (2004) Cancer and the chemokine network. Nat Rev Cancer 4:540–550

Bapat SA, Mali AM, Koppikar CB, Kurrey NK (2005) Stem and progenitor-like cells contribute to the aggressive behavior of human epithelial ovarian cancer. Cancer Res 65:3025–3029

Bonnet D, Dick JE (1997) Human acute myeloid leukemia is organized as a hierarchy that originates from a primitive hematopoietic cell. Nat Med 3:730–737

Cameron MD, Schmidt EE, Kerkvliet N, Nadkarni KV, Morris VL, Groom AC, Chambers AF, MacDonald IC (2000) Temporal progression of metastasis in lung: cell survival, dormancy, and location dependence of metastatic inefficiency. Cancer Res 60:2541–2546

Chambers AF, Naumov GN, Varghese HJ, Nadkarni KV, MacDonald IC, Groom AC (2001) Critical steps in hematogenous metastasis: an overview. Surg Oncol Clin N Am 10:243–255, vii

Chambers AF, Groom AC, MacDonald IC (2002) Dissemination and growth of cancer cells in metastatic sites. Nat Rev Cancer 2:563–572

Chiba T, Kita K, Zheng YW et al (2006) Side population purified from hepatocellular carcinoma cells harbors cancer stem cell-like properties. Hepatology 44:240–251

Cho RW, Clarke MF (2008) Recent advances in cancer stem cells. Curr Opin Genet Dev 18:48–53

Clarke M, Fuller M (2006) Stem cells and cancer: two faces of Eve. Cell 124:1111–1115

Collins A, Berry PA, Hyde C, Stower MJ, Maitland NJ (2005) Prospective identification of tumorigenic prostate cancer stem cells. Cancer Res 65:10946–10951

Croker AK, Allan AL (2008) Cancer stem cells: implications for the progression and treatment of metastatic disease. J Cell Mol Med 12:374–390

Dalerba P, Cho RW, Clarke MF (2007a) Cancer stem cells: models and concepts. Annu Rev Med 58:267–284

Dalerba P, Dylla SJ, Park IK, Liu R, Wang X, Cho RW, Hoey T, Gurney A, Huang EH, Simeone DM, Shelton AA, Parmiani G, Castelli C, Clarke MF (2007) Phenotypic characterization of human colorectal cancer stem cells. Proc Natl Acad Sci U S A 104:10158–10163

El Saghir NS, Elhajj II I, Geara FB, Hourani MH (2005) Trauma-associated growth of suspected dormant micrometastasis. BMC Cancer 5:94

Engl T, Relja B, Marian D, Blumenberg C, Muller I, Beecken WD, Jones J, Ringel EM, Bereiter-Hahn J, Jonas D et al (2006) CXCR4 chemokine receptor mediates prostate tumor cell adhesion through alpha5 and beta3 integrins. Neoplasia 8:290–301

Fidler IJ (2001) Seed and soil revisited: contribution of the organ microenvironment to cancer metastasis. Surg Oncol Clin N Am 10:257–269, vii–viiii

Fidler IJ, Talmadge JE (1986) Evidence that intravenously derived murine pulmonary melanoma metastases can originate from the expansion of a single tumor cell. Cancer Res 46:5167–5171

Folkman J (2002) Role of angiogenesis in tumor growth and metastasis. Semin Oncol 29:15–18

Fuchs E, Tumbar T, Guasch G (2004) Socializing with the neighbors: stem cells and their niche. Cell 116:769–778

Gil J, Bernard D, Peters G (2005) Role of polycomb group proteins in stem cell self-renewal and cancer. DNA Cell Biol 24:117–125

Hart IR (1982) 'Seed and soil' revisited: mechanisms of site-specific metastasis. Cancer Metastasis Rev 1:5–16

Hart CA, Brown M, Bagley S, Sharrard M, Clarke NW (2005) Invasive characteristics of human prostatic epithelial cells: understanding the metastatic process. Br J Cancer 92:503–512

Hedley BD, Allan AL, Chambers AF (2006) Tumor dormancy and the role of metastasis suppressor genes in regulating ectopic growth. Future Oncol 2:627–641

Hermann PC, Huber SL, Herrler T, Aicher A, Ellwart JW, Guba M, Bruns CJ, Heeschen C (2007) Distinct populations of cancer stem cells determine tumor growth and metastatic activity in human pancreatic cancer. Cell Stem Cell 1:313–323

Holmgren L, O'Reilly MS, Folkman J (1995) Dormancy of micrometastases: balanced proliferation and apoptosis in the presence of angiogenesis suppression. Nat Med 1:149–153

Jemal A, Clegg LX, Ward E, Ries LA, Wu X, Jamison PM, Wingo PA, Howe HL, Anderson RN, Edwards BK (2004) Annual report to the nation on the status of cancer, 1975–2001, with a special feature regarding survival. Cancer 101:3–27

Kalluri R, Zeisberg M (2006) Fibroblasts in cancer. Nat Rev Cancer 6:392–401

Kang Y (2005) Functional genomic analysis of cancer metastasis: biologic insights and clinical implications. Expert Rev Mol Diagn 5:385–395

Kang Y, Siegel PM, Shu W, Drobnjak M, Kakonen SM, Cordon-Cardo C, Guise TA, Massague J (2003) A multigenic program mediating breast cancer metastasis to bone. Cancer Cell 3:537–549

Kaplan RN, Riba RD, Zacharoulis S, Bramley AH, Vincent L, Costa C, MacDonald DD, Jin DK, Shido K, Kerns SA et al (2005) VEGFR1-positive haematopoietic bone marrow progenitors initiate the pre-metastatic niche. Nature 438:820–827

Kastan MB, Bartek J (2004) Cell-cycle checkpoints and cancer. Nature 432:316–323

Katoh M, Katoh M (2007) WNT signaling pathway and stem cell signaling network. Clin Cancer Res 13:4042–4045

Kiger AA, Jones DL, Schulz C, Rogers MB, Fuller MT (2001) Stem cell self-renewal specified by JAK-STAT activation in response to a support cell cue. Science 294:2542–2545

Kucia M, Reca R, Miekus K, Wanzeck J, Wojakowski W, Janowska-Wieczorek A, Ratajczak J, Ratajczak MZ (2005) Trafficking of normal stem cells and metastasis of cancer stem cells involve similar mechanisms: pivotal role of the SDF-1-CXCR4 axis. Stem Cells 23:879–894

Li L, Neaves WB (2006) Normal stem cells and cancer stem cells: the niche matters. Cancer Res 66:4553–4557

Li LC, Carroll PR, Dahiya R (2005) Epigenetic changes in prostate cancer: implication for diagnosis and treatment. J Natl Cancer Inst 97:103–115

Li C, Heidt DG, Dalerba P, Burant CF, Zhang L, Adsay V, Wicha M, Clarke MF, Simeone DM (2007) Identification of pancreatic cancer stem cells. Cancer Res 67:1030–1037

Liu Y, Hu T, Shen J, Li SF, Lin JW, Zheng XH, Gao QH, Zhou HM (2006) Separation, cultivation and biological characteristics of oral carcinoma-associated fibroblasts. Oral Dis 12:375–380

Lobo NA, Shimono Y, Qian D, Clarke MF (2007) The biology of cancer stem cells. Annu Rev Cell Dev Biol 23:675–699

Luzzi KJ, MacDonald IC, Schmidt EE, Kerkvliet N, Morris VL, Chambers AF, Groom AC (1998) Multistep nature of metastatic inefficiency: dormancy of solitary cells after successful extravasation and limited survival of early micrometastases. Am J Pathol 153:865–873

MacDonald IC, Groom AC, Chambers AF (2002) Cancer spread and micrometastasis development: quantitative approaches for in vivo models. Bioessays 24:885–893

Mimeault M, Batra SK (2006) Concise review: recent advances on the significance of stem cells in tissue regeneration and cancer therapies. Stem Cells 24:2319–2345

Minn AJ, Gupta GP, Siegel PM, Bos PD, Shu W, Giri DD, Viale A, Olshen AB, Gerald WL, Massague J (2005) Genes that mediate breast cancer metastasis to lung. Nature 436:518–524

Moore KA, Lemischka IR (2006) Stem cells and their niches. Science 311:1880–1885

Morrison SJ, Kimble J (2006) Asymmetric and symmetric stem-cell divisions in development and cancer. Nature 441:1068–1074

Morrison SJ, Spradling AC (2008) Stem cells and niches: mechanisms that promote stem cell maintenance throughout life. Cell 132:598–611

O'Brien C, Pollett A, Gallinger S, Dick JE (2007) A human colon cancer cell capable of initiating tumour growth in immunodeficient mice. Nature 445:106–110

Pantel K, Brakenhoff RH (2004) Dissecting the metastatic cascade. Nat Rev Cancer 4:448–456

Pardal R, Clarke MF, Morrison SJ (2003) Applying the principles of stem-cell biology to cancer. Nat Rev Cancer 3:895–902

Phadke PA, Mercer RR, Harms JF, Jia Y, Frost AR, Jewell JL, Bussard KM, Nelson S, Moore C, Kappes JC et al (2006) Kinetics of metastatic breast cancer cell trafficking in bone. Clin Cancer Res 12:1431–1440

Prince M, Sivanandan R, Kaczorowski A, Wolf GT, Kaplan MJ, Dalerba P, Weissman IL, Clarke MF, Ailles LE (2007) Identification of a subpopulation of cells with cancer stem cell properties in head and neck squamous cell carcinoma. Proc Natl Acad Sci U S A 104:973–978

Reya T, Clevers H (2005) Wnt signalling in stem cells and cancer. Nature 434:843–850

Reya T, Morrison SJ, Clarke MF, Weissman IL (2001) Stem cells, cancer, and cancer stem cells. Nature 414:105–111

Rodrigues VC, Moss SM, Tuomainen H (1998) Oral cancer in the UK: to screen or not to screen. Oral Oncol 34:454–465

Scadden DT (2006) The stem-cell niche as an entity of action. Nature 441:1075–1079

Schirrmacher V (2001) T-cell immunity in the induction and maintenance of a tumour dormant state. Semin Cancer Biol 11:285–295

Schofield R (1978) The relationship between the spleen colony-forming cell and the haemopoietic stem cell. Blood Cells 4:7–25

Singh S, Clarke ID, Terasaki M, Bonn VE, Hawkins C, Squire J, Dirks PB (2003) Identification of a cancer stem cell in human brain tumors. Cancer Res 63:5821–5828

Singh S, Hawkins C, Clarke ID, Squire JA, Bayani J, Hide T, Henkelman RM, Cusimano MD, Dirks PB (2004) Identification of human brain tumour initiating cells. Nature 432:396–401

Sneddon JB, Zhen HH, Montgomery K, van de Rijn M, Tward AD, West R, Gladstone H, Chang HY, Morganroth GS, Oro AE et al (2006) Bone morphogenetic protein antagonist gremlin 1 is widely expressed by cancer-associated stromal cells and can promote tumor cell proliferation. Proc Natl Acad Sci U S A 103:14842–14847

Song X, Wong MD, Kawase E, Xi R, Ding BC, McCarthy JJ, Xie T (2004) Bmp signals from niche cells directly repress transcription of a differentiation-promoting gene, bag of marbles, in germline stem cells in the Drosophila ovary. Development 131:1353–1364

Swartz MA, Skobe M (2001) Lymphatic function, lymphangiogenesis, and cancer metastasis. Microsc Res Tech 55:92–99

Tulina N, Matunis E (2001) Control of stem cell self-renewal in *Drosophila* spermatogenesis by JAK-STAT signaling. Science 294:2546–2549

Watt FM, Hogan BL (2000) Out of Eden: stem cells and their niches. Science 287:1427–1430

Weigelt B, Peterse JL, van 't Veer LJ (2005) Breast cancer metastasis: markers and models. Nat Rev Cancer 5:591–602

Weiss L (1992) An analysis of the incidence of myocardial metastasis from solid cancers. Br Heart J 68:501–504

Welch DR (1997) Technical considerations for studying cancer metastasis in vivo. Clin Exp Metastasis 15:272–306

Wicha MS, Liu S, Dontu G (2006) Cancer stem cells: an old idea – a paradigm shift. Cancer Res 66:1883–1890

Woodhouse EC, Chuaqui RF, Liotta LA (1997) General mechanisms of metastasis. Cancer 80:1529–1537

Woodward WA, Chen MS, Behbod F, Rosen JM (2005) On mammary stem cells. J Cell Sci 118:3585–3594

Index